HEALTH

and Health Care Delivery in Canada

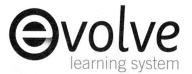
Evolve
learning system

Evolve provides online access to free learning resources and activities designed specifically for the textbook you are using in your class. The resources will provide you with information that enhances the material covered in the book and much more.

Visit the Web Address Listed Below to Start Your Learning Evolution Today!

http://evolve.elsevier.com/Canada/Thompson/health

Evolve® Student Learning Resources for Thompson, Health and Health Care Delivery in Canada *offer the following features:*

Student Resources

- **Multiple-Choice Review Questions** test your reading comprehension for each chapter.

- A **Glossary** lists all of the key terms found in the textbook.

- **WebLinks** allow you to link to Web sites carefully chosen to supplement the content of the textbook.

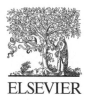
ELSEVIER

HEALTH

and Health Care Delivery in Canada

Valerie D. Thompson, RN, PHC, NP
Conestoga Institute of Technology and Advanced Learning

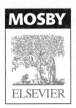

MOSBY

ELSEVIER

Library and Archives Canada Cataloguing in Publication

Thompson, Valerie D., 1948–
        Health and health care delivery in Canada / Valerie D. Thompson.

Includes index.
ISBN 978-1-897422-07-6

        1. Medical care--Canada. 2. Public health--Canada. 3. Medicine, Preventive--Canada. I. Title.

RA449.T46 2010   362.10971   C2009-903376-3

Vice President, Publishing: Ann Millar
Managing Developmental Editor: Tammy Scherer
Developmental Editor: Joanne Sutherland
Managing Production Editor: Roberta A. Spinosa-Millman
Substantive Editor: Lynda Cranston
Copy Editor: Cathy Witlox
Cover Design: George Kirkpatrick
Interior Design: Brett J. Miller, BJM Graphic Design & Communications
Cover Image: Don Farrall/Digital Vision/Getty Images
Typesetting and Assembly: BJM Graphic Design & Communications
Printing and Binding: Transcontinental

Elsevier Canada
905 King Street West, 4th Floor, Toronto, ON, Canada M6K 3G9
Phone: 1-866-896-3331
Fax: 1-866-359-9534

Printed in Canada

1 2 3 4 5   14 13 12 11 10

To the little ones in my life—Gregory, Russell, Lillian, and Bridgit—in the hopes that our health care system will remain sustainable and effective for their lifetimes.

To all the students entering the health care field, as well as existing health care professionals, who work tirelessly, adapt to continuous change, improvise, and overcome obstacles to ensure that health care in Canada is the best it can be.

PREFACE

Individuals working in any facet of health care must understand the components of health and wellness and how health care is delivered in Canada. This unique new text will provide a valuable foundation for understanding these important and challenging concepts.

While by no means exhaustive, *Health and Health Care Delivery in Canada* introduces various components of health and health care delivery. After introducing the concepts of health and illness, the book builds on population health principles in order to methodically examine the cost, structure, and function of the Canadian health care system at the federal, provincial, and municipal levels. The text also looks at human health resources, legal and ethical aspects of health care, and the future of health care in Canada.

The book's content has been carefully selected in order to highlight important, need-to-know material. Each chapter relates to and expands on ideas in the previous chapter so that common threads are carried throughout the book and material flows in an orderly and understandable manner.

By the end of this book, students will be able to say, "I understand health care issues in Canada and how different levels of government operate in terms of health care delivery. I understand how our health care system is funded and the future issues facing health and health care in Canada" and, most important, "I understand the system that I am choosing to work in." Intended to accompany postsecondary introductory courses in Canadian health care delivery, this book offers students a foundation with which they can easily move forward to other, more specifically focused courses.

CONTENT

Chapter 1 (Health and the Individual) sets the stage for the rest of the book by providing the student with an understanding of the key concepts of health, wellness, illness, disease, and disability. Among other things, students are encouraged to examine their own health beliefs and health behaviours and to consider how these contribute to maintaining health. Chapter 2 (Population Health: Introduction and Principles) explains how the government and other health care stakeholders evaluate the health of Canadians, identify risk factors, implement strategies to deal with current health problems, and predict problems that are likely to arise in the future. Chapter 3 (The History of Health Care in Canada) provides an interesting summary of the highlights in the history of our health care system, such as the *Canada Health Act*. Students are encouraged to examine the principles of this Act in terms of its relevance in the twenty-first century.

Chapters 4 (The Federal Government's Role in Health Care) and 5 (Provincial and Territorial Governments) focus on the division of powers and the implementation of health care from federal and provincial or territorial levels. Chapter 5 follows two families who have recently immigrated to Canada, highlighting some variations in the provincial and territorial health care plans and how these differences affect the families. Instructors are encouraged to expand on health care delivery in their own jurisdictions while comparing components of health care delivery in their own province or territory with those of other jurisdictions. Chapter 6 (The Dollars and "Sense" of Health Care Funding) looks critically at where the money for health care comes from and where it goes, and also examines what "strings" the federal government attaches to its funding for the provinces and territories. The chapter focuses on the cost of health care in general, as well as on the cost of specific procedures. It examines the sobering fact that real-life health care decisions are made based on who qualifies for treatment under a provincial or territorial plan and who does not—and who will opt to pay for services out-of-pocket.

Chapter 7 (Practitioners and Practice Settings) provides the student with a clear picture of our human health resources—who delivers the care, in what setting, and under what circumstances. It examines how primary health care reform is changing the way in which health care is delivered across Canada.

Chapter 8 (The Law and Health Care) analyzes legal issues, clarifying provincial, territorial, and federal boundaries in terms of legislation and the law. Considerable discussion is devoted to current laws regarding confidentiality and consent to treatment. Chapter 9 (Ethics and Health Care) highlights ethical principles and points out that health care professionals are held to a higher level of ethical accountability than are those in many other professions. The student will learn why this is and how to practise in a moral and ethical manner.

Chapter 10 (Current Issues and Future Trends in Health Care in Canada) considers current issues and looks at what Canadians can expect in the future. How can Canada maintain adequate health care services in the face of an aging population, complex medical problems, advancing and expensive technology, and less funding? Will electronic medical records and electronic health records be implemented at a national level, and how and when will this implementation take place? Although no concrete answers exist, the student will be prepared to look ahead, aware of the significant obstacles that we as a nation must overcome if we are indeed to salvage Medicare.

Learning Features

Each chapter contains several unique features meant to stimulate student interest. Learning outcomes outline the objectives for the chapter. Key terms define challenging concepts. Chapter summaries and review questions underscore key elements. Students can use discussion questions and annotated web resources to further research select topic areas.

Additional features include general interest, "Thinking It Through," "In the News," and "Case Example" boxes. These features encourage the student to think through facts and points of interest, as well as actual situations, statements of fact, or both, and to answer questions that promote personal views, general discussion, and, in some cases, further investigation. Additional Evolve® online resources to accompany the text can be found at **http://evolve.elsevier.com/ Canada/Thompson/health**.

ACKNOWLEDGEMENTS

Writing a book of this nature cannot possibly occur in isolation. I owe a great deal to so many people, from those working with the Canadian Institute for Health Information—particularly Jennie Hoekstra, Barbara Loh, Angela Allain-Levasseur, and Angela Baker—and provincial and territorial governments to colleagues representing individual professions. Those listed below have contributed essential information to this book and confirmed that information in their area of expertise is both correct and relevant:

Dr. Don Nixdorf
Executive Director
British Columbia Chiropractic Association

Dr. S. Brooke Milne
Department of Archeology
University of Manitoba

Shelagh Maloney
Executive Director, External Liaison
Canada Health Infoway/Inforoute Santé du Canada

Marcus Loreti
Program Lead, Decision Support Services
Acute and Ambulatory Care Information Services
Canadian Institute for Health Information

Richard Baker
Founder
Timely Medical Services

Deborah Cohen Richard
Manager, Health Human Resources
Canadian Institute for Health Information

Katherine Kelly
Director, Federal/Provincial/Territorial Secretariat
Prince Edward Island Department of Health

Dr. Richard Wedge
Director of Medical Programs
Prince Edward Island Department of Health

Nadeem Esmail
Director, Health System Performance Studies
Fraser Institute

Glenn Budgell
Regional Director, Medical Services Plan
Department of Health and Community Services

Keith Walls
Manager, Population Health Fund Section
Public Health Agency of Canada

Teresa D. Mrozek
Executive Director, Urban Regional Support Services
Manitoba Health

I would like also to acknowledge and thank Elsevier's reviewers, who provided helpful comments, constructive criticism, and suggestions for improvements during various stages of the manuscript:

Phil Bourget, MN
Faculty, Faculty of Nursing
Georgian College

Carrie de Palma, MEd
Faculty, Health Sciences Division
College of New Caledonia

Kim English, RN, BScN, MN
Faculty, Trent-Fleming School of Nursing
Trent University

Sharon A. MacKenzie, CHIM
Coordinator, Health Information Management Program,
School of Health Sciences
St. Lawrence College

Ursula Sinha, BScN, MSA, EdD
Course Writer and Tutor for Psychiatric Nursing, Faculty of Health and Community Studies
Grant MacEwan College

Lynn Smith, RN, BScN, MSN, PhD, NP (Paediatric)
Professor, Health Sciences
Northern College of Applied Arts and Technology

Charlotte Snyder, RN, BScN, MBA
Faculty, BScN Program (with McMaster University)
Conestoga College

Landa Terblanche
Chair, Department of Nursing
Trinity Western University

Paula Weisflock, BHA (HIM), CHIM
Program Coordinator, Health Information Management Program
Fleming College

I also owe a debt of gratitude to clear language consultant Susan Milne for her ongoing assistance in keeping me organized and in ensuring that the language of each chapter was clear and concise prior to the publisher's edit. A special thank-you goes out to Susannah Read, too, for continuously providing me with current news articles related to health care. I'd also like to acknowledge Carla Shapiro for her legal review of Chapter 8. As well, I cannot thank the editors from Elsevier—Ann Millar, Martina van de Velde, Joanne Sutherland, Lynda Cranston, Tammy Scherer, Roberta A. Spinosa-Millman, Lise Dupont, Cathy Witlox, and Claudia Forgas—enough for their expert advice, endless reviews, and constructive suggestions. Elsevier is an outstanding company to work with, and the result of its attention to detail is well evident in this publication.

Valerie D. Thompson
July 2009

CONTENTS

SPECIAL FEATURES

Health and the Individual

Learning Outcomes

1. Describe the concepts of health, wellness, illness, disease, and disability.

2. Explain the three models of health.

3. Explain how perceptions of health have changed over the past five decades.

4. Understand the health–illness continuum.

5. Identify factors that influence a person's attitudes toward health and wellness.

6. Examine the impact of sick role behaviour on clients, their families, and members of the health care team.

7. Summarize the stages of illness.

8. Examine the impact of self-imposed risk behaviours on a client's health.

9. Discuss the leading causes of morbidity and mortality in Canada today in terms of risk factors and prevention.

If you are entering a health care profession—physiotherapy, occupational therapy, respiratory therapy, laboratory technology, health informatics, nursing, pharmacology, or health administration, to name a few—you must understand the concepts of health and wellness. It is also important to know what makes Canadians ill. Many of the diseases you will encounter in your career are, to a large extent, preventable. Why, then, do people engage in behaviours that cause disease and illness? For one thing, many people take good health for granted until they are faced with illness or another incapacitating event.

Understanding your clients' health beliefs and health behaviours, and their corresponding response to treatment, will help you to maximize their health outcomes. Some clients will consider themselves well despite the presence of health problems. These individuals are often easy to treat and comply with treatment plans, such as taking medications, following a prescribed diet, and actively participating in rehabilitation regimes.

Definitions of *health, wellness, illness, disease,* and *disability* evolve constantly, along with social consciousness, the delivery of health care, the affordability of health care services, and medical science. This chapter will explore these issues, provide information on the leading causes of **morbidity** and **mortality** in Canada, and discuss the impact of self-imposed risk behaviours on the individual and on the health care system in terms of disease and cost. This chapter will also explain that your goal, as part of the health care team, is to support clients on the road to improved health, to help them maintain their existing health, and to assist them in coping with illness.

HEALTH, WELLNESS, AND ILLNESS: KEY CONCEPTS

For a long time, *healthy* meant "not sick," and *sick* meant "not well." Today, the key concepts of health, wellness, and illness are defined in less black-and-white, either–or terms. Health care professionals should understand the evolution of these definitions—how they have changed to become more multifaceted and inclusive over time.

HEALTH

The word *health* developed from the Old English word *hoelth*, which meant a state of being sound and generally suggested a soundness or wholeness of the body. That is, if the body was in good functioning order, one was considered to be in good health. Note that this definition primarily considers the physiological function of the body and nothing else.

This concept of health evolved from the early ages. Before Hippocrates (460 B.C.), health was viewed as a "divine gift," and illness was believed to be caused by the wrath of evil spirits or gods. Hippocrates, known as the father of modern medicine, introduced the idea that health and illness stemmed from more concrete causes. Based on reason and observation, he described the symptoms of various diseases. To this day, graduating doctors in some medical schools take the Hippocratic Oath upon receiving their medical degrees (see Chapter 9). The Oath, which has been updated over the years, is merely symbolic and holds no legal obligation. Today, many physicians choose not to take the Hippocratic Oath since parts of it fail to represent the standards of medical practice in the twenty-first century.

From Hippocrates' time to the 1800s, health simply meant the absence of disease, and the presence of disease usually entailed a threat to one's life. People often died from ailments that are treatable today, such as pneumonia and tuberculosis. On the other hand, being "healthy" (i.e., free of disease) meant being able to carry on with everyday activities and responsibilities, even if a

Morbidity

Disease, the occurrence of disease, or impairment resulting from accidents or environmental causes that adversely affects health.

Mortality

Death or the occurrence of deaths resulting from disease, accidents, or environmental causes.

person was not feeling entirely well. Throughout these centuries, unsanitary living conditions and lack of medical treatment resulted in high morbidity and mortality rates.

By the 1900s, researchers and doctors had developed an understanding of the **etiology** of diseases—discovering, for example, the link between infection and poor hygiene. From this development came the idea that if external factors caused disease, disease could possibly be avoided or controlled. For many people, however, health remained a black-and-white concept: A person was healthy or was ill.

Etiology
The study of causes. In medicine, *etiology* refers to the origin or cause of a disease.

In 1948, the World Health Organization (WHO) took the important step of acknowledging that health is multi-dimensional, and not merely the presence or absence of disease. A vast improvement over previous definitions, WHO's definition (Box 1.1) continues to evolve and to better encompass a broadening outlook on health.

Box 1.1   Health: An Evolving Definition

In 1948, the World Health Organization originally defined *health* as "a state of complete physical, mental, and social well-being and not merely the absence of disease or infirmity."

Over time, as perceptions of health have evolved, this definition has come into question. For instance, some suggest that the word *complete* is unrealistic: How many people can claim to be completely healthy—and what does *completely healthy* mean? The ambiguity of this term is particularly evident today, with individuals living much longer, sometimes with serious ailments, such as heart disease or respiratory disease, or with physical limitations. Many health care professions have struggled with this definition because it fails to include holistic concepts, such as spiritual wellness. Nurses, for example, must be aware of and respect the spiritual needs of their clients (e.g., by ensuring clients have access to a religious leader) when establishing a nursing diagnosis and implementing nursing interventions.

More recently, WHO developed a new concept for health that recognizes the strong link between individuals and their environment. Health encompasses "the ability to identify and to realize aspirations, to satisfy needs, and to change or cope with environment. Health is therefore a resource for everyday life, not the objective of living. Health is a positive concept emphasizing social and personal resources, as well as physical capabilities" (World Health Organization, 1986).

Sources: World Health Organization. (1948). *Preamble to the constitution of the World Health Organization as adopted by the International Health Conference.* New York; World Health Organization. (1986). *Health promotion: Concepts and principles in action—A policy framework.* Copenhagen: WHO Regional Office for Europe.

WELLNESS

Although often used interchangeably with *health*, **wellness** goes beyond having good health. Wellness considers how a person feels about his or her health and quality of life. For example, people may judge themselves to be well despite the presence of disease, sickness, sensory impairment, or physical disability. This personal perception reflects how individuals adapt to, cope with, and accept their state of health and, in turn, defines their view of wellness.

From a holistic perspective, to achieve wellness, a person must take responsibility for his or her own health by leading a balanced lifestyle and avoiding self-imposed risk behaviours. The path toward wellness is not static; it is continuous and must be a lifelong pursuit. Wellness develops from the decisions people make about how to live their lives with quality, good health (remember, good health is relative), and meaning.

Wellness
The way a person feels about his or her health and quality of life. People with a disability or a chronic disease may still consider themselves to be well and enjoying a good quality of life.

In the **News** Do You Remember Terry Fox?

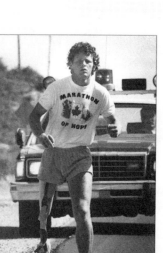

Terry Fox was born in Winnipeg, Manitoba, in 1958, and later moved to Port Coquitlam, British Columbia. A recognized athlete in high school, at 18 years old, Terry was diagnosed with bone cancer, which eventually resulted in the need for amputation of his right leg just above the knee.

Terry was so affected by the pain and suffering of people who had cancer and by the lack of funding for cancer research that he decided to run across Canada to raise money for this cause. Terry began his run—his "Marathon of Hope"—on April 12, 1980, starting in St. John's, Newfoundland. As Terry's run continued, it attracted more and more media attention and support from the public. By the time Terry reached Ontario, alarming symptoms appeared. He became short of breath, was easily fatigued, and experienced chest pains. Near Thunder Bay, Ontario, after 143 days and 5373 km, Terry announced he was postponing his run and returned to British Columbia for medical attention. The cancer had spread to his lungs. In the months that followed, donations kept coming.

Several months before Terry died, the president of the Four Seasons Hotel announced that she would ensure that Terry's run continued as an annual event called the Terry Fox Run. Terry died on January 28, 1981. Before he died,

Continued on next page

Terry received the Order of Canada, and on March 14, 2005, he became the first Canadian whose image has appeared on a general-circulation Canadian coin.

The Terry Fox Run continues annually in Canada and in more than 60 countries around the world, raising millions of dollars. In 2007, the Terry Fox Foundation donated $20 million to the National Cancer Institute of Canada for studies, including research on how viruses can be used to treat cancer.

Sources: The Terry Fox Foundation. (n.d.). Retrieved May 2, 2009, from http://www.terryfoxrun. org/english/about%20terry%20fox/default.asp?s=1; National Cancer Institute of Canada. (2007). *The Terry Fox Foundation research update.* Retrieved May 29, 2009, from http://www.terry foxrun.org/local/files/pdf_foundation/Research%20Update%2007%20EN%20FA3.pdf

Photo credit: Boris Spremo/GetStock.com.

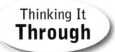

Thinking It Through

If you had been in Terry Fox's place, considering the nature of his illness and the enormous change it made to his life (e.g., having a leg amputated, learning to walk with a prosthesis, living with the knowledge that recurrence was a possibility), what do you think you would have done?

Dimensions of Wellness

The concept of wellness embraces several holistic elements, including, but not necessarily limited to, physical, emotional, intellectual, spiritual, and social health. Some models have more recently added environmental wellness. A fine line exists between some of these holistic categories, so some wellness models may group or label them differently.

Physical Wellness

The dimension of **physical wellness** entails maintaining a healthy body by eating a nutritious, balanced diet, exercising regularly, making intelligent, informed decisions about one's health, and seeking medical assistance when necessary. To do this, people must understand how lifestyle choices affect physical health.

Emotional Wellness

Emotional wellness and mental health are often but not necessarily interdependent entities. **Emotional wellness** involves people's ability to understand themselves, to recognize their strengths and limitations, and to accept who they are. The emotionally adapted person effectively handles and controls his or her emotions, communicates well, and seeks support when needed.

Good mental health allows a person to react proactively when things go wrong—to view adversity as an opportunity to learn and grow. Emotional health very much contributes to this ability. Mental illnesses, such as schizophrenia, bipolar disease, and depression, can affect a person's capacity to deal with situations effectively, especially when a situation poses challenges or problems. Mental illnesses usually have a physiological etiology and require treatment by a health care professional.

Intellectual Wellness

Intellectual wellness reflects a person's ability to make informed decisions that are appropriate and beneficial. From their experiences and learnings, intellectually well people are able to gather information throughout their lifespan and to use that information to make the best of situations. Moreover, these people apply critical thinking skills, prioritize data, and keep abreast of occurrences and current events.

Intellectual wellness may include occupational health—personal satisfaction from one's career and the ability to balance career with other activities like family and leisure time.

Spiritual Wellness

Spiritual wellness may include a commitment to a religion or some higher power that evokes a sense of belonging to something greater than "self." The spiritually well person seeks to contribute to society, plays an active role within the community, and displays gratitude and generosity. Spirituality may also involve solitude and reflection—focusing inward and reflecting upon feelings, actions, experiences, and ideas.

Thinking It Through

Spirituality has been linked to good health, from fewer illnesses to faster recovery from illness and an enhanced ability to deal with stress.

1. Why do you think spirituality may contribute to better health?

2. Do you think that to be spiritual, a person must be associated with a church or other religious entity?

Social Wellness

Social wellness is about relating effectively to others, including being able to form close, loving relationships, to laugh, to communicate effectively and empathically, to be a good listener, and to respond appropriately. Socially well individuals work agreeably in groups and within the community, are tolerant and accepting of others, and can form friendships and supportive networks. Confident and flexible, socially well people contribute to the welfare of others.

Environmental Wellness

Newer models of wellness take into account one's relationship with the environment (**environmental wellness**). An environmentally well person is one who engages in a lifestyle that is friendly to the environment. Friendliness to the environment can entail preserving the external world—walking or biking (instead of driving), recycling, and so on. It may also include creating a safe internal environment—for example, by protecting one's eyesight (e.g., using good lighting when reading or working) or limiting loud noises (controlling music volume).

ILLNESS

The term **illness**, often used to denote the presence of disease, can also refer to how a person feels about his or her health, whether or not a disease is present. Despite the absence of any pathology or disease, a person may feel ill as a result of tiredness, stress, or both. Although this state differs from feeling healthy and energetic, by definition, it is not a disease.

DISEASE

Disease
A disorder affecting a system or organ, which can be mental, physical, or genetic in origin. *Disease* also refers to a change in, or deviation from, how the body normally functions.

Disease typically refers to a condition in which a person's mental or bodily functions are different from normal. Usually biological in nature, disease may affect various organs of the body and have symptoms that are either observable or difficult to detect.

The term *disease* can also apply to behavioural or psychological alterations for which a biological or biochemical explanation exists. Schizophrenia is an example of such a disease.

The term *disease* may be used, too, to describe a group of symptoms (called a *syndrome*) that are not related to a clear-cut disease process. Although *disease* is often used interchangeably with the words *disorder*, *condition*, or *dysfunction*, these last terms are vague. *Disease* is also sometimes used incorrectly to refer to a disability.

A disease typically has an onset, follows an often predictable course, and then subsides. Some diseases, however, produce symptoms that may dramatically improve or even disappear for a time—the disease itself or the progression of the disease becomes dormant (i.e., it goes into a period of remission)—and then reappear. This reappearance of symptoms and reactivation of the disease is known as an **exacerbation** of the disease.

Remission of a disease can occur spontaneously or be induced by treatment. In the case of multiple sclerosis, for example, the use of immunosuppressive drugs can result in a treatment-related remission. A remission's length varies. The main aim of treatment for leukemia is a complete remission—that is, no signs of the disease from a symptomatic or pathological perspective. If a remission lasts more than five years, some consider the person to be cured. In the case of any kind of cancer, however, the word *cure* is used cautiously; some physicians avoid ever saying a person is cured, regardless of the length of time he or she has been cancer-free.

Exacerbation

A period of time when a disease (usually chronic) is active and the person has symptoms. *Exacerbation* may also refer to an increase in the severity of a disease.

Remission

A period of time during which a chronic disease is neither active nor acute and the person has no obvious symptoms.

Thinking It **Through**

Suppose you had a chronic disease like rheumatoid arthritis or multiple sclerosis but were managing reasonably well most of the time. Reflecting on your own definition of wellness:

1. Do you think you would consider yourself to be well?
2. Do you think your outlook would by influenced by periods of remission or exacerbation of the condition?

DISABILITY

A deviation from normal function, a **disability** can be physical, sensory (e.g., blindness, deafness), cognitive (e.g., Alzheimer's disease), or intellectual (e.g., Down's syndrome). A disability can occur in conjunction with, or as a result of, a disease or be caused by an accident or fall.

The language used to describe people with a disability has changed over the years, moving toward more sensitive, less hurtful terminology. Today, a person with a cognitive or intellectual disability is most likely to be deemed *mentally handicapped* or *intellectually impaired*.

Along with improved terminology has come the recognition that people with disabilities deserve the same rights and opportunities as all other members of society (Box 1.2).

Disability

A physical or mental incapacity that differs from what is perceived as normal function. A disability can result from an illness or accident or be genetic in nature.

Box 1.2	**People With Disabilities: Rights Are Formally Recognized**

Historically, people with disabilities have been viewed as individuals who need societal protection, evoking sympathy rather than respect. In an effort to change this perception and to ensure that all people have the opportunity to live life to their fullest potential, in December 2006 the United Nations formally adopted the *Convention on the Rights of Persons With Disabilities*, the first such inclusive human rights treaty of this century. The convention was opened for signature in March of 2007; Canada signed at that time.

This convention seeks to "promote, protect and ensure the full and equal enjoyment of all human rights and fundamental freedoms by all persons with disabilities, and to promote respect for their inherent dignity."

The convention covers a number of key areas, including accessibility, personal mobility, health care, education, employment, rehabilitation, participation in political life, equality, and nondiscrimination. Countries that agree to the conditions of this convention are required to adopt national laws that enforce equal rights for people with disabilities.

Source: United Nations. (2006). *Rights of persons with disabilities*. Retrieved May 29, 2009, from http://www.un.org/disabilities/

HEALTH MODELS

Defined as a design for delivering health care, a health model can influence both a health care professional's practice and his or her delivery of health care, which, in turn, affects treatment, priorities, and outcome measurements. The three most common types of health care models are the medical model, the holistic model, and the wellness model, all of which continue to evolve.

The principles of the wellness model—stressing wellness and illness prevention—are most commonly pursued in our current health care climate. Physicians are embracing evidence-based decision making and using best practices to deliver client-focused care in a team-oriented environment.

MEDICAL MODEL

The medical model was founded on a simple definition: Health is the absence of disease. More recently, this model has expanded to consider aspects of functioning, disability, and limitation of activity, thus accepting that a person with physical disabilities or limitations may nevertheless be healthy.

In the twenty-first century, critics of the medical model argue that the model's scope is too narrow and that the presence or absence of disease alone does not define one's health. This model does not consider social causes of disease that are beyond an individual's control (e.g., disparities in socioeconomic status and education). And, by emphasizing the diagnosis and treatment of disease, the medical model ignores the role of prevention—efforts to stop disease and disability before they occur (Larson, 1991).

HOLISTIC MODEL

The **holistic** approach to health considers all parts of the person. This approach has been used for some time by alternative practitioners, such as naturopaths; only recently has it been integrated into mainstream medicine.

Focusing on the positive aspects of health—not on the negatives of illness and disease that inform the medical model—the holistic model strives for a state of health that encompasses the entire person, rather than just aiming for a lack of disease and disability. Similar to the original WHO definition introduced in 1948 (see Box 1.1), the holistic definition of *health* goes much further by recognizing the impact of factors such as lifestyle, spirituality, economics, and culture on an individual's health.

Although initially described as "utopian" (i.e., impossible to achieve), the holistic model has become widely accepted as a better alternative to the medical model (Larson, 1991).

WELLNESS MODEL

The wellness model builds on the medical and holistic models. It considers health a process that continues to evolve and to progress toward a future state of improved health. Viewing health as a state of feeling, an experience based on an internal process rather than on external symptoms (Larson, 1991), the wellness model encompasses an individual's or a group's ability to cope with health-related challenges.

In the wellness model, people assume responsibility for their own health and make informed choices about such things as lifestyle and **self-imposed risk behaviours**. The wellness model also considers a person with a disability or illness to be healthy if that person can function, meet self-imposed goals, and is not incapacitated by pain.

The common thread linking the holistic and wellness health models is the inclusion of a broad spectrum of factors—physical, spiritual, social, emotional, economic, and cultural.

Holistic
Whole. In health care, a holistic approach treats the whole person, not an individual part of the person. For example, a holistic approach to treating a person with a heart condition would consider the client's emotional state, diet, and fitness level, not just his or her heart problem.

Self-imposed risk behaviours
Actions (such as smoking tobacco) that a person willfully engages in despite knowing they pose a danger to his or her health.

CHANGING PERCEPTIONS OF HEALTH

Perceptions of health vary. A person who is feeling happy and optimistic may pass off an illness as trivial or as something he or she can cope with. If that same person is feeling down, stressed, or otherwise vulnerable, however, an illness may seem more draining. Consequently, a positive frame of mind can help a person deal more effectively with stress and fight disease.

Until the early 1960s, Canadians, for the most part, held the attitude that if they were sick, they would seek medical care and the doctor would make them better. Few people recognized the impact of lifestyle on their health. Engaging in self-imposed risk behaviours, such as a sedentary lifestyle, poor nutritional habits, smoking, and alcohol abuse, was rarely directly linked to changes in health status. Canadians functioned very much within the realm of the medical model.

This way of thinking began to change in the 1960s and 1970s. With the help of government initiatives and the establishment of a population health approach to health care, Canadians started to see the value of prevention and to consider what they could do on a personal level to stay healthy—that is, they began to take more responsibility for their own well-being. Slowly, community and group involvement in health promotion and disease prevention emerged.

A federal public initiative, aptly called ParticipACTION, was launched in 1971 to promote a healthy lifestyle through increased physical activity. This initiative resulted from a 1969 study by the National Advisory Council for Fitness and Amateur Sport, which found Canadians to be largely sedentary (i.e., inactive), unfit, and, worse yet, uninterested in the concept of exercise and its health benefits (ParticipACTION, 1969).

One of the government's first nationally promoted health-related projects, ParticipACTION urged Canadians to get active so as to improve their health and prevent related health problems. Financial cutbacks shut down ParticipACTION in 2001. But, with renewed funding from the federal government, the program was revitalized in February 2007 to continue its efforts to encourage Canadians (particularly youth) to become active.

Other health initiatives have been delivered largely at the community level by the approval and under the direction of the provincial and territorial governments. Today, Canadians have a much broader-based understanding of the link between lifestyle and health. Most people recognize that smoking causes lung cancer and respiratory disease. And many know that being active can lower their chances of developing high blood pressure, osteoporosis, cardiovascular disease, and even some types of cancer.

Still, much work remains to be done. More than half of Canadian adults are considered inactive (Canadian Fitness and Lifestyle Research Institute, 2005), and only 9% of children and youth (aged 5 to 19) meet the recommendations in *Canada's Physical Activity Guide for Children and Youth* (Canadian Fitness and Lifestyle Research Institute, 2007). Physical inactivity is also costly, imposing a $2.1 billion burden on Canada's health care system (Katzmarzyk et al., 2000).

Thinking It Through

A close friend of yours, a very heavy smoker (two packs of cigarettes daily), is diagnosed with high blood pressure and has a family history of cancer. But he refuses to stop smoking, stating that "it's my life, and I love to smoke." You believe that he does not comprehend the consequences of his habit and feel very strongly that he should quit. How might you influence his decision?

THE HEALTH–ILLNESS CONTINUUM

A continuum is a method of measurement usually represented by a straight line with an opposing state at each end. The **health–illness continuum** measures one's state of health between "optimum health" and "poor health" or "death." In the middle is a section called **compensation** (Figure 1.1).

The health–illness continuum includes all of the dimensions of health and wellness, from physiological to spiritual and psychological health. Looking at health as a process, the wellness model supports the concept of the health–illness continuum.

Health–illness continuum
A method of measuring one's state of health at any given point in time. A person's health state may range from optimum health at one end to death at the other end.

Compensation
That part of the health–illness continuum in which a person is neither in good nor poor health, is able to accommodate a malady, and is continuing on with daily life.

Figure 1.1   Health–Illness Continuum

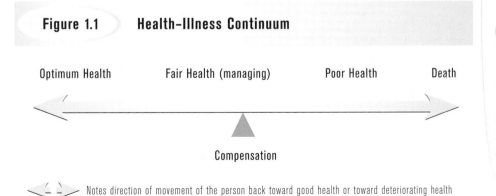

Optimum Health   Fair Health (managing)   Poor Health   Death

Compensation

Notes direction of movement of the person back toward good health or toward deteriorating health

Movement on the continuum is constant. An individual may wake up feeling good and then develop a headache two hours later, altering his or her perceived placement on the continuum. Also, one person may have a bad cold but not feel particularly ill so may place him- or herself on the "good health" part of the continuum. Someone else with a similar cold may feel unable to function and place him- or herself in compensation on the continuum.

Case Example 1.1

Angela has always enjoyed good health and, for the most part, eats sensibly and exercises regularly. Recently, however, she began to have a burning pain in her upper abdomen, as well as some bloating and nausea after eating. Her doctor thinks that she has a peptic ulcer (i.e., a sore in the lining of the stomach or upper small intestine), which likely developed when she was taking aspirin for several months to relieve pain from a knee injury. Angela is being treated, and her symptoms are starting to improve.

On the health–illness continuum, Angela considers herself to be in compensation but moving toward good health. For Angela, the direction of movement would be noted by an arrow moving toward optimum health (←). Figure 1.2 shows Angela on the continuum near "fair health" and moving toward "optimum health."

Figure 1.2　　　Health–Illness Continuum: Angela

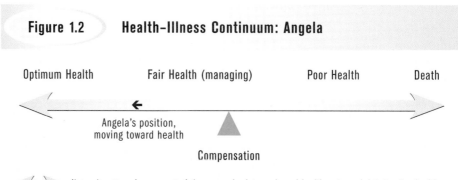

| Optimum Health | Fair Health (managing) | Poor Health | Death |

Angela's position, moving toward health

Compensation

Notes direction of movement of the person back toward good health or toward deteriorating health

THE PSYCHOLOGY OF HEALTH BEHAVIOUR

Health behaviour
The activities and actions a person engages in to acquire and maintain good physical and psychological health.

Demonstrated by a person's response or reaction to altered health, **health behaviour** has a significant impact on what a person does to maintain good physical and psychological health. Many factors, including what a person believes to be true about health, prevention, treatment, and vulnerability, influence how people act when they are ill or perceive they are ill. Health behaviour also depends on a person's level of health knowledge, personal motivation, cognitive processes, and perceived risk factors.

To explain human health behaviour, several models have been developed, including the transtheoretical model (Prochaska, 1979), the social–ecological model (Bronfenbrenner, 1979), the protection motivation theory (Rogers, 1975), and the health belief model (developed in the 1950s by the United States Public Health Service). Elements of the health belief model are relevant in one way or another to all of the others, so it is described in the most detail below.

TRANSTHEORETICAL MODEL

The transtheoretical model of health behaviour proposes that people must progress through the following series of steps before their health behaviour completely changes, modifies, or improves: precontemplation, contemplation, preparation, action, maintenance, and termination. Integrated into these steps are 10 cognitive and behavioural activities that further facilitate change. For example, during the precontemplation stage, although aware that a behaviour modification may improve his or her health, the person has no desire or motivation to make a change and may resist any attempts to help him or her to change. During the next step, the contemplation stage, the person is ready to think about making changes and may consider the risks and benefits of a behaviour change. The person moves through the remaining steps, ending in the termination stage. At this final stage, the person has established adaptive behaviour and has no desire to return to his or her previous behaviour. In this model, to be successful, a person must be able to make and commit to decisions.

SOCIAL–ECOLOGICAL MODEL

The social–ecological model maintains that many levels of influence shape one's health behaviour. Such influences include a person's education, occupation, or profession; the type of social support (personal, community) he or she has; his or her environment (e.g., workplace, availability of health care); and the public policies of various levels of government. The ideal environment is one that promotes good health, health education, and a healthy workplace, and welcomes government policies that support and endorse effective health care.

PROTECTION MOTIVATION THEORY

Building upon the health belief model (discussed below), protection motivation theory asserts that self-preservation is what motivates a person to change his or her health behaviour. The fear of illness, physical decline, or even death can encourage adaptive (or maladaptive) health behaviours. The person's actions depend on how severe he or she perceives a threat to be. For example, if a man fears that he will develop lung cancer, his health behaviours will be altered by how vulnerable he thinks he is (i.e., his likelihood of actually getting lung cancer), what he has to do to avoid this threat (e.g., quit smoking), and his ability (or motivation) to take action.

HEALTH BELIEF MODEL

People's **health beliefs** affect their health behaviour. Health beliefs are things people believe to be true about their personal health and susceptibility to illness, and about illness, prevention, and treatment in general. Beliefs are acquired largely through social interaction and experience. Around since the mid-1950s, the concept that health beliefs affect health behaviour is widely accepted and is based on a number of assumptions—for example, if people feel that by taking a certain action, they can avoid a negative outcome, they will take that action (Case Example 1.2).

Case Example 1.2

Marcy is 17 years old and sexually active. She is convinced that if she takes the birth control pill, she will avoid becoming pregnant.

Despite a family history of heart disease, Jacob, 30, smokes and does not exercise regularly. If he truly believes that he can prevent heart disease by quitting smoking and by taking up exercise, he will do so.

Many things can stop people from following a recommended course of action to avoid a negative health event—for example, how "at risk" a person feels. Consider Marcy. She may *know* that taking a birth control pill will prevent a pregnancy, but she may also feel that the chances of an unplanned pregnancy happening to her are so slim that she is inclined not to bother taking the pill. She may convince herself that using the withdrawal or rhythm method will be enough to prevent pregnancy. In other words, she does not believe that she is vulnerable.

Although Jacob may be aware of his vulnerability (due to his family history), he feels sure that he will not suffer heart disease. This feeling of security may be a result of his age. As well, he feels healthy and likes his current lifestyle. Some individuals have the sense that they are immortal and not vulnerable to developing health problems—a dangerous philosophy. This outlook affects one's health behaviour.

Another factor that influences people's choices and level of concern is the perceived seriousness of the condition or illness if acquired. Marcy may think that a pregnancy would be devastating, or she may believe that she and her boyfriend would marry and live happily ever after. She may also think that an abortion is a viable option if pregnancy were to occur. Jacob may feel that if he develops heart disease, it will be when he is old, and then who cares! He may feel that he will cross that bridge when he comes to it.

Experience and the emotions it produces (e.g., fear) can shape a person's health beliefs and behaviours, as is the case for Myra and Emiko (Case Example 1.3). For Günter (Case Example 1.4), beliefs about the quality of life and the inevitability of death have influenced his health behaviour—refusing a recommended treatment for his advanced cancer.

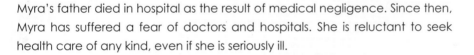

Case Example 1.3

Myra's father died in hospital as the result of medical negligence. Since then, Myra has suffered a fear of doctors and hospitals. She is reluctant to seek health care of any kind, even if she is seriously ill.

Emiko's best friend lost her first child at birth in the hospital. Emiko, when pregnant with twins, tried to find a midwife to deliver her babies at home. Despite the possible risks, Emiko believed a home birth was safer than going to a hospital.

Case Example 1.4

Günter, 57, has cancer of the bowel, which has spread to the lungs and bone. He has been told that he has six months to live. His family wants him to undergo treatment, but Günter believes that accepting treatment will only prolong a painful death and interfere with the time he has left with his family.

Culture and religion also influence health beliefs. As a multicultural country, Canada requires health care professionals to pay close attention to and respect cultural and religious traditions. The respect, or lack thereof, shown for such beliefs can affect how the client feels about seeking health care (timing and from whom) and following treatment plans (compliance).

SICK ROLE BEHAVIOUR

It is widely accepted that when people are ill, their behaviours, roles, and attitudes change. This response to illness is sometimes referred to as **sick role behaviour** or behavioural illness response (Thompson, 2005). The stress of being ill can alter people's perceptions and the way they interact with others, from those close to them to the health care professionals they deal with. A person's illness can also influence the behaviour of those associating with him or her, in large part because these people often have a burden placed on them. They may be required to provide extra support to the ill person or to assume his or her responsibilities, causing both a change in their daily routine and stress.

To better understand sick role behaviour, consider the fact that we all behave differently at different times, with different people, and in different situations. These varying behaviours affect, among other things, the diverse roles and responsibilities we assume throughout our lifetime. Persons who are ill are relieved from the roles and responsibilities they have in society—which ones and to what extent depend on the nature and severity of their illness.

The majority of clients you see will probably respond to their illness in an adaptive manner. Other clients, particularly those with a more serious illness or prolonged health problem, will respond by being "more of what they are." For example, people who consistently complain about their health, call frequently, and rely heavily on health care professionals will become more extreme in these behaviours. On the other hand, a normally easygoing client may become inwardly focused and quiet, even disagreeable and demanding (Case Example 1.5).

Although pronounced changes in attitude are more apt to be evident when a person suffers a serious illness, the stress of a relatively minor illness or accident (for example, a broken leg or pneumonia) can also be problematic—especially if the illness limits or alters the client's activities, role functions, or ability to work, even for a short period of time. Such limitations will invariably affect the client's attitude and outlook, as well as the attitudes of those close to the client (Case Example 1.6).

Case Example 1.5

Ashma, a student nurse, was looking after a young mother in labour and delivery. The mother was uncommunicative, almost passive, as labour progressed, making it impossible for Ashma to determine how much pain her client was experiencing and, therefore, to assess her needs accurately. The next day, when she went to see the new mother on the postpartum unit, Ashma was greeted by a big smile and an outgoing, chatty, and cheery demeanour. Ashma could not believe this was the same person.

Case Example 1.6

Jane has broken her leg, cannot put weight on it, and is unable to climb the stairs to the bedrooms. She is the main caregiver for her three small children. When her husband becomes almost paralyzed by the thought of assuming the responsibilities of bathing the children and putting them to bed by himself, Jane grows anxious and presses the doctor to do something so that she can resume these duties. Her husband becomes angry at both Jane and the doctor.

Health care professionals can do their part by maintaining their professional role and respecting the fact that clients will present moods and attitudes that differ from those they display in good health. Family members may also become upset, short-tempered, and demanding. It is important to remember that they, too, are coping with the stress of altered roles and functions and are probably frightened and concerned about their loved one who is ill. They, too, need support and empathy.

BEHAVIOUR IN HOSPITALIZED CLIENTS

Hospitalized clients are most likely to display visible changes in behaviour. While in the hospital, they must relinquish their responsibilities and may become passive and dependent or irritable and noncompliant. A person used to being independent can have difficulties adapting to the hospital environment. In most cases, the more serious a client's illness, the longer he or she is in the hospital, and the more his or her autonomy is restricted, the greater is the extent of behavioural changes.

Once a hospitalized client is released and sent home, he or she will likely require ongoing care. It is important that all health care professionals, regardless of their role in the client's care or recovery, show sensitivity for the client's demeanour and recognize that the client will need support and encouragement.

When clients are disagreeable and noncompliant with treatment, consider the nature and the severity of their illness and try to understand their viewpoint. Sometimes just asking why they are upset or refuse treatment can aid a situation. Clients' behaviour may relate to their previous experiences, a lack of knowledge, or some other problem that can be addressed. Importantly, do not mistake their sick role behaviour for their "normal" behaviour. Try to remain patient, good-humoured, and resourceful in creating a supportive environment, and do not take insults or criticism personally.

Sometimes it is necessary for you, as a health care professional, to seek the help of other team members to ensure optimal care and treatment. Involve the client in the treatment plan, explain the rationale and benefit for each step, and ask the client what he or she sees as realistic, as demonstrated in Case Example 1.7.

Case Example 1.7

Heidi, a physiotherapy assistant, has been asked to get Emily, a 76-year-old client, up and about after major abdominal surgery. The nurses have assured Heidi that Emily received medication for any pain she may feel when she tries to get up. Heidi carefully explains to Emily the benefits of early mobilization and asks her to walk to the door and back. Emily flatly refuses to move, bitterly complaining that nobody cares about her and no one will help her. She calls Heidi cruel and uncaring.

Heidi decides to make a "contract" with Emily about how far she can walk. She places a chair 1 m away from the bed and tells Emily she would settle for her going as far as the chair, resting, and then returning to bed. Heidi also reassures Emily that she will help her sit up on the bed and that she can move forward only when she feels she is ready. This solution is a compromise and gives Emily an element of control.

STAGES OF ILLNESS: INFLUENCE ON CLIENT BEHAVIOUR

A client's acceptance of a diagnosis and treatment plan normally follows a relatively predictable path through the stages of illness. But a person's response and choice of course of action depend on his or her health beliefs, health behaviours, and other variables discussed in this chapter. It must be noted that a person may have an illness "brewing" for some time before symptoms appear. How long the illness has been present will affect the nature and severity of the **signs** and **symptoms** of the illness once they do become apparent, as well as the outcome of the illness.

Preliminary Phase: Suspecting Symptoms

The preliminary phase of illness begins when an individual suspects that he or she is getting sick. Most people simply acknowledge the presence of symptoms (e.g., a headache or sore throat) and carry on with their activities, not dwelling on the possibility that they might be coming down with something. Others might spend more time analyzing their symptoms, perhaps looking them up online and even self-treating.

Acknowledgement Phase: Sustained Clinical Signs

If the symptoms persist and become so clearly defined that they cannot be ignored, most people will acknowledge that something is wrong. Some individuals may discuss the problem with a family member or friend. Others, depending on the severity of the complaint, will make an appointment to see their primary health care professional.

Action Phase: Seeking Treatment

During the action phase, a person decides to seek help from a health care professional, thereby taking the next step to deal with the illness.

Transitional Phase: Diagnosis and Treatment

Each person responds differently to a diagnosis. If the problem is simple and easily treated, the person will usually accept the diagnosis and its recommended treatment. But with an undesirable diagnosis, such as cancer, a person may initially deny the diagnosis and seek a second opinion.

In today's health care system, most clients participate in their own diagnosis and treatment. Health care professionals offer as many viable treatment plans as are reasonable (and, in some cases, affordable) for a given condition, and the client chooses one, usually with the support of the health care professional, his or her family, or both—but these two groups do not always agree. For example, a person may request aggressive treatment for a terminal illness, even when the health care professional feels that treatment is futile. Conversely, a person may refuse treatment, opting for a better quality of life without undesirable side effects.

Resolution Phase: Recovery and Rehabilitation

Once treatment has begun, the focus shifts toward getting better, preventing deterioration, and making the client comfortable. In the case of a short-term illness,

Signs

Those things related to an illness that a person or examiner can see (e.g., a rash).

Symptoms

Those things that a person feels that may relate to an illness (e.g., fatigue, a headache).

the client will quickly return to his or her normal position on the health–illness continuum. With a longer-term illness, the client will ideally focus on treatment until achieving recovery or until reaching his or her maximum potential if complete recovery is impossible or unrealistic.

Compliance with treatment can waver during the recovery phase. Some clients are proactive from the beginning to the end of the treatment regime and follow directions precisely. Others may follow directions until they begin to feel better and then become sporadic in adhering to treatment or give it up altogether. Health education from a primary health care professional or a nurse can go a long way toward persuading a client to properly complete a treatment plan.

For the most part, people accept their altered health state. Some, however, may vacillate between accepting their illness and denying it, and never come to terms with what has happened to them. When the client faces long-term disability or death, remember that family members and close friends will also go through a process before achieving acceptance. They, too, require support, patience, and understanding from the health care team.

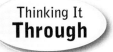

Thinking It **Through**

A hospitalized client has been diagnosed with diabetes and requires dietary adjustments and insulin injections. He refuses to eat his meals, opting for chips and candy brought in by friends. As a dietary assistant, you have been asked to review his meal plan with him. The client grumbles about the fuss everyone is making and does not understand the need for any changes to his lifestyle. What approach would you take with this client?

SELF-IMPOSED RISK BEHAVIOURS

Examples of self-imposed risk behaviours (see page 11) include smoking, unhealthy eating habits, inactivity, alcohol or drug abuse, and sexual promiscuity. People engage in risk behaviours for a number of reasons, including habit (which often becomes addictive behaviour) and thrill seeking. A common initiator among young people is peer pressure. For example, if a teen's friends smoke or take drugs, he or she will probably try it, rather than risk not fitting in. Risk behaviour includes indirect activity. For example, people who choose not to smoke may nevertheless place themselves in danger of inhaling second-hand smoke (often, however, this is not a choice, especially in a family environment). Or they may drive sensibly but voluntarily ride in a car with an impaired driver.

Health promotion and illness prevention initiatives undertaken by all levels of government aim to reduce self-imposed risk behaviour for two reasons: to ease the financial burden on our health care system and to promote the health and longevity of Canadians.

THE HEALTH OF CANADIANS TODAY

Today's Canadians are living longer. The **life expectancy** for both men and women continues to rise. On average, women are living 82.6 years and men are living 77.8 years, although this gap between the sexes is closing. The overall life expectancy for both men and women in Canada currently is 80.2 years (Table 1.1). Since 1979, men's life expectancy has increased 5.8 years, and women's, 3.3 years.

Life expectancy
The number of years a population or parts of a population is expected to live as determined by statistics.

Table 1.1	Life Expectancy[1] by Sex and Geography		
	Both Sexes (Years)	**Males (Years)**	**Females (Years)**
Canada	80.2	77.8	82.6
Newfoundland and Labrador	78.5	75.8	81.3
Prince Edward Island	79.2	76.8	81.6
Nova Scotia	79.1	76.5	81.6
New Brunswick	79.7	77.0	82.2
Quebec	80.1	77.5	82.6
Ontario	80.6	78.3	82.7
Manitoba	78.9	76.4	81.4
Saskatchewan	79.3	76.6	82.1
Alberta	80.2	77.8	82.6
British Columbia	80.9	78.7	83.1
Yukon Territory[2]	76.4	74.5	78.6
Northwest Territories[2]	79.1	78.4	81.7
Nunavut[2]	70.4	66.8	74.2

1. The population estimates used for the 2004 life expectancy calculations are July 1, 2004, updated postcensal estimates, adjusted for net census undercoverage, and include non-permanent residents. These population estimates appear in the publication "Annual Demographic Statistics, 2005" (catalogue number 91-213-XIB/XPB).

2. Life expectancy for Yukon Territory, the Northwest Territories, and Nunavut should be interpreted with caution due to small underlying counts.

Source: Statistics Canada. Canadian Vital Statistics, Birth and Death Database, and Demographic Division. (2009). *Life expectancy, abridged life table, at birth and at age 65, by sex, Canada, provinces and territories, annual (years).* CANSIM table 102-0511. Retrieved May 29, 2009, from http://cansim2.statcan.ca/cgi-win/CNSMCGI. PGM?Lang=E&ArrayId=102-0511&Array_Pick=1&Detail=1&ResultTemplate=CII/CII___&RootDir=CII/

A total of 230,132 people died in Canada in 2005, up 1.6% from the previous year. This rise was the largest annual increase since a 1.9% increase in 2002. Alberta, Ontario, and Newfoundland and Labrador suffered the largest increases in deaths (Statistics Canada, 2008). Reasons for higher death rates include an increasingly aging population and an escalation in obesity, which contributes to diabetes and cardiovascular disease.

Infant mortality
The death of an infant (i.e., within the first year of life).

The rate of **infant mortality** is often used as a measure of the effectiveness of a country's health care system. Prior to the late 1990s, the infant mortality rate had been declining steadily in Canada. Except for Japan, Canada had the most dramatic decline globally—in 1960, Canada's infant mortality rate was 27.3 per 1000 live births. This rate fell to 5.6 per 1000 live births by 1996 (Public Health Agency of Canada, 1999).

Aboriginal peoples
Broadly, individuals indigenous to a country or region. In Canada, the term applies to First Nations, Inuit, and Métis people.

From 1998 to 2005, infant mortality in Canada remained fairly stable at 5.4 infant deaths per 1000 live births, although Newfoundland and Labrador, Quebec, Saskatchewan, Alberta, British Columbia, and the Northwest Territories experienced an increase in male infant mortality. Infant mortality rates remain higher in areas that are populated predominately by **Aboriginal peoples**. These higher rates are due primarily to poorer than average living conditions and pre-natal care, and limited health care services (Statistics Canada, 2008).

More recently, with a mortality rate of 5.4 per 1000 live births in 2005, Canada has fared less well than the other G7 nations, with the exception of the United States (where the mortality rate is 6.8 per 1000 live births). On the other side of the scale, the United Kingdom showed an infant mortality rate of 5.1; Italy, 4.9; Germany, 3.9; France, 2.6; and Japan, the lowest, at 2.9 per 1000 live births (Human Resources and Skills Development Canada, 2009). It is important to note that countries may calculate infant mortality rates differently; Canada and the United States, for example, include in their rates very premature babies whose chances of survival are low, which thereby elevates their statistics.

Leading Causes of Death in Canada

Cardiovascular disease
Disease that affects the heart and vascular system (i.e., blood vessels).

Cardiovascular disease and cancer are the leading causes of death in Canada, with each claiming about 30% of the overall deaths in the country (Figures 1.3 and 1.4). According to 2004 statistics, the number of deaths due to cardiovascular disease fell sharply, while the number of deaths due to cancer rose; it is expected that, eventually, deaths from cancer will take the lead (Statistics Canada, 2007). The leading cause of death varies across differing age groups.

Cancer

Cancer results from abnormal cellular growth within the body. Along with familial or genetic causes, many cancers are associated with risk factors. Some risk

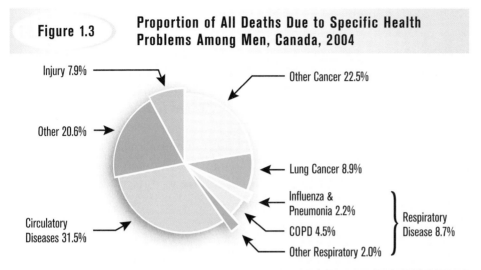

Figure 1.3 **Proportion of All Deaths Due to Specific Health Problems Among Men, Canada, 2004**

Injury 7.9%

Other 20.6%

Other Cancer 22.5%

Lung Cancer 8.9%

Influenza & Pneumonia 2.2%

COPD 4.5%

Other Respiratory 2.0%

Respiratory Disease 8.7%

Circulatory Diseases 31.5%

Source: Public Health Agency of Canada. (2008). *Chronic respiratory diseases facts and figures.* Figure 1-6. Retrieved October 7, 2009, from http://www.phac-aspc.gc.ca/cd-mc/crd-mrc/crd_figures-mrc_figures-eng. php. Adapted and reproduced with the permission of the Minister of Public Works and Government Services Canada, 2009.

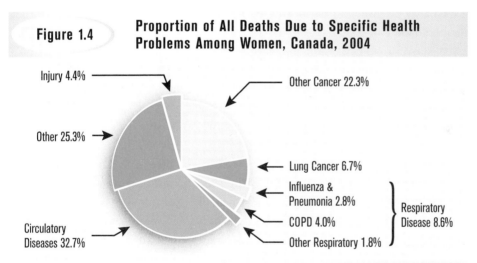

Figure 1.4 **Proportion of All Deaths Due to Specific Health Problems Among Women, Canada, 2004**

Injury 4.4%

Other 25.3%

Other Cancer 22.3%

Lung Cancer 6.7%

Influenza & Pneumonia 2.8%

COPD 4.0%

Other Respiratory 1.8%

Respiratory Disease 8.6%

Circulatory Diseases 32.7%

Source: Public Health Agency of Canada. (2008). *Chronic respiratory diseases facts and figures.* Figure 1-7. Retrieved October 7, 2009, from http://www.phac-aspc.gc.ca/cd-mc/crd-mrc/crd_figures-mrc_figures-eng. php. Adapted and reproduced with the permission of the Minister of Public Works and Government Services Canada, 2009.

factors are within our control (i.e., self-imposed risk behaviour); others we have little or no control over (e.g., a genetic propensity). Smoking tobacco, eating an unhealthy diet, abusing alcohol, and being exposed to toxic chemicals are risk factors that increase a person's chances of getting cancer.

In 2009, an estimated 117,000 new cases of cancer and 75,300 deaths will occur in Canada, an increase of 1500 deaths over 2008. Lung cancer remains the leading cause of all cancer-related deaths in both males and females, with an estimated 20,200 deaths annually in Canada. Morbidity and mortality rates from lung cancer in males are highest in Quebec and lowest in British Columbia; Nova Scotia is predicted to record the highest instance of lung cancer in females.

Breast cancer is the most common cancer among Canadian women, while prostate cancer is the most common among Canadian men. Overall, colorectal cancer is the second leading cause of death due to cancer (Canadian Cancer Society et al., 2008).

Cardiovascular Diseases

About one in four Canadians have or are at risk for cardiovascular disease, the leading cause of premature death in Canada (Canadian Institutes of Health Research, 2006). Cardiovascular diseases include ischemic heart disease (i.e., problems with circulation of blood to the heart), stroke, peripheral vascular disease (i.e., problems with circulation, primarily in the legs), heart failure, and coronary artery disease (caused by atherosclerosis, narrowing of the arteries) (Public Health Agency of Canada, 2008d).

A startling 90% of Canadians are aware that cardiovascular disease is preventable, but many do not appear to be aware of the associated self-imposed risk behaviours (MacDonald et al., 1992). The major risk behaviours for cardiovascular disease include tobacco smoke, lack of exercise, unhealthy eating, **obesity**, high cholesterol, high blood pressure, excessive dietary salt, and stress (Public Health Agency of Canada, 2008b).

Obesity
Excessive accumulation of body fat to the point that an individual's health is at risk; sometimes objectively defined as a person's weighing more than 30% of his or her ideal body weight as determined by individual height and build.

Men appear more likely to suffer from heart disease earlier in life, while women are more likely to develop heart disease around menopause. In its 2007 annual report, the Canadian Heart and Stroke Foundation reported that for a Canadian woman, the risk of dying within 30 days after a myocardial infarction (i.e., heart attack) was 16% higher than for a man. The risk for dying of a stroke was noted as 11% higher for a woman (Canadian Institute for Health Information, 2006). As well, women are less likely to be referred to and treated by a specialist and less likely to be recommended for testing, such as cardiac catheterization. Some literature suggests that women with heart disease who have strokes are also less likely to be diagnosed early and treated promptly.

At over $18 billion per year, the cost of treating cardiovascular disease is the highest health care cost in Canada (Canadian Institutes of Health Research, 2006).

Respiratory Diseases

Over 3 million Canadians suffer from respiratory diseases; the most common are asthma, **chronic obstructive pulmonary disease (COPD)**, lung cancer, tuberculosis (TB), and cystic fibrosis (Public Health Agency of Canada, 2008c).

Smoking tobacco remains the most significant preventable risk factor for chronic respiratory conditions. Environmental factors also cause respiratory diseases, with the quality of both indoor and outdoor air posing a continuing and serious problem (Public Health Agency of Canada, 2008a).

Since individuals over 65 are largely affected, Canada's aging population is contributing to increases in chronic respiratory diseases. Respiratory diseases cost the health care system over $8 billion annually (Public Health Agency of Canada, 2000).

> **Chronic obstructive pulmonary disease (COPD)**
> Persistent lung disease that interferes with normal breathing, including both chronic bronchitis (i.e., permanent inflammation of the main airways in the lungs) and emphysema (i.e., enlargement of the air sacs in the lungs).

In the **News**   **International Travel and Infectious Disease**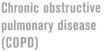

In Canada alone, about 1600 new cases of tuberculosis (TB) surface each year. Treating this disease presents a challenge, especially because certain strains of TB remain resistant to treatment. Although drug-resistant TB is not yet a major problem in Canada, it may become one due to the increase in and ease of international travel.

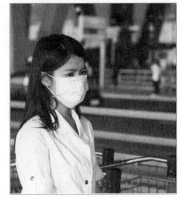

In May 2007, a US citizen with an extensively drug-resistant strain of TB arrived in Montreal from Prague, Czech Republic, and then drove across the border to New York. All of the passengers on his plane and anyone else who may have come into contact with him were followed up with to ensure they did not contract this serious and highly contagious disease.

Sources: Health Canada. (2009). *It's your health. Tuberculosis.* Retrieved May 29, 2009, from http://www.hc-sc.gc.ca/hl-vs/alt_formats/pacrb-dgapcr/pdf/iyh-vsv/diseases-maladies/tuberculosis-eng.pdf; Public Health Agency of Canada. (2007, June 1). *Infectious diseases news brief.* Retrieved May 29, 2009, from http://www.phac-aspc.gc.ca/bid-bmi/dsd-dsm/nb-ab/2007/nb2207-eng.php

Photo credit: © iStockphoto.com/macky_ch.

SUMMARY

❖ Differing definitions of terms like *health, disease, illness,* and *wellness* often relate to an individual's perceptions of good health and the absence of good health.

❖ The health–illness continuum is a measurement tool by which a person's level of health is measured. People move on this scale according to an interpretation of their health status.

❖ A person's perceptions of health—what a person believes to be true about health—will determine how that person deals with health issues and how he or she interacts with the health care system and with you as a health care professional. Your understanding of the client as a person (as much as time and opportunity will allow) will affect the quality of your professional relationship with that client and, possibly, the success of your interaction in terms of your role in the health care team.

❖ Overall, the health of Canadians has improved over the past decade, yet challenges remain in providing prompt and effective care, particularly for those with cancer, cardiovascular diseases, and diseases of the respiratory system—the leading causes of morbidity and mortality in the country. Aboriginal peoples are particularly at risk, for socioeconomic reasons and, for many, because of the lack of proximity to larger treatment centres.

❖ Focusing on disease prevention and health promotion is the best way to improve the health of Canadians. This approach involves educating people about self-imposed risk behaviours related to major diseases and encouraging healthy lifestyles. You, as a health care professional, can make an important difference.

REVIEW QUESTIONS

1. Describe the difference between a disease and a disability.

2. Compare and contrast the wellness, medical, and holistic models of health, identifying three key points of each.

3. Differentiate between health beliefs and health behaviours.

4. Briefly describe how someone's health behaviour can affect how you as a health care professional treat that person.

5. Considering the stages of illness, what issues must a client deal with in the resolution phase?

6. What are the leading causes of morbidity and mortality in Canada, as discussed in this chapter? Research current statistics to determine whether the three leading causes have changed over the past year.

DISCUSSION QUESTIONS

1. Construct your own definition of *health*. Compare it to the WHO definition and then to the definitions of four classmates. Discuss both similarities and differences in your personal definitions. Explain where you think the differences originate. Discuss your differences with the class in group format.

2. Select two self-imposed risk behaviours (e.g., smoking and inactivity) and, using Statistics Canada data, identify the related health statistics for your own province or territory. Compare these statistics with the statistics of a province or territory with a higher risk rate and one with a lower risk rate. What contributing factors do you think cause the statistics to vary?

3. You work in a large hospital. Several patients with the H1N1 virus have been admitted to a patient care unit. You have been asked, as a member of the health care team, to help attend to these individuals. A colleague has confided that she will call in sick rather than expose herself to anyone with this virus. How would you deal with this situation?

WEB RESOURCES

Public Health Agency of Canada
http://www.phac-aspc.gc.ca

The Public Health Agency of Canada provides research, information, and statistics on a wide variety of health-related issues, including diseases and conditions, healthy travel abroad, maternal health, and health and safety for all stages of life.

Canadian Cancer Society
http://www.cancer.ca

A community-based volunteer organization, the Canadian Cancer Society funds research on all types of cancer, offers information on cancer, and provides support for people living with cancer.

Canadian Institutes of Health Research
http://www.cihr-irsc.gc.ca/

The Canadian Institutes of Health Research (CIHR), consisting of 13 "virtual" institutes, is the Government of Canada's agency responsible for funding health research in Canada. The agency supports nearly 12,000 researchers and trainees in universities, teaching hospitals, and other health care organizations and research centres in Canada.

WEB RESOURCES

Heart and Stroke Foundation
http://www.heartandstroke.ca

Led and supported by more than 140,000 volunteers, the Heart and Stroke Foundation of Canada is a federation of 10 provincial foundations that promotes healthy living and works toward eliminating heart disease and stroke through research.

Statistics Canada
http://www.statcan.gc.ca

Statistics Canada is Canada's central, national statistical agency that collects data about virtually every aspect of Canadian life. In addition to about 350 active surveys, it conducts a census every five years.

Terry Fox Foundation
http://www.terryfox.org

The Terry Fox Foundation is an independent charitable organization that raises funds to finance cancer research. All money raised by the foundation is distributed through the National Cancer Institute of Canada.

United Nations Web Site for the Rights and Dignity of Persons With Disabilities
http://www.un.org/disabilities/

The United Nations World Program of Action is a global strategy to enhance disability prevention, rehabilitation, and equalization of opportunities. The program provides funding for building the capacity of nongovernment organizations to take part in the implementation of the *Convention on the Rights of Persons With Disabilities*.

Seven Dimensions of Wellness
http://wellness.ucr.edu/seven_dimensions.html

This article outlines the seven dimensions of wellness used in the wellness model of the University of California Riverside campus.

Spiritual Health Lectures
http://academic.cuesta.edu/wholehealth/Level2/Lecpages/sphlth.htm

The Spiritual Health Lectures discuss how spiritual health relates to physical health and offers definitions and questions to consider. The material is available in text, slide, and audio formats.

Wellness Wheel: The Seven Dimensions of Wellness
http://students.sfu.ca/health/healthpromotion/wheel.html

This Web page provides access to the wellness wheel developed by Simon Fraser University, which can be used to determine which areas of a person's life are balanced and which may need some improvement. Each dimension includes a list of resources. On this site, you will also find a link to a wellness quiz.

ADDITIONAL RESOURCES

Donatelle, R.J., Davis, L.G., Munroe, A.J., Munroe, A., & Casselman, M.A. (2005). *Health: The basics* (6th ed.). San Francisco: Benjamin Cummings.

Gochman, D.S. (1997). *Handbook of health behavior research I: Personal and social determinants*. Norwell, MA: Kluwer Boston, Inc.

Kubler-Ross, E. (1997). *On death and dying*. New York: Scribner.

Spurgeon, D. (2007). Gender gap persists in treatment of Canadians after heart attack. *British Medical Journal, 334*(7588), 280. Retrieved May 29, 2009, from http://www.bmj.com/cgi/content/extract/334/7588/280-b

REFERENCES

Bronfenbrenner, U. (1979). *The ecology of human development: Experiments by nature and design*. Cambridge, MA: Harvard University Press.

Canadian Cancer Society, National Cancer Institute of Canada, Statistics Canada, & Public Health Agency of Canada. (2008). *Canadian cancer statistics 2008*. Retrieved May 29, 2009, from http://www. cancer.ca/Canada-wide/About%20cancer/ Cancer%20statistics/~/media/CCS/Canada%20wide/ Files%20List/English%20files%20heading/pdf% 20not%20in%20publications%20section/Canadian% 20Cancer%20Society%20Statistics%20PDF%202008_ 614137951.ashx

Canadian Fitness and Lifestyle Research Institute. (2005). *2005 physical activity and sport: Encouraging children to be active*. Retrieved May 29, 2009, from http://www. cflri.ca/eng/statistics/surveys/documents/PAM2005. pdf

Canadian Fitness and Lifestyle Research Institute. (2007). *Kids CAN PLAY!* Retrieved May 29, 2009, from http://www.cflri.ca/eng/programs/canplay/documents/ kidsCANPLAY_b1.pdf

Canadian Institute for Health Information. (2006). *Health care in Canada*. Retrieved May 29, 2009, from http://secure.cihi.ca/cihiweb/products/hcic2006_e.pdf

Canadian Institutes of Health Research. (2006). *Health research—Investing in Canada's future 2003–2004*. Retrieved May 29, 2009, from http://www.cihr-irsc. gc.ca/e/24939.html

Human Resources and Skills Development Canada. (2009). *Indicators of well-being in Canada: Health— Infant mortality*. Retrieved July 29, 2009, from http://www4.hrsdc.gc.ca/.3ndic.1t.4r@-eng.jsp?iid=2

Katzmarzyk, P.T., Gledhill, N., & Shephard, R.J. (2000). The economic burden of physical inactivity in Canada. *Canadian Medical Association Journal, 163*(11), 1435–1440.

Larson, J.S. (1991). *The measurement of health: Concepts and indicators*. New York: Greenwood Press.

MacDonald, S., Joffres, M.P., Stachenko, S.J., Horlick, L., & Fodor, G. (1992). Multiple cardiovascular risk factors in Canadian adults. *Canadian Medical Association Journal, 11*(suppl.), 2021–2029.

ParticipACTION. (1969). *The ParticipACTION archive project*. Retrieved May 29, 2009, from http://www. usask.ca:80/archives/participaction/english/impact/ index.html

Prochaska, J.O. (1979). *Systems of psychotherapy: A transtheoretical analysis*. Georgetown, ON: Dorsey Press.

Public Health Agency of Canada. (1999). *Measuring up. A health surveillance update on Canadian children and youth*. Retrieved May 29, 2009, from http://www. phac-aspc.gc.ca/publicat/meas-haut/

Public Health Agency of Canada. (2000). *Economic burden of respiratory disease in Canada*. Retrieved May 29, 2009, from http://www.phac-aspc.gc.ca/ cd-mc/crd-mrc/crd_figures-mrc_figures-eng.php#t1-2

Public Health Agency of Canada. (2008a). *Chronic respiratory diseases. Risk factors*. Retrieved May 29, 2009, from http://www.phac-aspc.gc.ca/cd-mc/ crd-mrc/index-eng.php

Public Health Agency of Canada. (2008b). *Minimizing the risks of cardiovascular disease*. Retrieved May 29, 2009, from http://www.phac-aspc.gc.ca/cd-mc/ cvd-mcv/risk-risques-eng.php

Public Health Agency of Canada. (2008c). *Respiratory disease in Canada*. Retrieved May 29, 2009, from http://www.phac-aspc.gc.ca/publicat/rdc-mrc01/pdf/ rdc0901e.pdf

Public Health Agency of Canada. (2008d). *Six types of cardiovascular disease*. Retrieved May 29, 2009, from http://www.phac-aspc.gc.ca/cd-mc/cvd-mcv/ cvd-mcv-eng.php

Rogers, R.W. (1975). A protection motivation theory of fear appeals and attitude change. *Journal of Psychology, 91*, 93–114.

REFERENCES

Statistics Canada. (2007, April 27). *The Daily*. (No. 84F0209XWE). Retrieved May 29, 2009, from http://www.statcan.gc.ca/daily-quotidien/070427/tdq070427-eng.htm

Statistics Canada. (2008, January 14). Deaths. *The Daily*. (No. 84F0211XWE). Retrieved May 29, 2009, from http://www.statcan.gc.ca/daily-quotidien/080114/dq080114b-eng.htm

Thompson, V. (2005). *Administrative and clinical procedures for the health office professional*. Toronto: Pearson Prentice Hall.

World Health Organization. (1986). *Health promotion: Concepts and principles in action—A policy framework*. Copenhagen: WHO Regional Office for Europe.

CHAPTER TWO

Population Health:

Introduction and Principles

Learning Outcomes

1. Explain the key components of population health.

2. Compare and contrast *public health* with *population health*.

3. Describe the 12 determinants of health.

4. Describe the events leading up to the use of a population health approach in Canada.

5. List the partners instrumental in implementing population health in Canada.

6. Demonstrate an understanding of the purpose of the template for population health strategies.

7. Discuss how the determinants of health are used as indicators in the population health promotion model.

8. Explain the population health approaches used by British Columbia and Saskatchewan.

KEY TERMS

Determinants of health, p. 35

Disease prevention, p. 35

Epidemiology, p. 56

Health indicators, p. 56

Health promotion, p. 35

Inequities in health, p. 45

Intersectoral cooperation, p. 54

Population health, p. 34

Population-based surveillance, p. 56

Primary care, p. 42

Primary health care, p. 45

Public health, p. 35

Qualitative research, p. 57

Quantitative research, p. 57

SES gradient, p. 36

Upstream investments, p. 58

How healthy are Canadians? What is most affecting their health? What do they need to do to prevent illness in themselves and their children? What can they do now to improve their health? The answers are found in a population health approach to health care—collaborative efforts by various government departments, community groups, and individuals to promote health strategies, health, and well-being—and the development of public health strategies. In this chapter, you will learn about population health—what it is, how it was introduced in Canada, and the impact it continues to have on the health of Canadians. You will become familiar with the determinants of health, and you will better understand Canadians' current health status, where their health ought to be, and what Canadians need to do to raise their level of health. You will also see that, although many strategies for health promotion and disease prevention exist at a national level, each province and territory has its own agenda and timeline.

POPULATION HEALTH

Population health
A framework for gathering and analyzing information about conditions that affect the health of a population. The aim is to both maintain and improve the health of the entire population and to reduce inequities in health status among population groups.

A **population health** approach looks at health in broad terms—that is, it aims to improve the health status of the population, rather than that of the individual. It is a framework for gathering and analyzing data about the factors that affect a population's health and the causes behind some groups being healthier than others (Box 2.1). The population health approach also looks for ways to improve health and to reduce inequities in health status through reductions in material and social imbalance. The benefits of a population health approach, therefore, extend beyond improving population health to building a sustainable and integrated health care system, increasing national growth and productivity, and strengthening social cohesion and citizen involvement in health care.

Box 2.1	**Population Health Video**

An e-presentation from the Canadian Institute of Health Information provides a comprehensive introduction to the basics of population health. Visit http://secure. cihi.ca/cihiweb/en/downloads/intro_to_pop_health_e/Intro_to_Pop_Health_e.html to view this presentation.

Population health embraces the newer, broader definitions of health discussed in Chapter 1. It also moves away from the medical model of health and illness toward holistic concepts like the wellness model (also discussed in Chapter 1). Population health incorporates **public health** initiatives, **health promotion**, **disease prevention**, and the concept of wellness. These strategies are funded and implemented primarily by government, although health care professionals, industry, community agencies, and individuals play a role as well.

The terms *population health* and *public health* are often used interchangeably but are different entities with a common denominator—health information. Population health is a scientific, organized approach to health promotion and disease prevention that is both social and political in nature. It looks at how lifestyles and living conditions affect the health of individuals and population groups. Often using data from population health studies, public health focuses on the practice of promoting health and preventing disease.

KEY DETERMINANTS OF HEALTH

Since the Canadian Institute for Advanced Research (CIFAR) introduced the concept of population health in 1989, Health Canada has identified a number of factors known to influence the health of a population, called **determinants of health** (Box 2.2). Health is influenced not by one determinant in isolation but rather by the interaction of multiple determinants. How these determinants work together to affect the health of a population is not clearly understood.

INCOME AND SOCIAL STATUS

Income and social status appear to be the most important determinants of health. Extensive research demonstrates the link between income, social status, and

Public health
Public health uses health information to improve the health of communities. Public health programs often carry out recommendations made by population health studies, so they tend to focus more on applying measures than on gathering and analyzing information.

Health promotion
Initiatives that inform people about things they can do to remain healthy and to prevent disease and illness. These include the principles outlined in the *Ottawa Charter for Health Promotion*: building healthy public policy, creating supportive environments, strengthening community action, developing personal skills, and reorienting health services. Imparting such knowledge helps individuals take responsibility for their own well-being.

Disease prevention
Although used in conjunction with health promotion, disease prevention is a separate entity. It seeks to stop the development of a disease or to detect and treat a disease as early as possible when it does occur to control its spread and reduce the chances of it returning.

Determinants of health
The conditions (economic, social, environmental, etc.) in which people live that affect their current and future health.

Box 2.2 Determinants of Health

1. Income and Social Status

2. Social Support Networks

3. Education and Literacy

4. Employment and Working Conditions

5. Social Environment

6. Physical Environment

7. Personal Health Practices and Coping Skills

8. Healthy Child Development

9. Biology and Genetic Endowment

10. Health Services

11. Gender

12. Culture

Source: Public Health Agency of Canada. (2001). *Determinants of health: What makes Canadians healthy or unhealthy?* Retrieved May 29, 2009, from http://www.phac-aspc.gc.ca/ph-sp/determinants/index-eng.php#determinants

health (Health Canada, 1994). A lower socioeconomic status appears to be associated with poorer health, and a higher socioeconomic status with better health; in other words, an individual's health tends to be proportional to his or her position on the socioeconomic gradient, or **SES gradient** (Box 2.3).

Box 2.3 The SES Gradient

The socioeconomic gradient (SES gradient) is a measurement of health or health inequalities as they relate to a person's or population's socioeconomic circumstances. *SES gradient* is a term widely used in population health studies today. At the bottom of the gradient are people who are below the poverty line, perhaps unemployed, living in a poor socioeconomic environment, and, therefore, at risk for poor health. As an individual's or group's socioeconomic status improves, so does the individual's or group's health.

For example, those living in what we might consider a middle-class environment tend to be healthier than those in a lower-class group. Those living in the highest socioeconomic bracket, according to the SES gradient, enjoy the highest level of health. We also know, however, that people who are born into a lower socioeconomic environment can enjoy good health and be happy, productive individuals. So the theory is not absolute, and variables within and relationships among the determinants are not clearly understood.

Source: Keating, D.P., & Hertzman, C. (Eds.). (1999). *Developmental health and the wealth of nations: Social, biological, and educational dynamics.* New York: Guilford Press.

Poor living conditions, such as substandard housing and food, can, of course, negatively influence people's health. However, research indicates that the degree of control that people have over their lives and their ability to act also significantly affect their health status. Higher income and social status generally allow for more control. Lower income and social status are often accompanied by poor self-confidence and self-esteem, which diminish an individual's ability to make choices and exercise control, and, ultimately, increase his or her risk for poor health (Health Canada, 1994).

Thinking It Through

In many cases, individuals faced with continuing challenges, such as a limited income, alcoholism, or drug addiction, overcome these adversities. They are able to find opportunities, graduate from high school and postsecondary facilities, find rewarding employment, become financially secure, and be well adapted socially.

1. Is there something about an individual's character that carries that person through adversity to achieve goals beyond what would be expected for him or her?

2. Is there another common denominator that is responsible for some people moving up the socioeconomic scale?

SOCIAL SUPPORT NETWORKS

The opportunity to share feelings, discuss problems, and receive the clear support of others relieves stress and enhances a sense of well-being. It promotes the feeling of being wanted, supported, and valued and improves a person's physical and emotional health. Social support can come from family members, friends, or a community (i.e., a support group). The type and level of support a person has or seeks are influenced by many factors, including sex, gender, and culture. Typically, men are less likely to form supportive networks and share feelings. Similarly, in some more reserved cultures, sharing personal feelings with others is discouraged. Consider Case Examples 2.1 and 2.2.

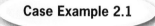

Case Example 2.1

Mary is 35 years old and has been married for five years. Her husband, Eric, is an alcoholic. They have two children. Mary is under great stress trying to cope with the effects of Eric's alcoholism on both herself and her family. She joins Al-Anon, a support group for friends and families of alcoholics. There she sees that she is not alone and learns coping mechanisms for dealing with her husband's drinking.

Case Example 2.2

Kumar is 50 years old and has been married to Reena for 15 years. They have been having marital problems for some time. Kumar is uncomfortable voicing personal problems and does not have a close friend with whom he could discuss such issues. He bottles up his feelings and, as a result, is bad tempered most of the time. His mood affects his family, friends, and colleagues. He has trouble sleeping, and his blood pressure is rising. Reena, on the other hand, is able to reach out for support and is learning to deal with her problems in a proactive way.

Kumar's behaviour is not unusual for many men. Statistically, men die at a younger age than women. This may be due, in part, to men's inability to access a social network for support and advice. In fact, recent reports show a link between the social environment and the risks of morbidity and mortality, exclusive of the effects of other health determinants. Findings also indicate that social environment can influence the course of a disease. For example, a person with cancer or cardiovascular disease will survive much longer if he or she accesses supportive social networks. This may relate, in part, to a reduction in stress and a positive, even optimistic, outlook generated by a loving and caring environment (Haydon et al., 2006; National Collaborating Centre for Determinants of Health, 2007; University of Waterloo, 2005).

EDUCATION AND LITERACY

Literacy and access to education often encourage a higher level of education, which, in turn, usually leads to jobs with higher social status and an established, steady income. Financial security increases opportunities for a person and his or her family on a number of different fronts. For example, children may benefit from participating in organized sports or taking lessons.

A higher level of education also widens people's knowledge base and their ability to think logically and to problem-solve. Higher education can develop right-brain activities such as enjoyment of the arts, creativity, philosophy, and politics, and it can motivate people to engage in meaningful relationships, become involved in the community, and, in general, become more satisfied.

EMPLOYMENT AND WORKING CONDITIONS

Individuals who are unemployed or work at menial jobs in which satisfaction is low and stress is high tend to have poorer health (Box 2.4). These people have a higher mortality rate at a younger age (e.g., from suicide—particularly among Canada's Aboriginal people living in isolated communities) and higher morbidity rates from chronic diseases (e.g., cardio-respiratory disease). Families of unemployed or underemployed individuals can also have poorer health, probably because of resulting high stress levels, related emotional problems, and a lower socioeconomic environment. Unemployment is cited as one of the largest stressors that a person or family can face. One study found that those who are unemployed experience significantly more psychological distress, anxiety, depressive symptoms, health problems, and hospitalizations, as well as take more disability days and face more activity limitations than do those who are employed (D'Arcy, 1986).

Box 2.4   **Landmark Studies Support the Link Between Employment and Health Status**

The Whitehall I Study, a classic study conducted at the British Civil Service from 1967 to 1977, demonstrated the link between health outcomes and levels of employment in the civil service. The study found that those at the lowest level of the employment scale (i.e., those with jobs that were menial and offered little job satisfaction and little control, such as messengers, doorkeepers) had a mortality rate three times higher than those in the highest employment bracket (e.g., supervisors and administrators). Furthermore, those at the lower end of the employment scale engaged in more risk behaviours (e.g., smoking, stress and unhealthy diet leading to obesity, inactivity) that contributed to the higher mortality rate. Interestingly, none

Continued on next page

of the individuals involved in the study was poor in the strict sense of the word. They each had a steady income and equal access to health care.

A follow-up study, Whitehall II, showed that individuals in high-status jobs at the British Civil Service did not have higher risks of heart disease. Whitehall II supported previous findings that employment status relates to health status but went further to suggest that the way a work environment is organized and the work atmosphere itself (e.g., how individuals are treated, relationships among employees, how much control individuals have over their work environment), along with other social influences, contribute to the SES gradient (see Box 2.3).

Sources: Marmot, M., Rose, G., Shipley, M.J., & Hamilton, P.J. (1978). Employment grade and coronary heart disease in British civil servants. *Journal of Epidemiology and Community Health, 32*, 244–249; Ferrie, J.E. (2004). *Work, stress and health: The Whitehall II Study*. London: Public and Commercial Services Union on behalf of Council of Civil Service Unions/Cabinet Office. Retrieved May 29, 2009, from http://www.ucl.ac.uk/whitehallII/findings/Whitehallbooklet.pdf

SOCIAL ENVIRONMENT

The social environment is constructed by how individuals behave; their relation-ships with others and their community; their gender, culture, and ethnic group; their education and roles in the workforce; the conditions and communities in which they live; and how they feel about themselves. These elements overlap with other determinants to influence health and life expectancy. Individuals in the same or similar social environments have been shown to demonstrate similar values, outlook on life, and ways of thinking.

The tighter knit and more organized a community, and the more involved the population is with activities within the community, the greater the health of that community. Volunteerism, for example, improves the well-being of the so-cial environment, apparently increasing a community's level of compassion, har-mony, and cohesiveness. Volunteers themselves generally live longer and suffer less from depression and heart disease (Public Health Agency of Canada, n.d.).

Thinking It Through

You have an opportunity to volunteer at your community health centre. You know it's a good cause but wonder if you can find the time with all your other commitments at school and home.

1. Do you believe that being a volunteer can contribute to your physical and social well-being?

2. Would volunteering in your chosen field add value to your résumé?

A well-organized community has agencies and resources that support community residents—for example, community- or government-sponsored child care. This affects the entire family positively by reducing stress and financial burden. Social stability fosters positive relationships, recognition and acceptance of cultural diversity, and unified communities that inspire confidence, a sense of being valued, and assurances of support—all of which have a powerful effect on reducing health risks.

Physical Environment

The physical environment consists of the "natural" environment and the "manufactured" environment. The "natural" environment includes the food people eat, the water they drink, the air they breathe, and the places they live—the outside or physical world. The "manufactured" environment refers to the homes people live in, the buildings they attend school or work in, the roads they travel, and the recreational areas such as parks and community structures they use. How this built environment is structured and constructed affects health status. For example, you may have heard the phrase "sick building syndrome." This term describes nonspecific illnesses that are attributed to time spent in a specific building. This syndrome appears to be a growing concern. In 1984, the World Health Organization (WHO) reported that up to 30% of buildings, particularly newer and remodelled structures that are airtight and well insulated, were associated with health-related complaints. The assumption is that these health issues are linked to poor air quality, although this is not an established fact in many cases (United States Environmental Protection Agency, 1991).

Currently, environmental issues are top of mind, with widespread concern over drinking water and related infrastructure, air pollution, environmental warming, pollution of agricultural land, and depletion of natural resources.

Personal Health Practices and Coping Skills

Personal health practices relate to self-imposed risk behaviours, health beliefs, and health behaviours (as discussed in Chapter 1). Personal health practices are often linked to a person's level of self-esteem, sense of control, and level of confidence. Coping skills help an individual deal with situations and problems and are, in part, a component of his or her genetic makeup. Some people are better able to deal with problems, stress, and daily challenges than others. Most health problems that are associated with this particular determinant of health relate to risk behaviour such as smoking, alcohol abuse, drug use, and poor dietary habits (e.g., eating when depressed, smoking when stressed, drinking alcohol when not wanting to face a problem) (Public Health Agency of Canada, 2003).

Thinking It
Through

As a student, you are likely faced with new challenges such as living away from home, meeting new people, and dealing with academic responsibilities.

1.   How do you respond to these stressors?

2.   Are you likely to approach a professor, friend, or family member for support?

3.   Are you aware of the resources at your university or college that can offer you support?

HEALTHY CHILD DEVELOPMENT

Many determinants of health affect the growth and development of a child, even before conception. The mother's nutritional intake, whether or not she engages in risk behaviours, and the quality and amount of her prenatal care all affect the baby during pregnancy and have lasting effects after birth. The formative years are influential in terms of the child's current and future health. Other influential determinants include socioeconomic status, biology and genetic endowment, and the physical environment. For example, babies born to mothers who have a lower position on the income scale are more likely to have a low birth weight (Child Poverty Action Group, 2005) (which, in itself, is associated with a variety of health problems), to eat a poor diet, and to experience both health and social problems throughout their lives.

BIOLOGY AND GENETIC ENDOWMENT

The phrase "biology and genetic endowment" refers to all the attributes that people inherit from their parents. These inherited attributes can make a person vulnerable to developing specific diseases and other health problems. The hereditary nature of some diseases, like cystic fibrosis, is now known (In the News: Canadian Researchers and Cystic Fibrosis); for others, the genetic link remains vague or unproven. CIFAR has recently delved into research about genetic endowment and other determinants of health, believing that significant interaction between them affects the health of both individuals and population groups.

HEALTH SERVICES

Health services include diagnosis, treatment, disease prevention, and health promotion. The type of health care services offered and their method of delivery affect the health of a population. Greater availability of **primary care** services

Primary care
Front-line care, direction, and advice provided by multidisciplinary health care teams. Primary care also involves initiatives that seek to improve access to, quality of, and continuity of care; client and health care professional satisfaction; and cost-effectiveness of health care services (Health Canada, 2006a).

In the **News**   **Canadian Researchers and Cystic Fibrosis**

Cystic fibrosis (CF) is the most common fatal genetic disease affecting young Canadians. While the exact mechanism behind the cause of cystic fibrosis remains unknown, the gene responsible for this disease was identified at Toronto's Hospital for Sick Children in 1989, a dramatic and groundbreaking discovery. Since then, scientists have been learning more about this gene and the way it works—knowledge that will ultimately lead to more effective treatments, maybe even a cure. In March 2008, it was announced that in a study led by Professor Igor Stagljar, University of Toronto scientists advanced research related to increasing the effectiveness of antibiotics used to treat chronic and acute bacterial lung infections in individuals with CF.

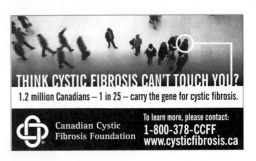

Source: Canadian Cystic Fibrosis Foundation. (2008). *About cystic fibrosis*. Retrieved May 29, 2009, from http://www.cysticfibrosis.ca

Photo credit: Courtesy of the Canadian Cystic Fibrosis Foundation.

and of health promotion and disease prevention programs (e.g., immunizations, preventive care such as breast screening, prenatal care, and well-baby initiatives) can lead to a healthier population.

Under the *Canada Health Act*, all Canadians are entitled to equal access to any and all medically necessary services. However, researchers are convinced that availability of health care plays only a small part in ensuring that a population's health is maximized, believing that the accessibility of the best health care services in the world would not guarantee a population overall good health.

GENDER

The word *gender* is often used interchangeably with *sex*, the latter of which indicates whether a person is male or female. However, *gender*, by definition, refers to social, not biological, differences. For example, gender identity is how a person perceives himself or herself socially (i.e., as a male or female). According to WHO, "Gender refers to the socially constructed roles and responsibilities assigned to women and men in a given culture. Thus, gender is distinct from sex, which is biologically determined" (Zaman & Underwood, 2003).

Gender, as a determinant of health, considers factors that produce inequities between men and women that affect the health of either sex, such as employment opportunities (e.g., men tend to have more opportunities, including greater opportunities for advancement) and income inequities (e.g., women tend to make less money). Gender also includes roles determined by society (e.g., until the late twentieth century, females were directed into such professions as teaching and nursing), attitudes, values, and personality traits.

CULTURE

Culture can be described as a way of life (e.g., behaviours, values, attitudes, geographic and political factors) that is attributed to a group of people. Ethnicity refers more to race, origin or ancestry, identity, language, and religion. Culture and ethnicity are often linked—and both affect health, particularly in terms of health beliefs, health behaviours, and lifestyle choices.

Those with different social, religious, value, and belief systems than others in their community are more likely to face inequities, marginalization, socioeconomic problems, and isolation. Minorities are especially at risk because the larger group's socioeconomic and cultural environments tend to dominate the community, and the needs of minorities can be overshadowed. Risk factors for minorities include health beliefs and health behaviours—for example, how and at what point they will approach the health care system. Barriers to seeking care may include fear, language struggles, and noninvolvement of family members. (Family members often contribute significantly by contacting a physician, providing transportation to the physician's office or hospital, explaining the rationale for treatments, and translating information when required.)

INTRODUCTION OF POPULATION HEALTH TO CANADA

The following reports and conferences were instrumental in the introduction and development of population health in Canada. The Lalonde Report, written in 1974, was the first that had Canadians looking at health differently, recognizing it as a resource that is influenced by a broad range of factors, rather than by biology alone.

THE LALONDE REPORT, 1974

In 1974, Marc Lalonde, then the minister of national health and welfare (now known as Health Canada), created a landmark document instrumental in introducing the concept of population health to Canada. This document, entitled *A New Perspective on the Health of Canadians* and informally called the Lalonde Report (Lalonde, 1974), is considered to be the first document acknowledged by a major industrialized nation to state that health is determined by more than just biology and that improved health could be achieved through changes in the following four key areas:

1. Human biology—physical and mental elements.

2. Environment—all elements related to health that are external to the body. The physical and social environments were integrated into one category.

3. Lifestyle—elements over which a person had control, such as self-imposed risk behaviours.

4. Health care organization—access to health care services within a given community.

Lalonde believed that governments at all levels should be involved in health promotion and be responsible for any increased expenditure associated with the delivery of health care. He suggested that lifestyle and self-imposed risk behaviours (see Chapter 1) should be addressed in health promotion strategies (e.g., by highlighting the dangers of smoking or impaired driving). Lalonde also outlined requirements for ongoing research and for various levels of government and community organizations to work together.

The Lalonde Report challenged traditional views about health and illness. Over the years, it has been significant in moving Canada away from the traditional medical model approach to health care. Shortly after the release of the Lalonde Report, in fact, a population health approach to health care was introduced by all levels of government and by various community groups across Canada, resulting in educational and public-awareness programs aimed at reducing risk behaviours and promoting a healthy lifestyle.

Alma-Ata Conference, 1978

In September 1978, the World Health Organization convened the international Alma-Ata conference in Kazakhstan to address the need for global cooperation on health issues and in health care reform. A slogan that emerged from that conference was "Health for All—2000," which reflected the shared goal to reduce **inequities in health** across the globe through an emphasis on primary care initiatives. **Primary health care**, as defined by the conference (Box 2.5), encompassed a broad range of concerns that paralleled those of the population health approach.

The conference's 10-point declaration (see Appendix, page 426) claimed health as a fundamental right and stated that attaining an optimum level of health should be given the highest priority by all nations. The declaration called

Inequities in health
Unfair and unequal distribution of health resources in relation to resources available and the population involved.

Primary health care
Health care with an emphasis on individuals and their communities. It includes essential medical and curative care received at the primary, secondary, or tertiary levels and involves health care professionals, as well as community members, delivering care within the community that is cost-effective, comprehensive, and collaborative (i.e., uses a team approach).

for the right of people and communities to be involved in participating in and planning their own health care and challenged governments to develop strategies to improve primary health care.

Thinking It Through

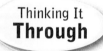

The *Declaration of Alma-Ata* identified primary health care as the key strategy for attaining universal health by the year 2000. "Health for All" was universally accepted as the main social goal (i.e., not merely a health goal) by the world health community. Today, efforts to improve the delivery of primary health care are underway in most regions across Canada, yet thousands of individuals remain without family doctors.

1. What improvements (if any) to health care have you seen in your own community?

2. If it were up to you, what changes to health care would you implement?

In the News

The World Health Organization: In Support of Primary Health Care

To commemorate the thirtieth anniversary of the Alma-Ata conference, WHO issued a new report in October 2008 entitled *Primary Health Care—Now More Than Ever.* This report documents the many failures that have left the health status of different populations, both within and among countries, dangerously out of balance. The inequities revealed by this report, listed below, are striking:

- Differences in life expectancy between the richest and poorest countries now exceed 40 years.

- Across the world, government spending on health ranges from as little as $20 USD per person to well over $600 USD per person.

- Personal spending on health now pushes more than 100 million people below the poverty line each year.

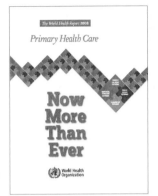

To improve the performance of health systems globally, this recent report calls for a renewal of the focus on primary health care that was originally launched at the Alma-Ata conference. "Primary health care brings balance back to health care and puts families and communities at the hub of the health system. With an emphasis on local ownership, it honours the resilience and ingenuity of the human spirit and makes space for solutions created by communities, owned by them, and sustained by them."

Source: World Health Organization. (2008). *World health report calls for return to primary health care approach* [News release]. Retrieved May 29, 2009, from http://www.who.int/mediacentre/news/releases/2008/pr38/en/index.html

Photo credit: World Health Organization. (2008). *The world health report: Primary health care—Now more than ever.* Reproduced by permisssion.

OTTAWA CHARTER FOR HEALTH PROMOTION, 1986

The 1986 WHO conference in Ottawa was convened to review and expand on the proposals put forward at the Alma-Ata conference and to determine what progress had been made toward assuring health for all by the year 2000.

At the Ottawa conference, the original factors affecting health, outlined in the Lalonde Report, were broadened and termed "health prerequisites" (Box 2.6), and the need for a collaborative approach to address health-related problems was reinforced.

Box 2.6	**Ottawa Charter for Health Promotion, 1986: Prerequisites for Health**		
Peace	Education	A stable ecosystem	Sustainable resources
Shelter	Food	Income/employment	Social justice and equity

Source: Canadian Public Health Association, Welfare Canada, and the World Health Organization. (2006). *Ottawa Charter for Health Promotion.* Charter adopted at the Move Towards a New Public Health international conference on health promotion, 17–21 November 1986, Ottawa, ON. Retrieved May 29, 2009, from http://www.who.int/hpr/NPH/docs/ottawa_charter_hp.pdf

The following five main strategies were identified at the WHO conference in Ottawa (some were repeated from previous conferences) and deemed essential for action in health promotion:

1. Develop public health policies for health promotion at all levels of government.

2. Create and maintain supportive environments—physical, social, cultural, spiritual, and economic.

3. Strengthen community action by setting priorities, making decisions, and planning and implementing strategies to achieve better health.

4. Develop people's personal skills so that they learn how to prepare themselves for all stages of life and to cope with illness and injury.

5. Redefine health services to better meet the health needs of the individual and the community (Public Health Agency of Canada, 2001).

The *Ottawa Charter* considered health care services important but supported the idea that many other factors outside of health care may play an even greater role in improving the health of large populations and groups. For example, government-funded day care was cited as a strategy that would benefit both the child and the parent. For the child, day care would facilitate intellectual and physical development and promote social skills; for the parent, day care would reduce the stress of working and caring for the child, reduce concerns about quality of care, and free up funds for other family priorities.

The *Ottawa Charter* has served as a template for health promotion around the world. Other international conferences with the same mandate followed: in Sweden in 1991, Indonesia in 1997, Australia in 1998, Mexico in 2000, and Thailand in 2005.

Thinking It **Through**

Some people believe government-funded day care should be available to everyone. Others feel that child care should be the responsibility of the family and that government involvement only adds to the taxpayer's burden.

1. If you were able to afford day care for your children, would you seek funded services if they were available?

2. Do you believe strict guidelines should exist regarding who should have access to funded day care services?

THE EPP REPORT, 1986

The Epp Report (Epp, 1986), *Achieving Health for All: A Framework for Health Promotion* by Jake Epp, minister of health and welfare, was released at the 1986 Ottawa conference and focused on the following three key areas:

1. Surveying the health status of disadvantaged groups and reducing inequities by, among other actions, enhancing people's ability to cope

2. Detecting and managing chronic diseases

3. Identifying diseases that were, by and large, preventable and focusing on prevention

The report stated that the government needed to be more active in providing support to groups and agencies within the community. The report also noted that the federal government received thousands of applications every year for financial resources that would be used for community health projects and proposed that these requests be dealt with promptly and equitably. At the same time, the report recognized that resources were limited and that distribution of those resources must be prioritized.

The Epp Report emphasized that health promotion initiatives must be supported at many levels—from the federal government to municipalities, local groups, and employers—and specifically underlined the responsibility of provincial, territorial, and federal governments in managing the cost of health care so that it was equally available to everyone. Finally, the report acknowledged that these initiatives would take time to implement but were achievable.

CANADIAN INSTITUTE FOR ADVANCED RESEARCH, 1987–2003

In 1987, the Department of Health and Welfare Canada asked CIFAR to design and implement an initiative called the Public Health Program to review determinants of health; analyze their impact on the health of the Canadian population; and assess the efficiency and effectiveness of the health care system. This project was completed in 2003. Through its research, CIFAR extended the idea that the determinants of health identified at previous conferences were linked—that is, that health outcomes were tied to multiple factors. For example, low income alone did not contribute to ill health, nor did a low position on the socioeconomic scale. Consider the potential outcomes in the life of Hinze (Case Example 2.3).

Remember the SES gradient in Box 2.3? While Hinze may develop a serious health problem, his friend Gus, who lives an almost identical lifestyle, is the picture of good health. This disparity has frequently been observed among groups of

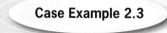

Case Example 2.3

If Hinze is in a low income bracket, chances are he will also be in a lower socioeconomic group, subject to less desirable living conditions, or both. As a result, Hinze may have less opportunity or motivation to advance his education or to obtain meaningful and satisfying employment. Perhaps he smokes or drinks alcohol to relieve stress. Cumulatively, he may then feel socially isolated or have low self-esteem and little confidence. He may also have poor nutritional habits perhaps because of a lack of knowledge about nutrition or maybe because he cannot afford nutritious food. Combine these factors, and Hinze is at risk for multiple health problems ranging from depression to cancer and heart disease.

people living in similar conditions. Why are some groups affected and some not, given common denominators? Research in this field continues today. One area under close scrutiny is the inequity in the health of Canadians despite universal access to health care.

TOWARD A HEALTHY FUTURE: THE FIRST REPORT ON THE HEALTH OF CANADIANS, 1996

The first *Report on the Health of Canadians* (Federal, Provincial and Territory Advisory Committee on Population Health, 1996) was released in September 1996 by federal Health Minister David Dingwall and Ontario Health Minister Jim Wilson. Its recommendations carried forward the proposals made by CIFAR in 1989. This was the first report to officially recognize and incorporate the determinants of health into its findings and recommendations.

The report concluded that Canadians were among the healthiest populations in the world and emphasized that collaboration among all levels of government, industry, and the private sector must be intensified to improve the health of Canadians. Box 2.7 lists strategies specified by the report to improve or maintain the health of Canadians, a further endorsement of the principles of the population health approach.

NATIONAL FORUM ON HEALTH, 1994–1997

The National Forum on Health was the blueprint for current Health Canada initiatives. The forum was launched by the Right Honorable Jean Chrétien in 1994 and wrapped up in 1997. An integral part of this forum was public input—the

---

Box 2.7　Strategies for Improving the Health of Canadians

- Create a thriving and sustainable economy, with meaningful work for all.
- Ensure an adequate income for all Canadians.
- Reduce the number of families living in poverty in Canada.
- Achieve an equitable distribution of income.
- Ensure healthy working conditions.
- Encourage life-long learning.
- Foster friendships and social support networks among families and communities.
- Create a healthy and sustainable environment for all.
- Ensure suitable, adequate, and affordable housing.
- Develop safe and well-designed communities.
- Foster healthy child development.
- Encourage healthy life-choice decisions.
- Provide appropriate and affordable health services, accessible to all.
- Reduce preventable illness, injury, and death.

Source: Health Canada. (1996). *Report on the health of Canadians.* Retrieved October 21, 2009, from http://dsp-psd.pwgsc.gc.ca/Collection/H39-385-1996-1E.pdf

---

beliefs and values of people across the country were sought through public discussion groups, conferences, meetings with experts, commissioned papers, letters, and briefs.

In February 1997, the forum published two final reports: *Canada Health Action: Building on the Legacy, Vol. I: Final Report* and *Canada Health Action: Building on the Legacy, Vol. II: Synthesis Reports and Issue Papers.* One of the key recommendations emerging from this forum was the need for more analysis and concrete evidence (i.e., an evidence-based approach) to support initiatives for improving health.

All of these reports, beginning with the Lalonde Report, were significant in initiating a united population health approach to achieving better health for Canadians. Recent reports—including *Toward a Healthy Future: The Second Report on the Health of Canadians,* 1999; *Building a Healthy Future,* 2000; *Final Report on the Health of Canadians,* 2002 (also known as the Kirby Report); and *Building on Values: The Future of Health Care in Canada,* 2002 (more commonly known as the Romanow Report) (see Chapter 3)—have analyzed the health of Canadians using a population health approach and offered recommendations for action.

PARTNERS IN POPULATION HEALTH ACTION

A number of departments, agencies, and organizations are instrumental in researching, gathering information, planning, and recommending strategies for Canada's population health approach. Discussed below are the roles that Health Canada, the Public Health Agency of Canada, the Canadian Institute for Health Information, the Canadian Institute for Advanced Research, Canadian Policy Research Networks, and Statistics Canada play in formulating Canada's population health approach.

Health Canada

Health Canada is the federal department responsible for helping Canadians maintain and improve their health. The department is "committed to improving the lives of all of Canada's people and to making this country's population among the healthiest in the world as measured by longevity, lifestyle and effective use of the public health care system" (Health Canada, 2006b, 12). Health Canada partners with other agencies and health care organizations to ensure its efforts meet the needs of all Canadians.

Public Health Agency of Canada

The Public Health Agency of Canada (PHAC) is a centralized agency under the umbrella of Health Canada. PHAC's role is to respond to national emergencies and to implement health promotion and disease and injury prevention initiatives. The agency—and the post of chief public health officer—was introduced by Prime Minister Paul Martin in September 2004 and created through a collaborative effort among the federal, provincial, and territorial governments. PHAC is part of a 10-year accord on health care reform signed by all of the premiers.

The unprecedented increase in global travel and international trade over the past 20 years has raised concerns about the re-emergence of infectious diseases once thought eradicated (or certainly controlled) and about the introduction of new diseases not indigenous to North America. PHAC is responsible for monitoring health risks as they appear to safeguard the health of Canadians.

Branches of PHAC include:

- Infectious Disease and Emergency Preparedness Branch
- Health Promotion and Chronic Disease Prevention Branch
- Public Health Practice and Regional Operations Branch
- Strategic Policy, Communications, and Corporate Services Branch

Canadian Institute for Health Information

The Canadian Institute for Health Information (CIHI), an organization that works collaboratively with Health Canada and PHAC, is an independent, nonprofit agency whose mandate is to provide information and analysis on the Canadian health care system and the health of Canadians. CIHI's data and reports focus on services, spending, and human resources in health care and on population health. For example, CIHI obtains information from hospitals, physicians, and public health agencies, which it uses to create reports on the number of deaths occurring in hospitals versus at home.

Canadian Institute for Advanced Research

A nonprofit organization relying on both public and private funds to sustain its research initiatives, the Canadian Institute for Advanced Research (CIFAR) brings together researchers from around the world to share ideas, thoughts, and theories concerning a wide variety of subjects. CIFAR specializes in advanced research, much of which is important to designing and implementing strategies used in population health. This agency remains a vital resource for both research and insight into health issues on national and international fronts.

Canadian Policy Research Networks

Founded in 1994, Canadian Policy Research Networks (CPRN) is a think tank whose main objective is to generate knowledge and discussion about socioeconomic issues in Canada. CPRN, which functions collaboratively with a variety of organizations, including all levels of government, and with industry, unions, educational institutions, and volunteer organizations, currently has the following four networks: family, health, public involvement, and work. The think tank conducts workshops, dialogues, and advisory committee meetings to generate information and debate in an impartial arena in which knowledge can be freely shared.

Statistics Canada

Statistics Canada is a branch of the federal government whose primary purpose is to gather information from every province and territory and to publish accurate statistics on almost every aspect of life imaginable. Statistics Canada is used extensively by government and agencies involved in public health and population health initiatives (e.g., for gathering data regarding births, deaths, and causes of morbidity and mortality).

Every five years, in the first and sixth years of every decade, Statistics Canada conducts a national census, which every household by law must participate in. The last national census, which, for the first time, offered participants the opportunity to complete the survey online, was in 2006; the next will be in 2011.

IMPLEMENTING POPULATION HEALTH IN CANADA

A population health approach seeks to improve the health and well-being of all Canadians. To increase the public profile of population health, Health

Canada recently developed a logo for use on all materials pertaining to population health. The design features a flower, which signifies growth and renewal, and suggests the complexity of health and health care in Canada and the efforts to encourage a healthier population.

The implementation of population health requires a formal plan, which ensures that steps are executed in a coordinated manner, that critical elements are identified, and that the role of agencies or individuals is clearly defined. Outlining a mission statement, goals, objectives, and methodology will help to ensure that all stakeholders understand the direction the approach will take. A clear plan is also necessary for the success and sustainability of **intersectoral cooperation**, a critical element of a population health approach. Planning should be transparent and flexible and should invite input from everyone involved.

Various agencies, particularly at the community level, act as valuable resources for ideas and suggestions related to the population health approach. The population health approach also energizes community members to be proactive, involved, and accepting of initiatives because they have been part of the planning process.

Intersectoral cooperation
Joint action among the public, the government, and nongovernment or community-based organizations.

Thinking It Through

In October 2009, the Public Health Agency of Canada set out guidelines for Canadians regarding getting the H1N1 flu vaccine. Among other recommendations, the guidelines advised that those in high risk groups get their vaccination first.

1.   If you are not in a high-risk group, would you wait?
2.   How many times have you been told to do something, and resisted, even though it may have been a good idea?
3.   If the decision-making protocol had been more transparent, do you think compliance would have been better?
4.   If you had been involved in making the decision, would you have been more likely to be a part of carrying out the plan?

HEALTH CANADA TEMPLATE

A template is much like a design or plan an architect would use to build a house. The Health Canada template has eight key elements, which appear in the shaded boxes in Figure 2.1. The white boxes in the figure indicate the basic steps necessary to link the key elements and to facilitate the entire population health process. In this process, the determinants of health are used as a means of analyzing the health of Canadians.

Figure 2.1 Template for Implementing a Population Health Approach in Canada

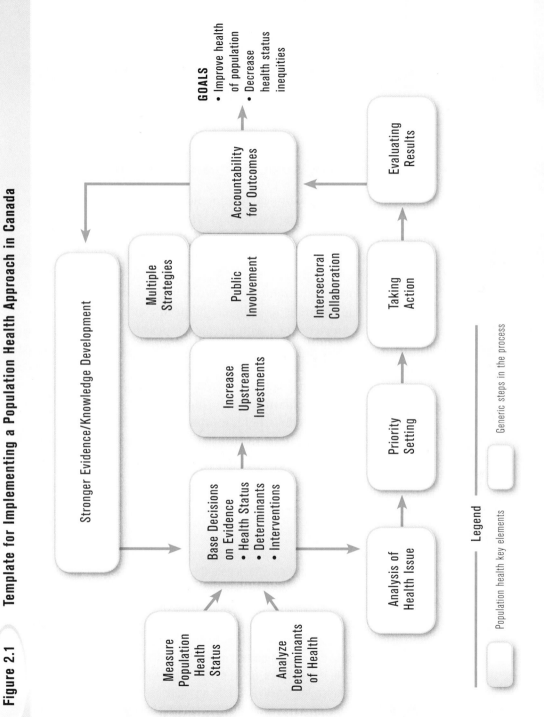

Source: Public Health Agency of Canada. (2001). *The population health template working tool.* Retrieved May 29, 2009, from http://www.phac-aspc.gc.ca/ph-sp/pdf/template_tool-eng.pdf. © 2001. Adapted and reproduced with the permission of the Minister of Public Works and Government Services Canada, 2009.

The Health Canada template can act as a guide for policymakers, program planners, health educators, evaluators, researchers, and academics.

Measure the Population Health Status

Measuring the health status of the population can answer the following key questions:

- How healthy is a population, and is its health improving?
- What can be learned about current trends in health status to help plan for future initiatives?
- What are the most important health issues (Health Canada, 2001)?

Health indicators
Measurements that help to gauge the state of health and wellness of a population.

The first step in measuring population health is to select indicators for gauging the health status of that population. **Health indicators** are standardized measures that assist in the comparison of health issues in a population and the identification of any change in health status. Traditionally, the most common health indicators have been mortality (e.g., infant death, life expectancy, death due to cancer) and hospitalization rates. While important, these indicators do not provide the whole picture where population health status is concerned. Instead, they need to be supplemented with enhanced measures of morbidity, with the effects of chronic disease or disability on the quality of life, and with measures of the positive factors that improve health.

Population-based surveillance
The collection and analysis of data that are needed to plan, implement, and evaluate population health initiatives.

Based on these health indicators, information is gathered in the form of **population-based surveillance**. Information for this surveillance comes from a range of sources, including **epidemiology** (Box 2.8), socioeconomic data, health indicators (e.g., cancer rates, life expectancy), and data on the use of health services.

Box 2.8   Epidemiology Explained

Translated literally from Greek, *epidemiology* means "the study of people"; however, the term is used more specifically to denote the study of diseases in populations.

Epidemiology describes disease patterns in human populations, identifies the causes of diseases, and then provides the information needed to plan, implement, and evaluate services to prevent, treat, and control diseases. Professionals who work in the field of epidemiology are known as epidemiologists.

Epidemiology is the most important method of studying and understanding population health. In recent years, it has played a key role in the study of epidemics and in identifying emerging health issues in populations, from infectious diseases like acquired immune deficiency syndrome (AIDS) to occupational hazards like asbestos.

Ongoing population surveillance is an excellent way to identify inequities in the health care system. For example, consider the inequities that exist between Canada's Aboriginal people living in the north and those Aboriginals living in urban areas. Most of the Aboriginal population in northern regions does not have immediate access to a wide range of medical services or even access to clean drinking water. An inequity previously discussed is the higher morbidity and mortality rates among individuals in lower socioeconomic groups.

Analyze the Determinants of Health

Population health considers all of the factors (determinants) that affect health status. As outlined in Box 2.2, determinants of health include social, economic, and physical environments, early childhood development, gender, personal health practices and coping skills, culture, biology and genetic endowment, and health services.

These determinants are scrutinized in terms of how they interact with each other and how they affect health status, which then forms the basis for developing and implementing population health interventions.

Use Evidence-Based Decision Making

All stages of a population health approach—selecting issues to be worked on, choosing interventions, deciding to implement and continue these interventions—are supported by decisions based on the most current best evidence available. This is called *evidence-based decision making (EBDM).*

An evidence-based approach utilizes the full range of data, both qualitative and quantitative in nature. **Qualitative research** examines the way a population group thinks, how it acts, and its health beliefs and health behaviours. Qualitative research is conducted in a number of ways, including the administration of surveys and holding of open forums. You may remember public debates on health and health concerns being held in your community to address issues like hospital closures, health care delivery choices (e.g., merging similar services in one location), doctor shortages, and long wait times for medical attention.

Quantitative research deals primarily with numbers, and numbers are interpreted most frequently as statistics. Data can be generated through epidemiological studies, databases, and surveys. No doubt you have had a telephone call from a surveyor during the supper hour asking you for "just a few moments of your time." This type of research generates data that are usually interpreted numerically. For example, "9 out of 10 people are more concerned with wait times than with doctor shortages."

Qualitative research
A method of research that examines the way a population group thinks and behaves. The analysis is largely subjective in nature.

Quantitative research
A method of objective research that deals with the measurement of data, such as the number of deaths from cancer.

Employ Upstream Investments

Upstream investments
Actions that can be taken to improve the health of a population or to prevent illness when the potential for a problem is first recognized.

The term **upstream investments** refers to the process of making decisions that will benefit the health of a population group *before* a problem occurs. Being pro-active regarding prevention gives a population "the best bang for its tax buck," as well as a healthier future. Short-term and long-term goals are set and priori-tized, and strategies are implemented, using evidence-based decision making. For example, encouraging Canadians to undergo periodic health exams, which is supported by most provinces, is a strategy to identify health problems at an early stage, and immunizations prevent an array of diseases, such as diphtheria, polio, measles, mumps, and hepatitis.

The most recent government-initiated upstream investment offers young women a vaccine to protect them from human papilloma virus (HPV), which causes precancerous changes to the female genitalia and can lead to cancer of the vulva and cervix. This investment has caused controversy (In the News: HPV Vaccinations).

In the **News**   **HPV Vaccinations**

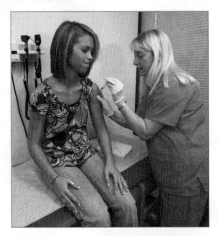

In 2007, the federal government announced a $300 million investment to offer a vaccination program for girls and women against the human papilloma virus (HPV) using Gardasil®. Critics of this program, who received significant media coverage, argued several points: invasive cervical cancer is slow moving and can be detected early by the widely available Pap smear; most HPV infections (at least 80%) clear up on their own; and not enough is known about the vaccine's effectiveness, side effects, or durability. These critics called for a reasoned, well-researched approach to "ensure a responsible and transparent evidence-based decision-making process" (Canadian Women's Health Network, 2007).

Despite this opposition, Health Canada continues to assert that widespread immunization will help to eradicate cervical cancer and to reduce the HPV-related financial burden on the health care system.

Source: Lippman, A., Melnychuk, R., Shimmin, C., & Boscoe, M. (2007). Human papillomavirus, vaccines and women's health: Questions and cautions. *Canadian Medical Association Journal*, *177*(5), 484–487.

Photo credit: THE CANADIAN PRESS/AP Photo/John Amis.

Use Multiple Strategies

Once a population health goal is set, the next step is to introduce interventions to achieve the goal. No one action is likely to accomplish this, so a multifaceted approach must be taken. Actions must relate directly to the situation; suit the age range, health status, and environment of the target population; and be implemented over a chosen time frame. Such interventions must also address all of the health determinants involved, recognizing that they are interrelated.

Those involved in implementing a population health strategy must accept both the goal and the plan of action. Collaboration is essential. It is up to the government, then, to work with all sectors deemed to have an influence on the success of the interventions (e.g., the individual, the community, industry, related agencies, and local, provincial, and territorial governments).

Consider the introduction of the Gardasil® vaccine. The upstream investment involved vaccinating all females at risk. The question was how to conduct the vaccination effectively and efficiently so that parents would allow their children to be vaccinated and so that those old enough to make their own decisions would understand and accept the rationale behind the vaccination program. The government launched a massive public relations campaign, primarily through radio and television advertising, and engaged schools, public health units, and family doctors to champion the program.

Engage the Public

Without public support, most health-care-related implementations will fail, in part because it is the public's health at issue and its tax dollars that fund implementation. Public involvement increases the likelihood that citizens will embrace a plan in a meaningful way. The key is to capture the public's interest early and in a positive manner. Plans to achieve positive public interest must be carefully considered and executed so as not to turn public opinion against the plan, especially because attempting to reverse public opinion can be difficult, if not impossible. For example, the concerns over Gardasil® illustrate how public opinion can dissuade a significant number of people within a population or community from participating in an immunization campaign. Engaging the public requires the establishment of trust and an open process of decision making and implementation. Questions must be addressed promptly, properly, and persuasively.

Another example of public engagement occurred when Ontario changed its approach to managing community health care. In 2005, the Ministry of Health and Long-Term Care (MOHLTC) decided to replace district health councils with local health integration networks (LHINs). The rationale for this change was the promise of better and more efficient coordination and use of health care services within communities. The plan had been researched, the information analyzed, and the decisions for implementation made.

When it came time to notify the public of the plan, MOHLTC posted a bulletin on its Web site explaining the plan and asked interested parties a series of questions, including the following: How could the plan best be implemented? What health integration initiatives were already in place within their community? What was necessary to make LHINs successful in their community? What role could individuals or organizations play in implementing the LHINs?

Interestingly, most of the respondents failed to answer the questions posted and instead offered general comments and expressed concern over the extent of the LHINs' responsibilities. Some respondents conveyed fear that the larger structure of the LHINs would result in smaller segments of a community not being heard and that the health-care-related problems of urban communities would overshadow those of rural communities. Opposition to this regionalization of power continues. On the whole, however, changes were implemented, and most Ontarians were brought onside when, through public forums, debates, and Web sites, they were given opportunities to voice concerns and have them addressed. The Ontario government divided the province into 14 LHIN regions, and, in April 2007, LHINs became fully operational.

Think Intersectoral Collaboration

Intersectoral collaboration involves developing partnerships between different segments of society—private citizens, community groups, industry, health and educational agencies, and various levels of government—to improve health. Each group comes to the table with its own values, outlook, opinions, and agenda. Harmonizing these variables is a challenge, but the benefits are profound: a commitment to common goals and an assurance that plans are implemented to meet these goals.

Efforts of the World Health Organization to control the AIDS epidemic, particularly in developing countries, are illustrative of this collaborative approach. Initially, most of the responsibility for treating and controlling the spread of the human immunodeficiency virus (HIV) rested with health care authorities. Subsequently, the involvement of other sectors was initiated through advertising campaigns on a number of fronts (e.g., educating populations on how HIV is contracted; involving schools and community agencies in the promotion of safer sex). Furthermore, a strategy to ensure a safe blood supply targeted all groups within the population and educated the public about behaviours that could reduce HIV transmission.

Demonstrate Accountability for Health Outcomes

A population health approach emphasizes the accountability for health outcomes—that is, the ability to determine if any changes in health outcomes can actually be attributed to specific policies or programs. The concept of accountability has an impact on planning and goal setting, since it encourages the selection of interventions or strategies that produce the greatest health results.

Important steps in establishing accountability, therefore, include dete
ing baseline measures (i.e., a standard against which to gauge progress), s
targets, and monitoring progress so that a thorough evaluation can be (
Evaluation tools provide criteria for determining the impact of policies or
grams on population health. Finally, making evaluation results public is cri
for gaining widespread support for successful population health initiatives.

POPULATION HEALTH PROMOTION MODEL

The population health promotion model (Figure 2.2) is a recently introduced
approach for promoting health on a population-wide basis. The model organizes
population health into three areas:

1. What—looking to the health determinants to measure the health of
   populations

2. How—creating and implementing prioritized strategies to improve health

3. Who—engaging multiple stakeholders to participate in health improvement
   strategies

Figure 2.2   Population Health Promotion Model

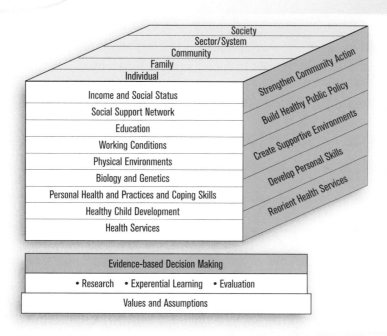

Source: Public Health Agency of Canada. (2008). *Population health promotion: An integrated model of
population health and health promotion*. Retrieved May 29, 2009, from http://www.phac-aspc.gc.ca/ph-
sp/php-psp/php3-eng.php. Public Health Agency of Canada 2009 ©. Adapted and reproduced with the
permission of the Minister of Public Works and Government Services Canada, 2009.

The population health promotion model demonstrates that health promotion is complex. The model emulates the population health approach by using the determinants of health as indicators to measure health and to gather information for health promotion initiatives.

Decisions about health promotion policies are made using three sources of evidence: research studies on health issues (i.e., the underlying factors, the interventions, and their impact); knowledge gained through experience; and evaluation of current programs to anticipate strategies needed in the future—in other words, upstream investments in health promotion.

Collectively, stakeholders should address the full range of health determinants when adopting a population health promotion approach. Particular organizations, however, may wish to focus on specific determinants.

The population health promotion model can be used by any level of government, community agency, or group and can be accessed from any point of entry, depending on the health issue. Consider an industry wanting to improve working conditions. It would conduct research, draw information from other industries in which similar working conditions exist, evaluate identified strategies, and recommend action.

Implementation Strategies: A Look at Two Provinces

The population health approach adopted by Health Canada has been implemented in all provinces and territories in some manner. Differences exist in each province's or territory's definitions of health, how health determinants are labelled and grouped, and the timelines and policies for implementing specific initiatives. Although each province and territory deals with its own specific health care issues, a broader emphasis on prevention, early detection, and prompt treatment exists across Canada.

One example of a province that developed its own health goals is British Columbia. In 1997, British Columbia adopted a set of health goals for its citizens based on a population health perspective (Box 2.9). These goals describe the province's vision for a healthy population and provide a reference point for both policy initiatives and health care practices.

Another example of a province that developed its own health goals is Saskatchewan. In 1999 (revised in 2002), the provincial government produced a paper called *A Population Health Promotion Framework for Saskatchewan Regional Health Authorities* to help regional health authorities understand their role in promoting the population health concept. A notation at the beginning of this report read, "A journey of a thousand miles begins with a single step," underlining that an organized approach to improving health in the province had begun. The re-

---

Box 2.9   British Columbia's Health Goals

Goal 1—Living and Working Conditions: Positive and supportive working conditions in all communities.

Goal 2—Individual Capacities, Skills, and Choices: Opportunities for all individuals to develop and maintain the capacities and skills needed to thrive and meet life's challenges and to make choices that enhance health.

Goal 3—Physical Environment: A diverse and sustainable physical environment with clean, healthy and safe air, water and land.

Goal 4—Health Services: An effective and efficient health service system that provides equitable access to appropriate services.

Goal 5—Aboriginal Health: Improved health for Aboriginal peoples.

Goal 6—Disease and Injury Prevention: Reduction of preventable illness, injuries, disabilities and premature deaths.

Source: Ministry of Health and Ministry Responsible for Seniors. (1997). *Health goals for British Columbia.* Retrieved May 29, 2009, from http://www.health.gov.bc.ca/library/publications/year/1997/healthgoals.pdf

---

port outlined a set of common values on which the province based its approach to population health (Box 2.10). Sharing these values provided a foundation of common interest and principles from which to build a progressive and cohesive partnership that would promote health in the province.

Box 2.10   Saskatchewan's Common Values for a Population Health Approach

- Respect for the worth and dignity of each individual, while at the same time giving priority to the common good when conflict arises

- Support for community participation in decision-making

- Sharing of resources, to meet the needs of all members of society

- Pursuing social justice to reduce health inequities

- Caring for the environment, so that the health and prosperity of the present generation are not purchased at the expense of future generations.

Source: Saskatchewan Health Population Health Branch. (1999). *A population health promotion framework for Saskatchewan Regional Health Authorities.* Retrieved May 29, 2009, from http://www.health.gov.sk.ca/health-promotion-framework

Currently, Canada has one of the healthiest populations in the world. Despite gains made through the application of population health initiatives, however, disturbing health-related inequities still exist. The Canadian Population Health Initiative (CPHI)—part of the Canadian Institute for Health Information—was created in 1999 to examine patterns of health among populations in Canada, as well as to determine what could be done to improve health when and where problems were identified. The CPHI acknowledges that due to the vastness of the field of population health, many areas still require research and analysis before a population health approach can be put into action.

CPHI's *Action Plan 2007–2010* focused on four areas: Healthy Weights (particularly in light of the current trend toward obesity in children); Place and Health (i.e., how our physical environment affects our health); Determinants of Mental Health and Resilience (with an emphasis on prevention of mental illness); and Reducing Gaps in Health (i.e., avoiding social exclusion by reinforcing strategies such as self-confidence and self-control) (Canadian Institute for Health Information, 2006).

The general consensus among Canadians seems to be that the population health approach has been relatively successful but that it requires ongoing funding and commitment by all levels of government to have a truly positive impact on the health of Canadians. In June 2008, Ted Bruce, the executive director of population health for the Vancouver Coastal Health Authority, addressed the Senate Subcommittee on Population Health. With respect to the issue of ensuring the continued success of population health strategies, he stressed the importance of collaboration, particularly with the federal government, in providing leadership in such areas as health assessment and surveillance and in analyzing the underlying causes of health inequities. He emphasized the importance of timely continued funding by the federal government, particularly for smaller communities, since, as previously discussed, smaller population groups and communities tend to have worse health outcomes than others (Vancouver Coastal Health, 2008).

Outside of Canada, although population health initiatives are used in most developed countries, they are almost nonexistent in developing nations. Information such as who is born, who dies, when, and of what cause is information that is not usually recorded. Consequently, the health profile of these developing nations (many of which have the highest burden of disease) is virtually absent.

Health care systems around the world were last ranked by the World Health Organization in 2000. At that time, Canada stood thirtieth, with France occupying the top position. The following five measures were used in WHO's assessment:

- Overall level of health or life expectancy
- Health fairness, or life expectancy as measured across various populations within a country
- Responsiveness, or how well people rated the performance of their health care system
- Fairness in responsiveness among different groups in the same country
- Fairness in financing among different groups, which looked at the proportion of income that is devoted to health care (World Health Organization, 2000)

The United States was thirty-seventh on the list. Last, at number 190, was Myanmar. Canada ranked seventh in overall health-system achievement and tenth in terms of health care spending but fell to thirtieth when these two measures were combined (Buske, 2001).

SUMMARY

❖ Population health is a framework for measuring the health status of groups of people. The framework has been around for many years but has only recently been applied in an organized manner in Canada.

❖ Several reports issued by the federal government were instrumental in launching the population health initiative, beginning with the Lalonde Report in 1974. Following this report, Canadians began thinking about health in terms of prevention, with campaigns at both the federal and provincial levels of government urging the population to look at lifestyle and risk behaviours.

❖ Since the late 1980s, promoting a healthy lifestyle has been coupled with the concept of health promotion and disease prevention. Definitions of health have been expanded. The impact of elements in our social and physical environments on our health status is emphasized. These variables are called *determinants of health* and are now the foundation on which to gather data, analyze them, and propose solutions for health problems at national, provincial, territorial, and community levels. That the determinants interrelate to influence health issues is well known; how they do so is not clearly understood.

❖ Public health, on the other hand, uses strategies developed by population health to measure the health of groups of people and to work toward improving the health of communities. Public health places more emphasis on action than on theory.

❖ A number of government agencies work together to gather data and develop strategies. These include the Public Health Agency of Canada, the Canadian Institute for Health Information, the Canadian Institute for Advanced Research, and Statistics Canada.

❖ Health Canada has developed a template and a logo for population health. The agency uses the template as a tool for the ongoing measurement of the health of Canadians and for the subsequent development of strategies to improve health.

REVIEW QUESTIONS

1. What are the differences between population health, health promotion, and public health?

2. What were Marc Lalonde's contributions to population health?

3. Explain the SES gradient.

4. What is the relationship between health care services and the health of a population?

5. What is equity in health?

6. State the advantages of engaging the public in developing population health initiatives.

7. How does the population health promotion model differ from population health itself?

8. Why did Saskatchewan develop a list of common values for use in its population health approach?

DISCUSSION QUESTIONS

1. Explain the concept of upstream investments in your own words. Identify recent upstream investments in your community and discuss their effectiveness.

2. Identify an area in your community or province in which you feel an upstream investment could be made. Develop a plan using the following headings: Problem Identification, Supporting Documentation, Recommended Actions, and Expected Goals.

3. "Health problems may affect certain groups more than others. However, the solution to these problems involves changing social values and structures. It is the responsibility of the society as a whole to take care of all its members." This statement is taken from the Population Health Approach Web site (see Web Resources). Discuss what you think it means, and explain the meaning of the statement using an example from your own community.

4. Using information from the Population Health Approach Web site (see Web Resources), compare and contrast the concepts of population health and public health. Summarize what the two concepts mean to you. Describe the public health and population health initiatives you see within your own community.

WEB RESOURCES

Canadian Institute for Advanced Research
http://www.cifar.ca

The Canadian Institute for Advanced Research is a non-profit organization that facilitates collaboration among its more than 350 affiliate researchers involved in 12 research programs in Canada and around the world.

Canadian Institute for Health Information
http://www.cihi.ca

An independent, nonprofit organization, the Canadian Institute for Health Information (CIHI) provides essential data and analyses on Canada's health care system and the health of Canadians, with a focus on services, spending, and human resources in health care and on population health.

Submission to the Senate Subcommittee on Population Health
http://www.cpha.ca/uploads/briefs/pophealth_e.pdf

This is the Canadian Public Health Association's written submission in response to the Senate Subcommittee's four reports on population health, issued on June 30, 2008.

WEB RESOURCES

Canadian Policy Research Networks
http://www.cprn.org

Canadian Policy Research Networks' main objective is to generate knowledge and discussion about socioeconomic issues in Canada. CPRN works collaboratively with a variety of organizations, including all levels of government, and with industry, unions, educational institutions, and volunteer organizations. It currently features the following four networks: family, health, public involvement, and work.

Determinants of Health
http://www.phac-aspc.gc.ca/ph-sp/determinants/determinants-eng.php#education

Health Canada has identified 12 key determinants of health, which are displayed on this Web site.

About Health Canada: About Missions, Values, Activities
http://www.hc-sc.gc.ca/ahc-asc/activit/about-apropos/index-eng.php

Health Canada is the federal department responsible for helping Canadians maintain and improve their health. The department partners with other agencies and health care organizations to ensure that its efforts meet the needs of all Canadians. This link provides information on Health Canada's mission, values, and activities.

Public Health Agency of Canada
http://www.phac-aspc.gc.ca

The Public Health Agency of Canada focuses on the health of the entire population at both the individual and community levels. The agency's role is to promote health, prevent and control chronic diseases and injuries, prevent and control infectious diseases, prepare and respond to public health emergencies, and strengthen public health capacity.

The Social Determinants of Health: Education as a Determinant of Health
http://www.phac-aspc.gc.ca/ph-sp/oi-ar/10_education-eng.php

This PHAC Web page discusses the role of education in a person's health. Education is one of the 12 key determinants of health as outlined by Health Canada.

Population Health Approach
http://www.phac-aspc.gc.ca/ph-sp/

This Web site discusses the population health approach taken by PHAC that has broadened the definition of *health* to include the entire range of factors that determine health. The approach also aims to improve the health of the entire population.

Statistics Canada
http://www.statcan.gc.ca

Statistics Canada is Canada's central, national statistical agency that collects data about virtually every aspect of Canadian life. In addition to about 350 active surveys, it also conducts a census every five years.

Vancouver Coastal Health Population Health Report 2008
http://www.bchealthyliving.ca/sites/all/files/VCH_Population_Health_Report.pdf

The purpose of this report is to facilitate an understanding of what determines the health of Vancouver's populations through the presentation of population health data; to identify and describe current priority areas for Vancouver Coastal Health population health activities; and to describe policy options for improving the health of Vancouver's populations.

ADDITIONAL RESOURCES

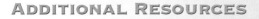

Evans, R.G. (1992). *Why are some people healthy and some people not?* Toronto: Canadian Institute for Advanced Research.

Gilmore, J. (2004). *Health of Canadians living in census metropolitan areas.* Ottawa: Statistics Canada, 89-613-MIE.

ADDITIONAL RESOURCES

McKinlay, J. (1990). The case for refocusing upstream: The political economy of illness. In P. Conrad & R. Kern (Eds.), *The sociology of health and illness: Critical perspectives* (3rd ed.) (pp. 502–504). New York: St. Martin's Press.

Public Health Agency of Canada. (1999). *The statistical report on the health of Canadians 1999.* Retrieved May 29, 2009, from http://www.phac-aspc.gc.ca/ph-sp/report-rapport/stat/over-eng.php

Wilkinson, R., & Marmot, M. (Eds.). (2003). *Social determinants of health: The solid facts* (2nd ed.). Copenhagen: World Health Organization.

World Health Organization. (1998). *Health promotion glossary.* Geneva: Author.

REFERENCES

Buske, L. (2001). Does Canada really rank 30th in world in terms of health care? *Canadian Medical Association Journal, 164*(1), 84. Retrieved May 29, 2009, from http://www.cmaj.ca/cgi/content/full/164/1/84-a

Canadian Institute for Health Information. (2006). *The Canadian population health initiative 2007–2010.* Retrieved May 29, 2009, from http://secure.cihi.ca/cihiweb/products/action_plan_2007_2010_e.pdf

Canadian Women's Health Network. (2007). *HPV, vaccines, and gender: Policy considerations.* Retrieved July 2, 2009, from http://www.cwhn.ca/resources/cwhn/hpv-brief.html

Child Poverty Action Group. (2005). *Mothers, babies and the risk of poverty.* Retrieved May 29, 2009, from http://www.cpag.org.uk/info/Povertyarticles/Poverty121/mothers.htm

D'Arcy, C. (1986). Unemployment and health: Data and implications. *Canadian Journal of Public Health, 77*(Suppl. 1), 124–131.

Epp, J. (1986). *Achieving health for all: A framework for health promotion.* Ottawa: Health and Welfare Canada (Focus Research Centre Publication). Retrieved May 29, 2009, from http://www.frcentre.net/library/AchievingHealthForAll.pdf

Federal, Provincial and Territory Advisory Committee on Population Health. (1996). *Report on the health of Canadians.* Ottawa: Health Canada.

Haydon, E., Roerecke, M., Giesbrecht, N., Rehm, J., & Kobus-Matthews, M. (2006). *Chronic disease in Ontario and Canada: Determinants, risk factors and prevention priorities.* Summary of full report. Ontario Chronic Disease Prevention Alliance and the Ontario Public Health Association. Retrieved May 29, 2009, from http://www.ocdpa.on.ca/docs/CDP-SummaryReport-Mar06.pdf

Health Canada. (1994). *Advisory committee on population health strategies for population health: Investing in the health of Canadians.* Ottawa: Author.

Health Canada. (2001). *The population health template: Key elements and actions that define a population health approach.* Strategic policy directorate of the Population and Public Health Branch. Ottawa: Author.

Health Canada. (2006a). *Health care system: About primary health care.* Retrieved May 2, 2009, from http://www.hc-sc.gc.ca/hcs-sss/prim/about-apropos-eng.php

Health Canada. (2006b). *Sustainable development strategy 2007–2010: A path to sustainability.* Retrieved June 27, 2009, from http://www.hc-sc.gc.ca/ahc-asc/pubs/sus-dur/strateg/sds2007-2010-sdd/appendix-a-annexe-eng.php

Lalonde, M. (1974). *A new perspective on the health of Canadians: A working document.* Retrieved May 29, 2009, from http://www.hc-sc.gc.ca/hcs-sss/com/fed/lalonde-eng.php

REFERENCES

National Collaborating Centre for Determinants of Health. (2007). *Determinants of health*. Retrieved May 29, 2009, from http://www.nccdh.ca/determinants.html

Public Health Agency of Canada. (n.d.). *Volunteering as a vehicle for social support and life satisfaction*, Factsheet, p. 1.

Public Health Agency of Canada. (2001). *Ottawa Charter for Health Promotion: An international conference on health promotion*. Retrieved May 29, 2009, from http://www.phac-aspc.gc.ca/ph-sp/docs/charter-chartre/pdf/charter.pdf

Public Health Agency of Canada. (2003). *What makes Canadians healthy or unhealthy?* Retrieved May 29, 2009, from http://www.phac-aspc.gc.ca/ph-sp/determinants/determinants-eng.php

United States Environmental Protection Agency. (1991). *Indoor air facts, No. 4 (revised): Sick building syndrome (SBS)*. http://www.epa.gov/iaq/pdfs/sick_building_factsheet.pdf

University of Waterloo. (2005). Health 102A, Lecture 4. Faculty of Applied Health Sciences. Retrieved May 29, 2009, from http://www.ahs.uwaterloo.ca/~hlth102/ModA_lec04.pdf

Vancouver Coastal Health. (2008). *Vancouver Coastal Health senate response.* Retrieved May 29, 2009, from http://www.vch.ca/public/docs/advocacy/VCH_SenateResponse.pdf

World Health Organization. (2000). *World Health Organization assesses the world's health systems* [News release WHO/44]. Retrieved May 29, 2009, from http://www.who.int/inf-pr-2000/en/pr2000-44.html

Zaman, F., & Underwood, C. (2003). *The gender guide for health communication programs*. Center Publication No. 102. Baltimore: Johns Hopkins Bloomberg School of Public Health/Center for Communication Programs.

CHAPTER THREE

The History of Health Care in Canada

Learning Outcomes

1. Describe early events in the evolution of the Canadian health care system.

2. Outline the introduction of formalized health care in Canada.

3. Discuss significant pieces of legislation relating to the introduction of socialized medicine in Canada.

4. Explain Tommy Douglas's role in the initiation of prepaid health care.

5. Summarize the state of the health care system in the post–World War II era.

6. Describe the events leading up to the *Canada Health Act* (CHA).

7. Describe the criteria and conditions of the CHA.

8. Discuss the key elements contained in the Romanow and Kirby reports.

9. Explain highlights of more recent significant accords and pieces of federal and provincial legislation.

KEY TERMS

Aseptic technique, p. 80

Block transfer, p. 86

Canada Health Act, p. 89

Catastrophic drug costs, p. 103

Delisted, p. 88

Eligible, p. 89

First ministers, p. 99

Gross national product (GNP), p. 87

Medically necessary, p. 95

Medicare, p. 84

Palliative care, p. 103

Prepaid health care, p. 84

Primary health care reform, p. 98

Quarantine, p. 73

Refugee claimants, p. 74

Royal assent, p. 89

Social movements, p. 82

"It isn't so much that this country needs a good and caring health care system; our health care system needs a good and caring country" (Wynne-Jones, 2002). What does this quote mean to you? Do you agree with it? Keep these words in mind as you read this chapter and as you answer the questions that appear at the end of it.

In this chapter, you will learn about the evolution of our health care system since before Confederation and about the struggles of Canadians to build the system into what it is today. Affected by social, economic, and technological growth, health care in Canada has transformed dramatically over the past 200 years. Every decade has brought changes to where and how people live, their views of and responses to illness, and the kind of treatment they expect. The level and quality of health care have, for the most part, adjusted accordingly, but change has not come easily.

As you read this chapter, note continuing parallels between the needs of the population and the adaptation and growth of health care services. When you reach the end, think about the criteria and conditions of the *Canada Health Act* in particular, and ask yourself if the Act still meets the needs of Canadians. Is health care universal? Is health care accessible to all? Is it provided to all Canadians on uniform terms? Is it delivered in a timely fashion to all? Continued debate about the quality and availability of our health care has generated repeated demands for system improvements and for increases in dedicated funds. Does the *Canada Health Act* need to be changed, or do the expectations and attitudes of Canadians need adjustment, as the opening quote suggests? Jot down your thoughts about these questions before you continue reading, and then compare your thoughts with those shared in this chapter.

HEALTH CARE SINCE CONFEDERATION: AN OVERVIEW

With the passage of the *British North America Act* in 1867 (renamed the *Constitution Act* in 1982), Confederation became a reality. The Dominion of Canada consisted of Ontario and Quebec (formerly Upper and Lower Canada, respectively), New Brunswick, and Nova Scotia, and Sir John A. Macdonald was the Dominion's prime minister. Each province had its own representation in government, its own law-making body (which evolved into a provincial government), and its own Lieutenant Governor to represent the Crown. The *British North America Act* also established a federal government comprising the House of Commons and the Senate—the same structure in place today. The first census for the new Dominion, in 1871, showed a population of 3,689,257—a large enough number to warrant closer attention to people's health care needs. Legislation regarding responsibilities for health care was vague at best, but, even at this early stage, responsibilities were divided between the federal and provincial governments.

DIVISION OF RESPONSIBILITIES FOR HEALTH

Health matters received little attention in the *British North America Act*. The federal government was charged with responsibilities for the establishment and maintenance of marine hospitals, the care of Aboriginal populations, and the management of **quarantine**. Relatively common, quarantines were imposed to prevent outbreaks of such diseases as cholera, diphtheria, typhoid fever, tuberculosis (TB), and influenza (Health Canada, 2006).

Quarantine
The enforced isolation of people having, or suspected of having, a contagious disease.

Provinces were responsible for establishing and managing hospitals, asylums, charities, and charitable institutions. Many of the health-care-related responsibilities of the provinces—including social welfare, which, broadly speaking, encompassed health and public health matters—were assumed by default since they were not clearly outlined in the Act as federal responsibilities.

In 1919, the federal government created the Department of Health, largely to assume the health-care-related responsibilities of the federal government, which included working collaboratively with the provinces and territories in health care matters and promoting new health care initiatives. Early projects undertaken by this new department reflected the issues faced by Canadians at that time—specifically, the increase in sexually transmitted infections (STIs) and the recognition of the importance of keeping children healthy and safe. In response, venereal disease clinics were established across the country, and campaigns promoting child welfare were launched.

In 1928, the Department of Health became known as the Department of Pensions and National Health. The name changed again in 1944 to the Department of National Health and Welfare, and federal responsibilities expanded to include food and drug control, the development of public health programs, health care for members of the civil service, and the operation of the Laboratory of Hygiene (a precursor to Canada's current Laboratory Centre for Disease Control). In the late 1990s, the department was renamed Health Canada. Today, the federal government retains responsibility for health care for members of the RCMP and the armed forces. As well, under the Interim Federal Health (IFH) program, the federal government will pay for temporary health insurance for **refugee claimants** and their dependants who cannot afford medical insurance and who are not yet covered by a provincial or territorial health insurance plan.

Refugee claimants
People who, feeling unsafe in their home country, seek protection in another country.

THE ORIGINS OF MEDICAL CARE IN CANADA

With the European settlers (primarily from England and France) came the first doctors in Canada, a combination of civilian and military physicians. These doctors cared for the sick initially in their homes, and then in hospitals once they were built. In the eighteenth century and early nineteenth century, only the wealthier settlers were able to afford medical attention from a doctor and to seek care in a hospital when required. The less fortunate received care through religious and other charitable organizations or from family and friends, who provided in-home care using botanical remedies and other natural medicines shared with them by the Aboriginals.

Canada's first medical school was established in Montreal in 1825. By the time of Confederation, the country had a steadily increasing number of doctors, hospitals, and medical schools, resulting in medical and hospital care that was more accessible to all sectors of the population.

ABORIGINAL MEDICINE AND THE SHAMAN

The medicine practised by Aboriginal peoples in North America (i.e., First Nations, Métis, Inuit) has a long and rich history. Sometimes referred to as shamans or medicine men (note, however, the role of healer was not exclusive to men; women in many Aboriginal cultures have long been recognized as equally powerful healers), traditional Aboriginal practitioners were believed to have a strong connection to the spirit world and to Mother Earth. Many of the shamans' teachings and remedies attempted to maintain balance and harmony among spiritual and natural elements and the human populations that depended on these elements for survival.

Like many traditions, an understanding of healing and the use of herbal medicines was passed down through generations via oral teachings and observances. While attributing some ailments to the presence of evil spirits, traditional healers nevertheless knew how to use local plants, herbs, roots, and fungi to remedy common sicknesses that are still prevalent today. For example, Aboriginal healers used willow bark (which contains salicylic acid, one of the base elements in aspirin) to treat headaches; blood-wort with rosebuds to treat sore throats; and dandelion to treat skin irritation and rashes. Today, many traditional medicines have been incorporated into contemporary Western medicinal practices.

Thinking It Through

Traditions still play a significant role in Aboriginal health care and will affect how an individual responds to a diagnosis as well as to a treatment plan. Research some of the significant traditions of an Aboriginal population in your geographic area. Bearing these traditions in mind, how could you enhance the delivery of culturally sensitive health care?

THE CONCEPT OF PUBLIC HEALTH IS INTRODUCED

At the beginning of the nineteenth century, the prevalence of infectious diseases peaked. In 1834, William Kelly, a British Royal Navy physician, suspected a relationship between sanitation and disease and deduced that water was possibly a major contaminant. Although how disease spread was not clearly understood, many recognized the effectiveness of quarantine practices in limiting the spread.

Upper and Lower Canada each established a board of health, in 1832 and 1833, respectively. These boards of health enforced quarantine and sanitation laws, imposed restrictions on immigration (to prevent the spread of disease), and stopped the sale of spoiled food. Some health care measures met tremendous public opposition. For example, in the mid-1800s, a doctor in Nova Scotia attempted to introduce a smallpox vaccine, which had been discovered and proven successful in England around the turn of the century. Public resistance was strong despite proof that the vaccine protected individuals from the disease. Consequently, the value of smallpox vaccinations was not fully appreciated until the 1900s.

In the early 1900s, the provinces began establishing formal organizations to manage public health matters. A bureau of public health was established in Saskatchewan in 1909 and became a government department in 1923. The provinces of Alberta, Manitoba, and Nova Scotia likewise established departments of health in 1918, 1928, and 1931, respectively. These public health units assumed responsibility for public health matters, including activities such as pasteurizing milk, testing cows for tuberculosis, managing TB sanatoriums, and controlling the spread of sexually transmitted infections. Maternal and child health care became a focus of public health initiatives at the beginning of the twentieth century. Both doctors and nurses actively promoted such things as immunization clinics and parenting education.

THE ROLE OF VOLUNTEER ORGANIZATIONS IN EARLY HEALTH CARE

In the eighteenth and early nineteenth centuries, Canadians' health care needs were attended to largely by volunteer organizations, which were also relied upon heavily for raising funds for health care. These groups are discussed below. Many you will recognize because they still function today.

The Order of St. John

The Order of St. John (later known as St. John Ambulance) was introduced to Canada in 1883 by individuals from England with knowledge of first aid, disaster relief, and home nursing. The organization and its volunteer responsibilities expanded over the years, providing invaluable assistance and health care to Canadians. During the 1918 flu epidemic, which killed 50,000 Canadians, St. John Ambulance volunteers served in hospitals and cared for the sick. Today, more than 11,000 members provide health care services at public events and participate in community health initiatives across Canada (St. John Ambulance, 1995).

The Canadian Red Cross Society

The Canadian Red Cross Society was founded in 1896. In the early 1900s, the Red Cross established a form of home care designed to keep families together during times of illness. The Red Cross trained interested women to take care of families in need—their own and others. These volunteers also assumed household duties (much like stay-at-home parents today) when a family member was too ill to manage them.

The Red Cross gradually became involved in other public health initiatives, establishing outpost hospitals, nursing stations, nutrition services, and university courses in public health nursing. In 1939, it set up more than 2000 branches, nine provincial divisions, and a national headquarters in Toronto in preparation for World War II. The Red Cross also launched a first aid program at this time. In the 1940s, the first blood depot was opened in Vancouver to provide blood to those in need in that province (In the News: Blood Collection Services in Canada) (Canadian Red Cross, 2008).

For over 40 years, the Canadian Red Cross Society supervised the collection of blood from volunteer donors across Canada. The society was stripped of this responsibility in the late 1990s, following the contaminated blood crisis—from 1980 to 1985, at least 2000 people who had received blood and blood products contracted HIV; another 30,000 people were infected with hepatitis C between 1980 and 1990.

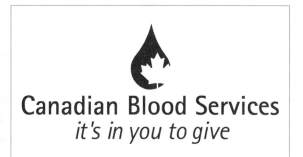

Following the publication of the conclusions of Mr. Justice Krever in his *Final Report: Commission of Inquiry on the Blood System in Canada* (released in 1997), a new national blood authority, Canadian Blood Services, was created in an effort to assure the safety and security of Canada's blood supply system. On September 26, 1998, Canadian Blood Services assumed full responsibility for the Canadian blood system outside of Quebec, and continues in that role today.

Sources: Canadian Blood Services. (n.d.). Retrieved May 29, 2009, from http://www.bloodservices. ca; Krever Inquiry. (n.d.). In *The Canadian Encyclopedia*. Retrieved May 29, 2009, from http://www.thecanadianencyclopedia.com/index.cfm?PgNm=TCE&Params=A1ARTA0009152; Krever Commission. (2004). *Final Report: Commission of Inquiry on the Blood System in Canada*. Retrieved May 29, 2009, from http://www.hc-sc.gc.ca/ahc-asc/activit/com/krever-eng.php

Photo credit: Courtesy of the Canadian Blood Services.

Victorian Order of Nurses

Founded in 1897 by Lady Ishbel Aberdeen, wife of Canada's Governor General at the time, the Victorian Order of Nurses (VON) was one of the first groups to identify the health care needs of the population (particularly women and children) in remote areas of the country and to provide services to these groups. The Order admitted 12 nurses in November of 1897 and shortly thereafter had established VON sites in Ottawa, Montreal, Toronto, Halifax, Vancouver, and Kingston (Victorian Order of Nurses, 2009). Today, the VON offers prenatal education, well-baby clinics, school health services, and nursing home care services.

YMCA, YWCA

The Young Men's Christian Association (YMCA) was founded in London, England, in 1844 by George Williams. The first YMCA in North America opened in

Montreal in 1851 with the goal of assisting young men in health and social matters (Young Men's Christian Association, n.d.).

In 1870, Agnes Blizzard opened the first Canadian Young Women's Christian Association (YWCA) in Saint John, New Brunswick (Young Women's Christian Association, 2004). The YWCA sought to instill self-confidence in young women and to promote physical, economic, and spiritual well-being (Forster, 2004, pp. 112–113).

Thinking It Through

Volunteers have played a major role in the development of health care in Canada over the years. Today, in the face of widespread shortages in health care services, both in hospitals and in the community, the health care system increasingly depends on volunteers.

1. What roles do you think volunteers can continue to play in health care? Identify four areas that would benefit from the contributions of volunteers.

2. How do you think social and demographic trends will affect the roles of volunteers and volunteer organizations?

Children's Aid Society

Until the late 1800s, help for Canadian children in need came either from poorly funded, volunteer-driven private organizations or from the government-funded criminal system (children convicted of crimes were cared for by the government). In some regions, apprenticeship programs arranged for orphaned or abandoned children to work for an individual or family in return for food and shelter.

The *Act for the Protection and Reformation of Neglected Children*, passed in Ontario in 1888, allowed volunteer organizations to intervene when a child was thought to be at risk for abuse or mistreatment. The child could be made a ward of the organization, which would receive funding from the local government for the child's care. Similar acts were passed in other provinces.

The Children's Aid Society of Toronto, created in 1891, was the first of many such volunteer organizations to be established across Canada over the next 10 years (Ontario Association of Children's Aid Societies, 2008). Originally, Children's Aid Society volunteers acted as board members and assumed duties that paid professionals perform today. The Children's Aid Society initially focused on providing food and shelter to disadvantaged children, with little thought given to maintaining the family unit. Children at risk for harm or abuse and needing protection were removed from the family environment and placed in foster homes or orphanages. Today, the provision of a secure and caring environment for the child is still paramount, but keeping families together is also a priority.

Canadian National Institute for the Blind

Established in 1918, the Canadian National Institute for the Blind (CNIB) provides support and health care assistance for people with visual impairment and vision loss. In its first year, with only 27 employees, CNIB served 1521 people in need, many of whom were veterans returning from World War I. In 1930, the organization was instrumental in the passing of the *Blind Voters Act*, which permitted blind people to vote with the assistance of a sighted person. Today, the organization focuses on helping visually impaired people lead productive, healthy, and happy lives by offering them emotional support, as well as assistance obtaining food, clothing, and shelter (Canadian National Institute for the Blind, n.d.).

THE ROLE OF NURSING IN EARLY HEALTH CARE

Nursing care has been an essential element of the Canadian health care system since the 1600s, when the Hôtel-Dieu Hospital in Quebec launched the first structured training for North American nurses in the form of a nursing apprenticeship (Canadian Museum of Civilization, 2004).

Seven years after Confederation, in 1873, the first school of nursing (which differs from an apprenticeship) was established at Mack's General and Marine Hospital in St. Catharines, Ontario (Mount Saint Vincent University, 2005). Another nursing school opened at Toronto General Hospital in 1881. Soon thereafter, nearly every major hospital across Canada offered a school of nursing. In 1908, the Canadian National Association of Trained Nurses (CNATN) was formed to provide support for nurses graduating from formal programs. Not long after, nursing as a professional program was introduced to the school system. At this time, nursing programs taught strategies for disease prevention and health promotion, not unlike the concept of population health in use in Canada and around the world today. Nurses' responsibilities included promoting sanitation, mental health, and vaccinations and establishing well-baby clinics (Mount Saint Vincent University, 2005).

THE DEVELOPMENT OF HOSPITALS IN CANADA

An order of Augustinian nuns from France, who worked as "nursing sisters," established Canada's first hospital, the Hôtel-Dieu de Quebec, which opened in Quebec City in 1639. The nuns set up several other hospitals in the days before Confederation. In fact, with government funding often limited and unreliable, all of Canada's early hospitals were charitable institutions that relied on financial support from wealthy people and well-established organizations. It was not until the already-established Toronto General Hospital closed from 1867 to 1870 due to lack of funds that the Ontario government passed an act providing yearly grants to hospitals and other charitable institutions, laying the groundwork for the present-day provincial government funding of hospitals.

Hospitals of the early 1800s were crowded places focused on treating infectious diseases primarily in the poorer classes, who could not afford private care. At this time, the wealthier segment of the population avoided hospitals, instead hiring doctors, who would visit the client's home to provide treatment. With the introduction of anaesthesia, the **aseptic technique**, and improved surgical procedures in the 1880s, hospitals were finally regarded as places to go to get well, and the use of hospital facilities increased.

In the early 1900s, tuberculosis sanitariums were developed to isolate and care for tuberculosis patients. The disease was difficult to treat, with surgical removal of diseased organs often the only viable cure, and many tuberculosis patients died in hospital. Institutions to care for mentally ill people were also established. Because of the shame associated with mental illness at the time, those who suffered from it were often forcibly admitted to these institutions by family members. Most patients never emerged.

With grants from federal and provincial governments and advances in medical care, the number of hospitals increased over the next several decades. Physician and hospital services remained as out-of-pocket expenses, although some had insurance protection through their employers. Charitable and religious organizations continued to assist those who could not afford care.

During this time, governments made some efforts to improve access to medical care and to provide an affordable fee structure for it (Box 3.1).

Aseptic technique
A procedure performed under sterile conditions to reduce the risk of infection.

Box 3.1   **Innovation in Newfoundland: The Cottage Hospital System**

In the 1930s, approximately 1500 communities in Newfoundland were scattered across 7000 miles of coastline. To service these communities, in 1934, the provincial government developed the Cottage Hospital and Medical Care Plan, which funded the building of a network of small hospitals and paid doctors and nurses to travel to port communities along the extensive coastline. One hospital was even built on a boat.

Intended primarily to provide outpatient care, these small hospitals were equipped with minimal inpatient facilities (20 to 30 beds), an operating room, diagnostic facilities, and a well-equipped emergency department, and were staffed mostly by physicians and nurses with surgical and emergency care experience.

An annual fee of $10 provided a family with health care and use of the cottage hospitals, including transfer to the nearest base hospital when necessary. The cottage hospitals offered other outpatient services, such as immunizations, prenatal and infant care, and client follow-up at home.

Not only was Newfoundland's cottage hospital system innovative and progressive for its time; to this day, provincial and territorial systems draw on some of its key elements, such as small clinics and points of service for rural communities.

Source: Connor, J.H.T. (2007). Twillingate: Socialized medicine, rural doctors and the CIA. *Newfoundland Quarterly, 100*(424). Retrieved May 29, 2009, from http://www.newfoundlandquarterly.ca/issue424/twillingate.php

The Road Toward Health Insurance

Concerned about the continued shortage of physicians within their community, in 1914, without government approval, the residents of the small municipality of Sarnia, Saskatchewan, devised a plan to offer a local doctor $1500 (from municipal tax dollars) as an incentive to practise medicine in the community rather than join the army. The scheme proved successful and, over the next several years, attracted a number of doctors to the area. In 1916, the provincial government passed the *Rural Municipality Act*, formally allowing municipalities to collect taxes to raise funds for retaining physicians and administering and maintaining hospitals. By 1931, 52 municipalities in Saskatchewan had enacted similar plans. Not long afterward, the provinces of Manitoba and Alberta followed suit.

In 1919, the first federal attempt to introduce a publicly funded health care system formed part of a Liberal election campaign. However, once in power, the Liberals were unsuccessful in their negotiations for joint funding with the provinces and territories, so the plan was not carried out.

In the aftermath of the Depression in the 1930s, public pressure for a national health program mounted. Canadians had realized that a more secure, affordable, and accessible health care system was necessary.

First Attempts to Introduce National Health Insurance

In 1935, the Conservative government of R.B. Bennett pledged to address social issues such as minimum wage, unemployment, and public health insurance. Bennett's government proposed the *Employment and Social Insurance Act* on the advice of the Royal Commission on Industrial Relations. Under the Act, the federal government would gain the right to collect taxes to provide social benefits. The

Act, however, was declared unconstitutional by the Supreme Court of Canada and the Privy Council of Great Britain on the grounds that it violated provincial and territorial authority.

In 1937, employment and social insurance was deemed the responsibility of provincial and territorial governments. The federal government nevertheless secured some gains in social programs. In 1940, under Prime Minister Mackenzie King, the provincial and federal governments agreed to amend the *British North America Act* to allow the introduction of a national unemployment insurance program. This program became fully operational in 1942. In 1944, the federal government passed another piece of legislation introducing family allowances for each child aged 16 and under (often referred to as "the baby bonus"), paving the way for more social programs, the modification of existing ones, and formalized health insurance.

POST–WORLD WAR II: THE POLITICAL LANDSCAPE

Major changes in Canada's political landscape followed World War II. Provinces and territories began to exercise more authority over the social and economic lives of their populations. A shift in thinking, largely due to the devastating effects of the Depression, resulted in the idea that governments were responsible for providing citizens with a reasonable standard of living and acceptable access to basic services, such as health care. Canadians wanted the security and equity that a publicly funded health care system would bring.

Canadians, particularly the middle class, had felt the impact of not having access to appropriate health care. The rich could afford proper care; the poor could turn to charities. The expanding middle class was caught in between.

At the same time, medical discoveries were advancing treatment, care, and diagnostic capabilities. A shift from home- to hospital-based care, particularly when complex medical procedures were involved, created a perceived need for a

Social movements
Advancements by a collective of people to promote a common interest by acting together to influence public policy.

more organized approach to health care. Various **social movements** advanced this agenda, believing the involvement of the federal government would result in more stable and equitable funding, which would, in turn, support and promote medical discoveries and treatment options.

In 1948, the federal government set up a number of grants to fund the development of health care services in partnership with the provinces. In 1952, these grants were supplemented by a national old age security program for individuals 70 years of age or older. That same year, the provinces and territories introduced financial aid for people between the ages of 60 and 69, provided on a cost-sharing basis with the federal government. In 1954, legislation permitted the federal government to finance allowances for adults who were disabled and unable to work. All of these measures contributed to Canadians' health and well-being.

Yet, despite increasing public requests for a nationally funded health care system, the provinces, the territories, and the federal government continued to struggle over how the system would be implemented. Who would be in charge of what, and how much power would the federal government hold over matters under provincial and territorial control?

Looking for a workable solution, the federal government ultimately decided to offer funds to the provinces and territories to help pay for health care costs; however, it also set restrictions on how the funds could be spent.

PROGRESS TOWARD PREPAID HOSPITAL CARE

The National Health Grants Program of 1948 marked the first step the federal government took into the provincial and territorial jurisdictions of health care. Through this program, the federal government offered the provinces and territories a total of $30 million to improve and modernize hospitals, to provide training for health care professionals, and to fund research in the fields of public health, tuberculosis, and cancer treatments. Welcomed in all jurisdictions, these grants resulted in a hospital building boom that lasted nearly 30 years.

The next decade saw little progress in the introduction of comprehensive insurance plans in the provinces and territories. Then, in 1957, the federal government under John Diefenbaker introduced the *Hospital Insurance and Diagnostic Services Act*. The Act proposed that any province or territory willing to implement a comprehensive hospital insurance plan would receive federal assistance in the form of 50 cents on every dollar spent on the plan, literally cutting in half the province's or territory's expenses for the cost of insured services—an appealing offer indeed! Five provinces, along with the Northwest Territories and Yukon, bought into the plan immediately. All remaining jurisdictions were on board by 1961.

Even with the financial aid of the federal government, some provinces and territories were not able to implement comprehensive services, primarily because of population distribution. To rectify this problem, the federal government introduced an equalization payment system through which richer provinces would share revenue with poorer provinces to ensure all could offer equal services.

The *Hospital Insurance and Diagnostic Services Act* stated that all residents of a province or territory were entitled to receive insured health care services upon uniform terms and conditions. The Act provided residents with full care in an acute care hospital for as long as the physician felt necessary. It also included care provided in outpatient clinics, but not in tuberculosis sanitariums, mental institutions, or homes for the aged.

Prepaid health care
Access to "medically necessary hospital and physician services on a prepaid basis, and on uniform terms and conditions" (Health Canada, 2005).

Services for some allied health (e.g., physiotherapists) and other nonmedical professionals, as well as diagnostic procedures, were covered by provincial and territorial health insurance plans only if the care was provided in a hospital setting and under the direction of a physician. This coverage paved the way for a huge increase in hospital admissions, some more necessary than others. If **prepaid health care** was available with no out-of-pocket fee in the hospital, why would a client go elsewhere, where he or she would have to pay? As a result, spending for hospital services increased dramatically.

PROGRESS TOWARD PREPAID MEDICAL CARE

Medicare
The informal name for Canada's national health insurance plan. Note that the term's use in Canada differs from that in the United States, where *Medicare* refers to a federally sponsored program for individuals over the age of 65 (Health Canada, 2004).

Tommy Douglas, known as the father of **Medicare** (although this remains controversial—Justice Emmett Hall is also sometimes referred to as Canada's father of Medicare), was the premier of Saskatchewan from 1944 to 1961 (Tommy Douglas Research Institute, n.d.). Douglas long campaigned for a combined comprehensive hospital and medical insurance plan that everyone could afford. He firmly believed that the implementation of a social health insurance plan was a government responsibility and that private insurance plans, while useful, discriminated against those with lower incomes, disabilities, and serious health issues.

In 1939, the Saskatchewan government enacted the *Municipal and Medical Hospital Services Act*, permitting municipalities to charge either a land tax or a personal tax to finance hospital and medical services—a precursor to comprehensive hospital insurance in the province. Eight years later, in 1947, Tommy Douglas's government passed the *Hospital Insurance Act*, guaranteeing Saskatchewan residents hospital care in exchange for a modest insurance premium payment.

Then, in 1960, Douglas was ready to take the next step of providing Saskatchewan citizens with comprehensive, publicly funded medical care in addition to hospital insurance. His initial attempts to introduce medical care insurance inspired fierce opposition from Saskatchewan doctors, who worried they would be controlled by the province. Douglas fought an election campaign with a platform promising to introduce the health insurance program and was re-elected in 1960. The following year, Douglas left Saskatchewan to lead the NDP party in Ottawa. Under his successor, Premier Woodrow Lloyd, the *Saskatchewan Medical Care Insurance Act* was passed in 1961 and took effect in July 1962.

On the day the Medicare law came into effect, the doctors in Saskatchewan launched a province-wide doctors' strike. The provincial government recruited doctors from Great Britain and the United States to cope with the emergency. Fortunately, the strike was short-lived, lasting only 23 days, but it left bitterness and discontent in its wake.

In early August of 1962, the Saskatchewan government revised the *Medical Care Insurance Act* in an attempt to repair the relationship with the province's doctors. One amendment allowed doctors the option of practising outside the medical plan. By 1965, however, most doctors were working within the plan, finding it the easier route to follow. (Billing clients separately and collecting money owed proved expensive and time-consuming and resulted in only a marginal difference in remuneration.) Most other provinces and territories adopted similar plans over the next few years.

Thinking It **Through**

The *Saskatchewan Medical Care Act*, which enforced socialized medicine and imposed fee schedules, prompted outrage and strike action among Saskatchewan doctors. Even today, with changing fee structures and changes in fee-for-service remuneration, some physicians feel that their independence is threatened.

Assume that you were a physician in Saskatchewan in 1962, self-employed in a sector that was considered free enterprise. Feeling that your independence as a health care professional was threatened, what would you do in response to the Medicare proposals? Would you go on strike? How else might you respond?

The Hall Report (1960)

Still committed to introducing a comprehensive health insurance program, the federal government authorized the *Royal Commission on Health Services* (also known as the Hall Report) in 1960. Headed by the Honourable Justice Emmett Hall, this committee investigated the state of health care in Canada and was instrumental in passing the *Medical Care Act* of 1966. Hall supported the introduction of a national Medicare program and suggested that Canada construct new medical schools and hospitals and provide scholarships to doctors and dentists. He recommended that the number of physicians in the country—at the time estimated at 19,000—be doubled by 1990 in preparation for caring for the growing and aging population of Canada. Hall predicted that, if these steps were not taken, Canada's health care system would suffer a shortage of doctors, dentists, and nurses, as well as inadequate health care facilities to care for the population. Hall's prediction became a reality.

When confronted with the question of whether Canadians would rely too much on free health care if implemented, using it as a welfare benefit, Hall declared that free health care was not "welfare" but rather an economic invest-ment in the country—and that healthy people meant a healthy economy.

Hall urged that private health insurance companies in the country (some 145 of them) be replaced by 10 provincial public health insurance plans. He also recommended that the federal government retain strong control over health care financing but that the provincial and territorial governments retain a degree of authority over the implementation of their health care services. Introduced to the provinces in 1965, Hall's recommendations were the final layer in the foun-dation of the *Medical Care Act*.

The *Medical Care Act* (1966)

The *Medical Care Act* was introduced to Parliament in December 1966 and imple-mented on July 1, 1968. Although Ontario and Quebec objected to the Act on the grounds that it would have an impact on provincial priorities, both provinces put medical insurance plans in place by 1969 and 1970, respectively. The last jurisdictions to create medical insurance plans were New Brunswick (1971), the Northwest Territories (1971), and Yukon (1972).

Each province and territory was free to administer the plan in its own way as long as the criteria outlined in the Act were met. To be eligible for federal funds, provincial and territorial health plans had to meet the criteria of *universality*, *por-tability*, *comprehensive coverage*, and *public administration*. These criteria mirror those of the *Canada Health Act* and will be discussed in detail later in this chapter.

Importantly, the *Medical Care Act* reinforced physicians' position as the pri-mary health care professionals within Canada. The services of any other health care professional would cost a fee. Understandably, a doctor became the first choice for most people.

After implementation of the *Medical Care Act*, provincial and territorial ex-penses soared. Hospitals continued to grow, as did their expenditures. Since funding from the federal government was restricted to hospital-based and physician-oriented services, and the provinces and territories were recognizing the need for community-based services outside of the hospital environment, the need for alternative funding arrangements became evident. As well, with the rapidly growing health expenditures, the federal government decided that pro-vincial and territorial spending had to be curbed.

The *Established Programs Financing Act* (1977)

Block transfer
One payment to cover all services.

In 1977, a new funding mechanism, called the *Established Programs Financing (EPF) Act*, was implemented to allocate money to health care and to postsec-ondary education. This arrangement replaced the previous 50/50 cost-sharing formula with a **block transfer** of both cash and tax points (Box 3.2) to the

Thinking It
Through

With the implementation of the *Medical Care Act*, health care costs rose dramatically, fuelling the claim that health care in Canada is consumer-generated—meaning that because health care is perceived as being free, many have sought care indiscriminately, going to the doctor for almost any complaint.

1. Do you think consumers should bear more responsibility for system costs by being more discriminating about when and why they access health care?

2. Do you think Canadians as a whole regard health care as "free," without recognizing they are paying for it (indirectly or otherwise)?

provinces and territories every two months. The funding amount was relative to the **gross national product (GNP)** and population growth.

Under this new funding formula, provinces and territories enjoyed fewer restrictions on how they could spend the money. For example, the provinces and territories could now use the federal money for community-based services and other health care services and products that they deemed beneficial.

The *EPF Act* also included a new transfer of money to the provinces and territories for the Extended Health Care Services Program, which covered intermediate care in nursing homes, ambulatory health care, residential care, and some components of home care that related directly to health issues (e.g., administering medications). This funding formula remained in effect until 1996.

Gross national product (GNP)
The total value of all the goods and services produced by a country within a year.

Box 3.2   Tax Points Explained

Tax points are a reduction in the amount the federal government taxes the provinces and territories. Provinces and territories, in turn, can increase their taxes by the amount of their tax points and use the money earned from provincial or territorial taxes to pay for health care services. The result is that individuals pay the same amount in taxes; however, the tax money is distributed differently. For example, if the federal government taxed a province $200,000 less, that province could tax its residents an additional $200,000 (in place of what the residents had to pay the federal government) and use that money for health care services.

Sources: Government of Canada. (2002). *The transfer of tax points to provinces under the Canada health and social transfer*. Retrieved May 29, 2009, from http://dsp-psd.tpsgc.gc.ca/Collection-R/LoPBdP/BP/bp450-e.htm; Department of Finance Canada. (2008). *Tax points transfer*. Retrieved May 29, 2009, from http://www.fin.gc.ca/transfers/taxpoint/taxpoint-eng.asp

EVENTS LEADING UP TO THE *CANADA HEALTH ACT*

In the few years following the introduction of the *EPF Act*, health care spending continued to increase dramatically, faster than the GNP. And since the funds from the federal government were relative to the GNP, provinces and territories ended up paying more for health care services than the federal government was giving them. The only way to control costs was to cut back on health care services.

Hospitals, therefore, began cutting back on staff, services, and the number of beds. Some medical services were **delisted** from provincial and territorial coverage; others were eliminated altogether. In 1977 and 1978, the governments also imposed restrictions on the fees paid to doctors. In response, in 1978, outraged doctors began billing clients over and above what the provincial or territorial plan paid (in accordance with the negotiated fee schedule). For example, if the public insurance plan paid $25 for a doctor's visit, the doctor added an extra amount—say $10—and asked the client to pay out-of-pocket for that service. This was called *extra billing* and contravened the principles of the *Medical Care Act*.

Opposition to extra billing was swift, with the public claiming that the fees unfairly limited access to health care. Tensions rose between physicians and the public sector. About to launch yet another investigation into the state of health care, the federal government added the issue of extra billing to the agenda. Once again, Justice Emmett Hall was asked to lead the health care services review, with the assistance of Dr. Alice Girard from Quebec.

This review explored a number of items related to the current state of and the progress of health care since the original Hall Report. The review scrutinized the principles set out under the *Medical Care Act*: Were the provincial and territorial governments following the principles, and were they achieving the related objectives? Hall was asked to consider whether changes should be made to the *Hospital Insurance and Diagnostic Services Act*, the *Medical Care Act*, or both. He was also asked to examine the legality of extra billing by physicians.

Hall's conclusions were released in 1980 in a report called *Canada's National–Provincial Health Program for the 1980s*. The report stated that extra billing violated the principles of the *Medical Care Act* and created a barrier for those who could not afford to pay. Hall recommended an end to extra billing and suggested that, instead, doctors be allowed to operate entirely outside of the *Medical Care Act*. That way, clients had the choice of avoiding a doctor who was not working within the boundaries of the provincial or territorial insurance plan.

Physicians opting out of the public insurance plan would bill clients directly for their services; clients would then have to collect money from their provincial or territorial insurance plan. Alternatively, the doctor could bill the plan for

Delisted

The removal of an item from a list or a registry. In Canada, the term is frequently used when a medical service is no longer considered medically necessary and is removed from the government's list of insured services (Canadian Broadcasting Corporation, 2009; Sibbald, 2002).

services, the plan would pay the client, and the client would pay the doctor with the money received, plus any amount the doctor charged above the plan's allowances. It was a lengthy and cumbersome process.

Hall also advised that national standards be created to uphold the principles and conditions of the *Medical Care Act*, that the criterion of *accessibility* be added to the Act, and that an independent National Health Council be established to assess health care in Canada and to suggest policy and legislative changes when needed.

The recommendations from the second Hall Report were taken seriously but put on hold until the Parliamentary Task Force on Federal–Provincial Arrangements completed its review the following year. This task force was to review the funding arrangements under the *EPF Act* and other subsidies the federal government provided to the provinces and territories. The task force's recommendations included adjusting equalization payments, introducing federal responsibility for income distribution, and separating health care funding from higher education funding.

Together, the Hall Report and the report of the Parliamentary Task Force on Federal–Provincial Arrangements prompted the *Canada Health Act*, new and comprehensive legislation that replaced both the *Hospital Insurance and Diagnostic Services Act* and the *Medical Care Act*.

THE *CANADA HEALTH ACT* (1984)

The *Canada Health Act* became law in 1984 under Prime Minister Pierre Trudeau's Liberal government. It received **royal assent** in June 1985 and is still in place today, governing and guiding—and perhaps limiting—our health care delivery system. The Act's primary goal is to provide equal, prepaid, and accessible health care to **eligible** Canadians (Box 3.3) and thereby meet the objectives of Canadian health care policy (Box 3.4).

Box 3.3	Eligibility for Health Care Under the *Canada Health Act*

To be eligible for health care in Canada, a person must be a lawful resident of a province or territory. The *Canada Health Act* defines a resident as "a person lawfully entitled to be or to remain in Canada who makes his home and is ordinarily present in the province, but does not include a tourist, a transient or a visitor to the province" (*Canada Health Act*, 1985, s. 2). Each province or territory determines its own minimum residence requirements.

Source: *Canada Health Act*, R.S.C., c. C-6 (1985).

Canada Health Act
Legislation passed in 1984 that governs and guides the delivery of equal, prepaid, and accessible health care to Canadians.

Royal assent
The final stage a bill passes through before becoming law. Largely symbolic in nature, this approval is given by the Governor General as a representative of the Crown.

Eligible
To be qualified for something by meeting certain criteria or requirements.

> ### Box 3.4   The Primary Objective of Canadian Health Care Policy
>
> "To protect, promote and restore the physical and mental well-being of residents of Canada and to facilitate reasonable access to health services without financial or other barriers."
>
> Source: Health Canada. (2004). *What is the Canada Health Act?* Retrieved May 29, 2009, from http://www.hc-sc.gc.ca/hcs-sss/medi-assur/cha-lcs/overview-apercu-eng.php

CRITERIA AND CONDITIONS OF THE CANADA HEALTH ACT

The *Canada Health Act* established criteria for the delivery of health care. To qualify for federal payments, the provinces and territories must adhere to the five criteria discussed below, as well as to two additional conditions (Box 3.5).

> ### Box 3.5   The *Canada Health Act*: Criteria and Conditions
>
> #### Criteria
>
> 1. Public administration
> 2. Comprehensive coverage
> 3. Universality
> 4. Portability
> 5. Accessibility
>
> #### Conditions
>
> 1. Information
> 2. Recognition
>
> Source: Library of Parliament. (2005). *The Canada Health Act: Overview and options.* Retrieved May 29, 2009, from http://www.parl.gc.ca/information/library/PRBpubs/944-e.pdf

Public Administration

The *Canada Health Act* stipulates that each provincial and territorial health insurance plan be managed by a public authority on a nonprofit basis. That is, the health insurance plan must not be governed by a private enterprise and must not be in the business of making a profit. The public authority answers to the provincial or territorial government regarding its decisions about benefit levels and services, and must have all records and accounts publicly audited.

To meet the criteria of the Act, health plans must be overseen by the Ministry of Health, the Department of Health, or the equivalent provincial or territorial government department. Services provided under the umbrella of the Ministry or Department of Health are distributed via different vehicles, primarily via regional health authorities or the equivalent.

Comprehensive Coverage

Provincial and territorial health insurance plans allow eligible persons with a medical need to access prepaid services provided by physicians and hospitals. Select services offered by dental surgeons, when delivered in the hospital setting, are also covered. Services included under the plan must be available to all residents of the province or territory. All insured individuals must be given equal opportunity to seek all insured services—there must be no barriers to access.

Each province or territory has the latitude to select which services will be covered under its specific plan. Coverage may include components of home care or nursing home care, chiropractic care, eye care under specific conditions, and pharmacare for designated population groups. Comprehensive coverage of these provincially or territorially tailored services must be offered to every eligible resident in the jurisdiction.

Universality

All eligible residents of a province or territory are entitled, on uniform terms and conditions, to all of the insured health services that are provided under the provincial or territorial health insurance plan. The previous legislation, the *Medical Care Act*, had required that 95% of the population be covered under provincial or territorial health insurance. The *Canada Health Act* orders 100% coverage.

The federal government allowed the provinces and territories to decide whether they would charge their residents insurance premiums. If premiums were charged, however, a citizen's inability to pay could not prevent his or her access to appropriate medical care. The province or territory was allowed to subsidize premiums for those with low incomes but could not discriminate on any basis—for example, on the individual's previous health record, current health status, race, or age.

Portability

Canadians moving from one province or territory to another are covered for insured health services by their province of origin during any waiting period in the province or territory to which they have moved. Most jurisdictions enforce a three-month wait before public health insurance becomes active. Under the Act, the waiting period cannot exceed three months. Individuals moving to Canada may also have to endure a waiting period of up to three months and are, therefore, encouraged to have private insurance in place for that time.

Canadians who leave the country will continue to be insured for health services for a prescribed period of time. Every province or territory sets its own time frame (usually about six months, or 183 days). Ontario states that a person may be out of the country for a maximum of 212 days in any given year, while Alberta, British Columbia, Manitoba, and New Brunswick state that a person must remain in the province for at least six months to retain coverage. In Nova Scotia, with permission and under certain conditions, a temporary absence of up to one year is allowed. Newfoundland and Labrador offers out-of-province coverage for individuals who remain in the province for only four months of the calendar year. This is the lowest residency requirement of all jurisdictions and is, in part, due to the number of migrant workers in the province. As well, every jurisdiction offers coverage for special situations, such as absences for educational or work purposes. Although Canadian residents are covered for necessary care (i.e., urgent or emergency care) while absent from their home province (e.g., for business or a vacation), they are not permitted to seek elective surgeries or other planned care in another province or territory. In some cases, prior approval for coverage may be granted for elective nonemergency surgery (Case Example 3.1). The Web sites of the provincial and territorial ministries of health offer information about the particulars of each jurisdiction's health care coverage.

Case Example 3.1

At 69 years old, Nancy is booked for elective hip replacement surgery in six months in her home province of Nova Scotia. However, she decides to visit her sister in British Columbia and have her hip replaced there because surgical wait times are shorter. To ensure that the Nova Scotia government will cover the cost of Nancy's surgery in British Columbia, she has to contact the Nova Scotia Department of Health for prior approval.

If Nancy has the surgery without requesting approval from the Nova Scotia Department of Health, or if she is denied approval, she will have to pay for the surgery out-of-pocket. However, if she falls down the stairs and breaks her hip while she is visiting her sister, the surgery would be done in British Columbia, and the total cost would be covered by her province of origin without question.

Insured services received outside the person's province of origin will be paid at the host province's rate, except by Quebec (Case Example 3.2).

Case Example 3.2

Jeremy, a 20-year-old living in Ontario, is visiting friends in Saskatchewan. While there, he develops a severe and persistent sore throat and pays a visit to a local doctor. If the cost of a visit to the family doctor in Saskatchewan is $20 but is only $15 in his home province of Ontario, the Ontario health plan will pay the $20 required by the doctor in Saskatchewan.

Now consider the situation if Jeremy is from Quebec. If the fee for the same doctor's visit is $15 in Quebec, the Quebec health plan will pay only $15 to the doctor in Saskatchewan and Jeremy will have to pay $5. Quebec does not honour the host province's or territory's fee schedule if it is higher than its own.

Accessibility

The criterion of accessibility was added to the *Canada Health Act* in an attempt to ensure that eligible individuals in a province or territory have reasonable access to all insured health services on uniform terms and conditions. *Reasonable access* means access to services when and where they are available, as they are available. Therefore, individuals living in an area where a required service is not available must be granted access to that service in the closest location it is offered (Case Example 3.3). Note, however, that a province or territory would only pay for a client to receive an available service at the closest location, not a location farther afield.

Case Example 3.3

Monique is a 40-year-old woman living in Sioux Lookout, Ontario. She has just been diagnosed with breast cancer. Her community does not have access to radiation therapy, but this therapy is available in Thunder Bay, Ontario. In accordance with the accessibility criterion, Monique would be sent to Thunder Bay for her treatments. If radiation therapy was not available in Thunder Bay—or if the wait time was excessive—Monique would be sent to Winnipeg, Manitoba.

A recent real-life case in Alberta (In the News: Care: Access and Cost) highlights the promise of accessibility, even if it means going across the border.

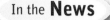

In the **News**   **Care: Access and Cost**

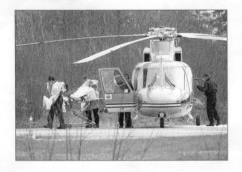

In August 2007, a Calgary woman, pregnant with identical quadruplets, unexpectedly went into labour at 31 and a half weeks' gestation. At that time, no neonatal facility was available in the province to support the babies after their births. In fact, no adequate facility in Canada was available. The woman was flown to Montana in the United States, where the babies were born and safely cared for. Within a few days, the mother and babies were returned to Alberta by air ambulance. The staggering cost of $170,000 was paid by the Alberta government. Imagine if the family had been expected to cover that cost themselves!

Source: Lang, M. (2007, August 17). Calgary's quads: Born in the U.S.A. *Calgary Herald*. Retrieved July 13, 2009, from http://www.canada.com/topics/news/story.html?id= 78b28230-d3ff-47d3-ab04-fff760931f1a

Photo credit: THE CANADIAN PRESS/The Timmins Daily Press—Arron Pickard.

The criterion of accessibility specifies that the province or territory must provide reasonable payment to doctors and dentists who are eligible to bill provincial and territorial plans for insured services. The province or territory must also cover the costs of hospitals' insured health care services.

The interpretation of *reasonable access* is controversial. A person living in Churchill, Manitoba, will not have the same access to health care as a person living in Halifax, Toronto, or Vancouver. Today, service availability even varies between rural and urban settings. For the purposes of the *Canada Health Act*, accessibility has been interpreted as access to services where and when available. It does not, in the true sense of the word, guarantee "equality" of services across Canada.

The following two conditions were included in the *Canada Health Act*:

- *Information*. Each province or territory must provide the federal government with information about the province's or territory's insured health care services and extended health care services for the purposes identified in the *Canada Health Act*.

- *Recognition*. The provincial and territorial governments must publicly recognize the federal financial contributions to both insured and extended health care services.

Interpreting the *Canada Health Act*

Medically necessary is a subjective term that has been hotly debated within the context of the *Canada Health Act* (also see Chapter 8). Typically, a physician or other health care professional eligible to bill the provincial or territorial plan makes a clinical judgement to provide the client with specific "medically necessary" services, which usually include assessment, diagnostic tests, and treatment. Note, however, that jurisdictions may not cover all diagnostic tests and treatments. Since the *Canada Health Act* does not detail which services should be insured, the range of insured services varies among provinces and territories.

Medical services must not be provided simply for the convenience of the client or physician (e.g., Caesarian section). And when more than one treatment is available, a physician must consider cost effectiveness. For example, when faced with two treatment options that have similar outcomes, a physician must recommend the less expensive option.

What one doctor considers medically necessary another doctor may not. Consider breast reduction: A surgeon in Manitoba might determine that this surgery is medically necessary for a particular client with large breasts because of the backaches and muscle strains she suffers. Another surgeon may not think breast reduction is medically necessary for this client, meaning that the client would have to pay for the surgery since it would be then considered a cosmetic procedure.

Medically necessary
A clinical judgement made by a physician regarding a service provided under a provincial or territorial health plan that is necessary to maintain, restore, or palliate (i.e., ease symptoms, such as pain, without curing the underlying disease).

Thinking It Through

The term *medically necessary* appears in the *Canada Health Act* to identify procedures and services that are covered by provincial and territorial insurance.

1. Do you think that the term is too subjective?
2. Are there health services in your province or territory that you feel should be covered but are not?

Physicians, through their governing body, and government officials, usually from the Ministry or Department of Health, select which services are medically necessary and are, therefore, insured. At designated intervals, the provinces and territories review their lists of insured services, sometimes adding services, sometimes removing them.

A few years ago, for example, many jurisdictions removed elective newborn circumcision from the list of insured services because evidence showed no medical reason for this procedure and found other reasons (e.g., a belief that a circumcised penis is cleaner or that the baby should resemble his father) to be invalid. However, circumcision is still insured when a valid medical reason exists for doing it.

Also addressed in the *Canada Health Act* are extra billing and user charges. Under the Act, extra billing (see page 88) and user charges (Box 3.6) are not allowed. If a province or territory permits extra billing or user charges, the federal government will total the amount of money the province or territory has collected and will take back that amount from the next transfer of funds.

Box 3.6   User Charges Explained

User charges are fees billed directly to an individual for a medically necessary service that is insured by the provincial or territorial health plan. Like extra billing, user charges are not permitted under the *Canada Health Act* because such fees create a barrier to seeking medical care. Proponents of user charges believe they play a useful role in today's health climate—for example, charging people who use the emergency department for nonurgent complaints may ultimately improve emergency department wait times.

Additional Components of the Act

The *Canada Health Act* specifically outlines extended health care services that are considered medically necessary and are thus insured. Extended health care services insured under the Act include intermediate care in nursing homes, adult residential care services, home care services, and the services provided in ambulatory care centres.

A number of services, such as certain components of home care, however, are not covered under the Act and are subject to each province's or territory's health insurance plan. Some jurisdictions, for example, will provide a certain number of home care hours per week. Once the limit is reached, the client must pay a home care agency for additional care. The legislation prohibiting user charges and extra billing, therefore, does not apply to extended health care services.

Each province and territory chooses which optional services (i.e., services that are not medically necessary) will be covered under its health plan. Optional services may include chiropody (i.e., foot care), massage therapy, physiotherapy, dental care, drug plans, and assistive devices coverage. (Note: Services supplied within a hospital or other insured facility are usually covered.)

The amount of coverage for optional services will vary. For example, a province's plan may cover up to $200 per month in physiotherapy services. Services in excess of this amount are subject to user charges and extra billing, which, as mentioned, are permitted for services deemed not medically necessary under the Act.

AFTER THE *CANADA HEALTH ACT*

Most of the resistance to the Act came from physicians and those affected directly by the restrictions set out in the Act. In 1986, Ontario physicians participated in a 25-day strike in opposition to the Act, arguing that the key issue was not money but professional freedom, a claim not well received by the public. That same year, the Canadian Medical Association opposed the implementation of the *Canada Health Act* on the grounds that it violated the *Constitution Act* of 1982. The case went to the Supreme Court of Canada but did not proceed.

Just prior to the introduction of the Act, most of the provinces and territories had established some form of extra billing, user charges, or both as a result of

---

In the **News** **Doctors Striking for Autonomy**

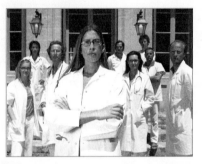

On June 12, 1986, Ontario doctors took strike action on the grounds that banning extra billing violated their right to contract directly with clients and undermined the quality of care. Doctors saw this ban as an end to their independence, a means of essentially turning them into civil servants. For the first time, Ontarians turned on the news to see militant doctors marching with picket signs in hand.

While the strike was supported by nearly all regions and specialties, a majority of doctors did not participate. Furthermore, public opinion remained firmly opposed to the doctors' arguments. In fact, the strike was widely viewed as a public relations disaster. The Ontario Medical Association later admitted that, to a large degree, hostile public opinion prompted the end of the strike.

Ultimately, the strike failed to stop the ban on extra billing. The true outcome? Bitter feelings that persist even today.

Sources: Kravitz, R.L., Shapiro, M.F., Linn, L.S., & Froelicher, E.S. (1989). Risk factors associated with participation in the Ontario Canada doctor's strike. *American Journal of Public Health*, 79, 1233–1277; Brennan, R. (1986, December 27). Doctor's strike memories linger. *The Windsor Star*, p. A3.

Photo credit: Ghislain & Marie David de Lossy/GetStock.

events leading up to the implementation of the *Canada Health Act* (e.g., the regulation of services and fees doctors could charge). These extra fees could not be removed overnight. Over the next two years, the federal government imposed monetary penalties to noncompliant jurisdictions, again fuelling resentment and opposition. The government decided, however, to reimburse provinces that took corrective action against extra billing and user charges within three years. Most jurisdictions complied, but these practices were not entirely eliminated. Even today, some provinces and territories defy this part of the Act, resulting, each year, in withheld funding primarily related to user charges at private clinics deemed by the federal government to be operating outside of the law.

In the decade following the implementation of the *Canada Health Act*, the health care system in Canada experienced increasing difficulties that persist today. At first, hospitals had trouble functioning within their allotted budgets. Provinces and territories pushed for more money to sustain reasonable levels of care, yet federal funding continued to dwindle. In the early 1990s, hospitals restructured, downsized, redistributed beds, laid off staff, cut services, and closed. Doctors and nurses left the country, and fewer graduates pursued careers in these roles, leading to widespread staffing shortages.

Some provinces and territories responded proactively by establishing innovative and alternative health care strategies (Box 3.7). Home care became a priority across Canada, the concept of "health care teams" (i.e., the physician working with other health care professionals to deliver more comprehensive, client-oriented care) was introduced, increased access to primary care services (e.g., through after-hours clinics, telephone helplines, and extended office hours) was implemented, and **primary health care reform** began to take place (Table 3.1).

Primary health care reform
Changes to the delivery of primary health care with the goal of providing all Canadians access to an appropriate health care professional 24 hours a day, 7 days a week, no matter where they live.

Box 3.7   New Brunswick Leads the Way in Community Care

New Brunswick was one of the first jurisdictions to predict the problems related to funding shortfalls, cutbacks, population changes, and an increased need for hospital beds. The province led the move toward community-based care, called "hospital without walls," and established the Extra-Mural Program, which focused on shortening hospital stays and providing the appropriate care and support to meet health care needs in the home and community settings. This concept was actually introduced in 1979, five years before the *Canada Health Act* was passed.

Throughout the 1980s and 1990s, various provinces and territories completed investigations into the state of health care—the Royal Commission on Health Care in Nova Scotia (1989), Advisory Committee on the Utilization of Medical Services in Alberta (1989), Premier's Commission on Future Health Care in Alberta (1989),

New Brunswick Commission on Selected Health Care Programs (1989), Commission on Directions in Health Care in Saskatchewan (1990), Premier's Council on Health Strategy in Ontario (1991), Royal Commission on Healthcare and Costs in British Columbia (1991), and the Health Services Review in British Columbia (1999).

National reports were also commissioned—for example, the first and second reports on the health of Canadians, released in 1996 and 1999, respectively, examined and summarized the health status of Canadians.

By 2002, public confidence in health care was at an all-time low, with health care topping the list of Canadians' concerns. Only recently have Canadians become more concerned about the environment than health care. Ironically, environmental concerns (e.g., pollution, contaminated drinking water, and poor air quality) squarely interact with health care concerns.

Source: South East Regional Health Authority. (n.d.). *Extra-Mural Program*. Retrieved May 29, 2009, from http://www.serha.ca/extra_mural/htm/english/about_us.htm

Table 3.1	The Goals of Primary Health Care Reform

Medical Model of Health Care	Primary Health Care Reform Goals
Physician-based care	Team-oriented care
Illness-focused	Emphasis on health
Hospital-based care	Community-based care
Curative (in relation to disease)	Focus on health promotion and disease prevention
Problems are isolated	Care is comprehensive and integrated (i.e., holistic)
Health care professional–dominated	Collaborative care involving client, family, and loved ones

SOCIAL UNION

In 1997, the provincial and territorial **first ministers** met with their federal counterparts to form a social renewal program that would bind all governments to a commitment to move forward collaboratively on what the first ministers called a social union (Social Union, 1999). First ministers from all jurisdictions, except Newfoundland and Quebec, gathered to press Ottawa for a funding increase. Over the next several months, negotiations became increasingly confrontational, with the federal government wanting a voice in how money would be spent and on what services (e.g., cancer treatments, improvements to emergency

First ministers
The premiers of the provinces and territories.

rooms, long-term care). However, in 1999, Prime Minister Jean Chrétien put forth a plan that offered the provinces and territories more spending flexibility. On January 22, 1999, all of the provinces (including Quebec) and territories agreed to commit to the prime minister's proposals. Quebec, however, did not sign the final agreement on February 4, 1999 (Government of Canada, 1999). The province opposed any arrangements that implied the federal government would have any authority over provincial social policy. As well, Quebec was unwilling to sign any agreement that did not clearly support the province's right to unconditionally opt out of programs supported by or initiated by the federal government, which the social union did not provide for.

The social union was a significant move forward in harmonizing federal–provincial and federal–territorial relationships. The union's goal was to clarify the role of the federal government with respect to funding and commitment and to work collaboratively to improve health care and social programs for Canadians.

The union agreed to maintain the five criteria of the *Canada Health Act* and to work continuously to improve health care by sharing information and innovations. The ministers also pledged to report ongoing government activities to keep Canadians informed about their health status and public programs. The union was committed to working collaboratively with Aboriginal people, their governments, and their organizations to improve health care and social programs for Aboriginals. The federal government promised to boost health care spending by $11.5 billion over the next five years, starting in the 1999–2000 fiscal year.

COMMISSIONED REPORTS

By the end of 2002, three major reports on the status of health care in Canada had been commissioned and released: The Mazankowski Report, the Kirby Report, and the Romanow Report.

The Mazankowski Report: *A Framework for Reform*

A Framework for Reform, known as the Mazankowski Report (Mazankowski, 2001), examined health care in the province of Alberta; however, the report's findings bore noteworthy similarities to the Romanow and Kirby reports, which looked at health care on a national level.

The Mazankowski Report was commissioned by former Alberta premier Ralph Klein in August 2000 and was chaired by Donald Mazankowski, former Cabinet member in the Mulroney government. Mazankowski and his team were to scrutinize health care in Alberta and provide recommendations on both short- and long-term reform. The final report was submitted in December 2001.

One of the most controversial recommendations concerned the role of private health care and private insurance in Alberta. The report suggested that doctors be required to work for a specified length of time in the public sector and then be allowed to devote the rest of their time to private health care if they chose to do so.

The report recommended reviewing medically necessary services and delisting a portion of these services. It also emphasized the need for a province-wide electronic health record system to enhance continuity of client care and an electronic health card to help the government track service access. The report suggested that taxes be used as a source of increased revenue and that Albertans pay higher health premiums—not a particularly popular recommendation.

By 2003, Alberta had implemented a province-wide electronic health record initiative, becoming the first Canadian province to do so.

The Kirby Report: *The Health of Canadians—The Federal Role*

An independent report, released in October 2002, just two months before the Romanow Report, *The Health of Canadians—The Federal Role* (Kirby, 2002) examined the state of the Canadian health care system and the role of the federal government in it. Led by Senator Michael J. Kirby, this report identified a number of problems and made recommendations to resolve them. As in the Mazankowski Report, support for the role of private health care figured as a key component.

Kirby argued that Canada's current health care system was not sustainable given existing funding levels and suggested other avenues of funding, such as new taxes or insurance premiums based on income—Canadians with lower incomes could pay as little as 50 cents per day, while Canadians with higher incomes might pay as much as $4 per day.

The report acknowledged the problem of wait times and called for the government to set limits on them. Once the limit was reached, the report stated, the government should pay for the health care client to receive treatment elsewhere, even in the United States if necessary.

The report recommended that the government provide financial assistance to cover the cost of medications under certain circumstances. For example, a person whose medication costs topped $5000 per year should have 90% of this cost covered by the federal government and the remaining 10% by the province or territory in which the person lived.

Further, the report recommended an immediate outlay of $2 billion for information technology, including the development of a national system for electronic health records, and another $2.5 billion over five years for advanced medical equipment.

Kirby wanted the government to offer incentives, such as short-term tax breaks, to encourage health care professionals to return to Canada, as well as funds to recruit, train, and retain doctors and nurses.

Most of Kirby's recommendations have not been adopted, nor was his report considered in the same context as the Romanow Report. The Romanow Report garnered more public interest, publicity, and government involvement. Ontario did adopt a health tax in the form of premium payments, but, by and large, funding for health care initiatives has come from other resources.

The Romanow Report: *Building on Values: The Future of Health Care in Canada*

Roy Romanow, former premier of Saskatchewan and chair of the Commission on the Future of Health Care in Canada, released his final report in November 2002 (Romanow, 2002). Its purpose was to present recommendations to ensure the survival of Canada's health care system while continuing to provide Canadians with a high level of health care. The report was to consider health promotion and disease prevention initiatives. In preparing his report, Romanow criss-crossed the country, holding public forums and meetings to gather information and advice from Canadians.

Unlike Kirby, Romanow believed that health care *was* sustainable, but only with appropriate and immediate action on the part of governments (all levels), communities, and individual Canadians. Fundamentally, Romanow opposed privatization of health care but acknowledged that a level of private health care was already operating in some parts of Canada. He believed, however, that privatization should be limited and new initiatives in this area discouraged.

The Romanow Report, *Building on Values: The Future of Health Care in Canada*, provided 47 recommendations for both health care reform and renewal of the *Canada Health Act*. Key proposals included the following:

- A Canadian Health Covenant, an agreement by the government to clearly state how the health care system could be approved and a commitment to ensuring such improvements happen, should be created. The covenant would give the government the responsibility of regularly reviewing the performance of the health care system and reporting results to the public. This responsibility would be among the duties and mandate of a proposed Health Council of Canada.

- The proposed Health Council of Canada would monitor the progress of health care initiatives (or lack thereof) and report to the public any progress, barriers, and specific issues related to both health care and population health. Key issues for reporting would include home- and community-based care, primary care reform initiatives, human health resources, implementation of drug plans, and wait times.

- Health care reform should be paid for with funds from the federal surplus or by raising taxes.

- The federal government should provide predictable and sustained funding for long-term care and home care services.

- Injury and disease prevention and health promotion strategies should be continued and enhanced.

- The criterion of accountability should be added to the *Canada Health Act*.

- Insured services, including home care and diagnostic testing, should be extended. Programs for training home care providers should be extended to address the shortage of these workers. Individuals discharged from hospital and recovering from acute illnesses or surgery should have full health care at home for a period of no less than 14 days and up to 28 days if rehabilitation is necessary. Coverage and services related to **palliative care** and mental health care should be expanded in the home and community.

- Employment Insurance benefits and job security should be extended to family members and friends who choose to care for sick or dying loved ones at home.

- **Catastrophic drug costs** should be covered. The report suggested that the federal government pay $1 billion annually toward drug coverage and, above that, reimburse provinces and territories 50% of the cost of any drug plans in excess of $1500 per person per year. The report also recommended that co-payments and deductions paid for prescription drugs be reduced for Canadians needing the assistance.

- The price of drugs should be monitored and controlled under a national drug agency, which could provide a centralized list of all drugs to be covered by provincial and territorial drugs plans. This agency would also be responsible for "ensuring the safety, quality, and cost-effectiveness of all new drugs before they are approved for use in Canada" (Romanow, 2002). Romanow further added that of equal importance was the task of "reviewing drugs on an ongoing basis, monitoring their use and outcomes across the country, and sharing high quality, timely information" (Romanow, 2002). The report recommended that another agency, independent of the government, be established to review and approve prescription drugs and to ensure that the Canadians have clear and concise information about the drugs they are taking (Canadian Labour Congress, 2002).

- While it did not recommend a maximum wait time for services, the report did advocate the organization of a central body to monitor and streamline waiting lists.

- The federal government should establish a dedicated, cash-only Canada Health Transfer to replace the health care component of the current Canada Health and Social Transfer (CHST).

Palliative care
Care for the dying. Palliative care services, offered in the home or another facility (e.g., palliative care unit in a hospital or a hospice), may include nursing care, counselling, and pain management and may involve those close to the client.

Catastrophic drug costs
Prescription drug costs that cause undue burden on individuals suffering with serious health conditions or illnesses.

Following the release of the Romanow Report, the federal government under Prime Minister Jean Chrétien stated that the report would provide the foundation for the direction of health care over the next several years. In 2004, the federal government earmarked $10 billion for health care to be distributed over a 10-year time frame to address the problems identified in the report.

Several of Romanow's recommendations have been implemented. The Canada Health Transfer has been put in place. Health promotion campaigns have been maintained and further promoted by all levels of government. Wait lists are being addressed. The Health Council of Canada was created as a result of the 2003 First Ministers' Accord. At the 2004 first ministers' meeting, Canada's first ministers agreed on more funding and initiatives for health care renewal, including funding for family members to remain at home to care for ill relatives. Primary health care reform initiatives have been tested, implemented, and revised across Canada. Funds have been made available for information technology and electronic health records in all jurisdictions. A national drug plan, however, has not been implemented.

Thinking It Through

Introducing a national drug plan and increased coverage for home care, two of the recommendations made in the Romanow Report, would cost billions of dollars.

1. Do you think that health care as we know it is sustainable?
2. Are Canadians expecting too much, or do Canadians need to change their expectations?
3. Do you think initiatives as those noted above would be cost effective?

ACCORDS

The following summaries of first ministers' meetings highlight the latest agreements on health care between the federal government and the provincial and territorial governments.

First Ministers' Meeting, 2000

In September 2000, the first ministers met and agreed to work together to identify the significant issues facing health care in each province and territory, to prioritize these concerns, and to pledge to work collaboratively to address these concerns on both a provincial or territorial and national level (First Ministers, 2000).

The major issues identified at this meeting included the following:

- Timely access to health care
- Health promotion and disease prevention
- The structure and function of primary care services (access and wait times)
- The shortage of health care professionals across Canada
- The cost and availability of home and community health care services
- The cost and management of medications, health information, and electronic health records
- Inadequate diagnostic equipment
- Lack of accountability to Canadians regarding the implementation and function of health care services

A number of meetings followed. Agreements were achieved, commitments were made, and funding was pledged to address concerns. The renewed commitment at each subsequent meeting built on the promises made at the September 2000 first ministers' gathering. Each meeting addressed the same general concerns but extracted more specific promises regarding various health care services and federal funding.

First Ministers' Accord on Health Care Renewal, 2003

In February 2003, the prime minister and the premiers of seven provinces met in Ottawa to outline the immediate direction for health care in Canada (First Ministers, 2003). The overriding commitment made was to preserve universal health care under the current *Canada Health Act*.

A key component of this accord was the outlining of standards of care for Canadians, including access to health care providers 24 hours a day, 7 days a week; prompt access to diagnostic services and treatments; the implementation of a nationwide electronic health record system; and financial assistance for those who needed medications but could not afford them.

Created at this meeting, the Health Reform Fund, over a five-year time frame, would channel money into primary care, a catastrophic drug plan, and home care services. The federal government would transfer money to the provinces and territories so that they could address the specific needs of their residents.

The ministers also addressed the unique needs of Aboriginal people. The federal government pledged to work more closely with provincial and territorial governments and Aboriginal leaders to bring health care services for Aboriginal people on par with those provided to other Canadians.

The equalization payment program was re-examined to ensure that all provinces had adequate funding to provide comparable health care services to their citizens. It was through this accord that the Canada Health Transfer was created, separating the funding formula that had combined federal funding for both health care and postsecondary education.

In this accord, the federal government also pledged to introduce a compassionate care benefit package through the Employment Insurance program, along with job protection through the Canada Labour Code (as recommended in the Romanow Report), to provide financial security and job protection for individuals who temporarily leave their place of employment to care for a seriously ill or dying parent, spouse, or child.

First Ministers' Meeting on the Future of Health Care, 2004

The First Ministers' Meeting on the Future of Health Care was convened to follow up on agreements made in 2003, discuss progress, and move forward with other proposals (First Ministers, 2004). At this meeting, the prime minister and premiers signed a second agreement, with the federal government pledging $41 billion for health care services over a 10-year time frame. Once again, the first ministers renewed their commitment to building on the criteria of the current *Canada Health Act* and to working together in a constructive and open manner. They promised to share information and to be more accountable to the public about progress being made. The Canada Health Council was given increased responsibilities to report to Canadians on health outcomes.

The prime minister, first ministers, and Aboriginal leaders established the Aboriginal Health Transition Fund, which provided $200 million for improving Aboriginal health care services to meet the needs of Aboriginal people across Canada.

Annual Conference of Ministers of Health, 2005

At the Annual Conference of Ministers of Health in 2005, particular consideration was given to the catastrophic drug coverage mentioned at previous meetings (First Ministers, 2005). The ministers of health discussed measures to move forward with previous recommendations to standardize the price of drugs across Canada and pledged to have better control over the pharmaceutical industry's relationship with provincial and territorial health insurance plans.

The Kelowna Accord, 2006

The first ministers met again in Kelowna, British Columbia (Kelowna Accord, 2006), where the federal government promised to spend $5 billion over five years to improve health, housing, and education for Aboriginal people.

The ministers also established the *Blueprint on Aboriginal Health*, a plan aimed to bring the health outcomes of Aboriginal people in line with those of the general Canadian population—although provinces and territories have yet to commit to the plan.

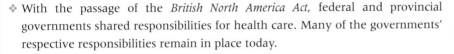

SUMMARY

❖ With the passage of the *British North America Act*, federal and provincial governments shared responsibilities for health care. Many of the governments' respective responsibilities remain in place today.

❖ European settlers, primarily from England and France, brought doctors and nurses with them. Many of the first doctors were employed by the military but cared for civilians as well.

❖ Before the arrival of Europeans, Aboriginal shamans ("medicine men") practised medicine in their communities for millennia, handing down remedies through their oral traditions.

❖ First Nations people played a healing role as well—their herbal and spiritual remedies were often incorporated into treatments used by settlers and physicians.

❖ Over time, the semblance of a formalized health care system emerged. Early on, volunteers played a significant role in both delivering and developing health care, as did organized charitable groups, many religious in origin. St. John Ambulance, the Victorian Order of Nurses, and the Red Cross all made early appearances and remain important contributors and supporters of health care today.

❖ Initially, hospitals were viewed as dens of infection, so much of the necessary care was delivered at home. As technology advanced and hospitals modernized, the reverse happened—more care became hospital-based.

❖ Following World War II, Saskatchewan spearheaded an organized push to implement prepaid medical and hospital care and a public health care system. This goal was achieved in 1984 with the passing of the *Canada Health Act*, which remains in place today—although not without controversy. Some critics believe the Act is outdated and fails to meet the needs of Canadians in the twenty-first century.

❖ Recent initiatives in health care include implementing primary health care reform, expanding insured services to home and community care, building a nationwide computerized system for electronic health records and information sharing, and ensuring sufficient health care professionals are available to meet the needs of Canadians in the future.

❖ At the same time, the health care system must cope with a growing need for more funding, an aging population, advancing but expensive technologies, and the expectation of entitlement among Canadians. It appears the cost of universal services will only increase.

❖ Many Canadians find the prospect of widespread private health care services unappealing, although privatization may happen out of necessity. If so, the challenge will be to preserve a high standard of care and services and to work with private enterprise as a parallel but unobstructive system.

REVIEW QUESTIONS

1. What were the responsibilities of the federal and provincial governments outlined in the *British North America Act*?

2. Who first introduced the concept of prepaid hospital care to Canada?

3. How did Newfoundland deal with providing services to its sparsely populated geographic areas?

4. What two pieces of legislation combined to produce the *Canada Health Act*?

5. What is meant by *medically necessary*?

6. What were the principal goals of the social union (1999)?

7. What was the primary objection of the government to user charges and extra billing?

8. What is the Canadian Health Covenant?

DISCUSSION QUESTIONS

1. Review the criteria of the *Canada Health Act*. Which criteria mean the most to you? Do an Internet search for articles criticizing the principles and conditions of the *Canada Health Act* as it now stands, and validate your opinion of its effectiveness in today's society. Do you feel that the criteria of universality, accessibility, and comprehensiveness meet the needs of Canadians today?

2. Compare and contrast the recommendations of the Romanow Report and the Kirby Report. Investigate which measures the federal, provincial, and territorial governments have implemented from each report. Do you feel that these measures are improving health care? What recommendations

would you make to improve health care in your own community? In your province or territory?

3. Interview five people in their 60s, and five in their 30s. Ask them what they remember about health care in the 1980s, 1990s, and in the past 10 years. Write a summary of their impressions.

4. Review in detail the 2003 and 2004 first ministers' accords and the Hall Report. Summarize the proposals, promises, and commitments in each. What suggestions made in the Hall Report were carried forward to 2004? Have they been acted on? What more do you think should be done to renew health care in your jurisdiction? What matters should be added to the first ministers' list of concerns?

WEB RESOURCES

An Interview With Supreme Court Justice Emmett Hall
http://archives.cbc.ca/health/health_care_system/clips/447/

This Web page provides access to the National Farm Radio Forum, November 2, 1964, broadcast—an interview with Justice Emmett Hall, making the case for national health care.

Public vs. Private Health Care
http://www.cbc.ca/news/background/healthcare/public_vs_private.html

This Web page discusses the differences among public, private, and two-tier health care and explains the forms of private health care and their presence in Canada today.

WEB RESOURCES

Union Hospital and Municipal Hospital Care Plans
http://esask.uregina.ca/entry/union_hospital_and_
municipal_hospital_care_plans.html

This *Encyclopedia of Saskatchewan* article offers historical background to the union hospital and municipal hospital care plans in Saskatchewan from 1916 to 1957.

Canada Health Act: Federal Transfers and Deductions
http://www.hc-sc.gc.ca/hcs-sss/medi-assur/
cha-lcs/transfer-eng.php

This article discusses federal transfers and deductions and outlines how Health Canada determines provincial and territorial compliance. It also provides the history of deductions under the *Canada Health Act* and the history of federal transfers related to health care from 1957 to 2003.

Canada Health Act: Frequently Asked Questions
http://www.hc-sc.gc.ca/hcs-sss/medi-assur/res/
faq-eng.php

This Web page provides frequently asked questions and answers regarding the *Canada Health Act*, including such topics as eligibility, health care services provided, health care premiums, and coverage of alternative services.

REFERENCES

Canada Health Act, R.S.C., c. C-6 (1985).

Canadian Broadcasting Corporation. (2009). No delisting of health services for now: Alberta health minister. *CBC News*. Retrieved May 29, 2009, from http://www.cbc.ca/canada/edmonton/story/2009/02/05/edm-delisting-liepert.html

Canadian Labour Congress. (2002). *CLC preliminary analysis of the Romanow Commission report on the future of health—*Building on Values. Retrieved May 29, 2009, from http://www.healthcoalition.ca/CLC-Romanow.pdf

Canadian Museum of Civilization. (2004). *A brief history of nursing in Canada from the establishment of New France to the present.* Retrieved May 29, 2009, from http://www.civilization.ca/cmc/exhibitions/tresors/nursing/nchis01e.shtml

Canadian National Institute for the Blind. (n.d.) *Understanding CNIB.* Retrieved May 29, 2009, from http://www.cnib.ca

Canadian Red Cross. (2008). *Historical timeline 1900–1950.* Retrieved May 29, 2009, from http://www.redcross.ca/article.asp?id=7834&tid=019

First Ministers. (2000). *Details of the first ministers' conference, Ottawa.* Retrieved May 29, 2009, from http://www.scics.gc.ca/cinfo00/800038004_e.html

First Ministers. (2003). *First ministers' accord on health care renewal, Ottawa.* Retrieved May 29, 2009, from http://www.hc-sc.gc.ca/hcs-sss/delivery-prestation/fptcollab/2003accord/nr-cp_e.html

First Ministers. (2004). *First minister's meeting on the future of health care 2004: A 10-year plan to strengthen health care.* Retrieved May 29, 2009, from http://www.hc-sc.gc.ca/hcs-sss/delivery-prestation/fptcollab/2004-fmm-rpm/index-eng.php

First Ministers. (2005). *Annual conference of federal-provincial-territorial ministers of Health, Toronto, Ontario.* Canadian Intergovernmental Conference Secretariat [News release]. Retrieved May 29, 2009, from http://www.scics.gc.ca/cinfo05/830866004_e.html

Forster, M. (2004). *100 Canadian heroines: Famous and forgotten faces.* Toronto: Dundurn Press Ltd.

Government of Canada. (1999). *Intergovernmental relations—social union issues.* Prepared by Jack

REFERENCES

Stilborn, Political and Social Affairs Division. Retrieved May 29, 2009, from http://dsp-psd.pwgsc.gc.ca/Collection-R/LoPBdP/BP/prb9937-e.htm

Health Canada. (2004). *Canada's health care system (Medicare)*. Retrieved May 29, 2009, from http://www.hc-sc.gc.ca/hcs-sss/medi-assur/index-eng.php

Health Canada. (2005). *Canada Health Act. Frequently asked questions*. Retrieved May 29, 2009, from http://www.hc-sc.gc.ca/hcs-sss/medi-assur/res/faq-eng.php

Health Canada. (2006). *Health care system: Background*. Retrieved May 29, 2009, from http://www.hc-sc.gc.ca/hcs-sss/pubs/system-regime/2005-hcs-sss/back-context-eng.php

Kelowna Accord. (2006). *Aboriginal roundtable to Kelowna Accord: Aboriginal policy negotiations, 2004–2005*. Retrieved May 29, 2009, from http://parl.gc.ca/information/library/PRBpubs/prb0604-e.htm

Kirby, M.J.L. (2002). *The health of Canadians—The federal role. Final report*. Retrieved May 29, 2009, from http://www.parl.gc.ca/37/2/parlbus/commbus/senate/Com-e/soci-e/rep-e/repoct02vol6-e.htm

Mazankowski, D. (2001). *A framework for reform: Report of the Premier's Advisory Council on Health*. Retrieved May 29, 2009, from http://www.health.alberta.ca/resources/publications/PACH_report_final.pdf

Mount Saint Vincent University. (2005). *Formal training for nurses, the beginning*. Retrieved from http://www.msvu.ca/library/archives/nhdp/history.htm

Ontario Association of Children's Aid Societies. (2008). *History of child welfare*. Retrieved May 29, 2009, from http://www.oacas.org/childwelfare/history.htm

Romanow, R. (2002). *Building on values: The future of health care in Canada*. Retrieved May 29, 2009, from http://www.cbc.ca/healthcare/final_report.pdf

Sibbald, B. (2002). BC takes ax to budget of a health system "in danger." *Canadian Medical Association Journal, 166*(4). Retrieved May 29, 2009, from http://www.cmaj.ca/cgi/content/full/166/4/492

Social Union. (1999). *A framework to improve the social union for Canadians: An agreement between the Government of Canada and the governments of the provinces and territories*. Retrieved May 29, 2009, from http://socialunion.gc.ca/news/020499_e.html

St. John Ambulance. (1995). *Our history*. Retrieved July 14, 2009, from http://www.kwsja.com/history.html

Tommy Douglas Research Institute. (n.d.). Retrieved May 29, 2009, from http://www.tommydouglas.ca/

Victorian Order of Nurses. (2009). History: A century of caring. Retrieved July 14, 2009, from http://www.von.ca/en/about/history.aspx

Wynne-Jones, T. (2002). Whose health: Who cares? [Editorial]. *Canadian Medical Association Journal, 167*(2). Retrieved July 20, 2009, from http://www.cmaj.ca/cgi/content/full/167/2/156

Young Men's Christian Association. (n.d.) *History of the YMCA*. Retrieved May 29, 2009, from http://www.ymca.net/about_the_ymca/history_of_the_ymca.html

Young Women's Christian Association. (2004). *Our history in Canada*. Retrieved June 25, 2009, from http://www.ywcacanada.ca/public_eng/national_office/index.cfm?Heading1_link=who_we_are&Heading2_link=who_we_are_history&Heading3_link=who_we_are_history&Heading4_link=who_we_are_history&Hlinks=3&Date=1870

The Federal Government's Role in Health Care

Learning Outcomes

1. Outline the federal government's responsibilities related to health care.

2. Describe Health Canada's mission statement and philosophy.

3. Summarize the health care roles played by the departments and agencies of the federal and provincial governments.

4. Discuss the structure, function, and role of the World Health Organization (WHO) in health care.

5. Explain how WHO collaborates with Health Canada.

6. Summarize the function of two of the international organizations (other than WHO) that Health Canada collaborates with regarding health issues.

KEY TERMS

The federal, provincial, and territorial governments all play a part in health care. The responsibilities of each were originally outlined in the *British North America Act* in 1867. Today, the federal government possesses little power over the health care of individual Canadians and absolutely no legal power over health care in provincial and territorial jurisdictions. The provinces and territories continually guard their authority over health care, causing strain in their individual relationships with the federal government. On the other hand, the provinces and territories want and need federal financial support, which comes with stipulations. In fact, it is through the federal government's control over medical and hospital care funding that it exerts most of its influence.

The federal government also provides leadership, advice, and direction on health care issues on a national and international front. International issues require Health Canada to interact regularly with global organizations, particularly the World Health Organization (WHO). For this reason, this chapter includes an overview of WHO, which has been more visible to Canadians since the **severe acute respiratory syndrome (SARS)** crisis in April 2003. WHO played a significant role in tracking the disease and in making efforts to contain outbreaks, ultimately naming Canada as a destination to avoid during the worst of the crisis. More recently, WHO has been instrumental in tracking the H1N1 virus.

This chapter examines the role of the federal government in health care, the hierarchical structure of Health Canada, and the functions of the various government departments and agencies. The chapter begins by looking at Health Canada's mission statement, philosophy, and commitment to health care in Canada. These pledges provide the foundation upon which the ministry was built and the

Severe acute respiratory syndrome (SARS)
A severe form of pneumonia that first swept across parts of Asia and the Far East before spreading worldwide in 2003.

values with which it strives to function. Despite the best of intentions, however, many issues are not addressed effectively and consistently, so problems with the Canadian health care system persist today.

HEALTH CANADA: OBJECTIVES AND RESPONSIBILITIES

Health Canada, formerly known as the Department of Health and Welfare, is the federal government department responsible for federal health matters. Headed by a minister of health, it consists of a number of sub-departments organized into functional and administrative branches, agencies, offices, and sub-organizations. Since Health Canada's organizational structure changes frequently, this chapter discusses only the ministry's major components, with a focus on the responsibilities of each and the impact of each on Canadians. Refer to the Health Canada Web site for information about any recent changes to the organizational structure.

Health Canada's detailed mission statement (available on its Web site; see Web Resources at the end of this chapter) includes information about its purpose, values, and activities. Under "Mission and Vision," Health Canada states that it is "committed to improving the lives of all of Canada's people and to making this country's population among the healthiest in the world as measured by longevity, lifestyle and effective use of the public health care system" (Health Canada, 2007).

With a mandate to provide national leadership for health care and to maximize health promotion and disease prevention strategies, Health Canada has committed to working collaboratively with the provinces and territories on joint ventures such as creating policies and financing projects. The ministry manages funding policies and oversees the transfer of money and tax points to the provinces and territories for health, education, and social programs. Health Canada also plays an authoritarian role, ensuring the provinces and territories remain compliant with the *Canada Health Act* and enforcing penalties on those that function outside of the principles within the Act. Health Canada may restrict funding to noncompliant provinces and territories.

As a service provider, Health Canada is responsible for health care coverage for members of the Royal Canadian Mounted Police, **Inuit**, **Innu**, **First Nations** Canadians living on reserves, veterans, refugee claimants, the men and women employed in the military, and inmates of federal penitentiaries. First Nations Canadians on reserves and Inuit receive supplemental benefits, including medications, dental care, vision care, medical transportation, medical supplies and equipment, crisis intervention, and health counselling. Health Canada also provides primary care services in remote and isolated areas when the provincial or territorial government cannot meet these needs.

Inuit
Aboriginal people in northern Canada living generally above the treeline in the Northwest Territories, Northern Quebec, and Labrador.

Innu
Naskapi and Montagnais First Nations (Indian) peoples who live in Northern Quebec and Labrador.

First Nations
A Canadian term of ethnicity referring to indigenous Canadians. The First Nations comprise a group (usually registered as "Indians" under the *Indian Act*) of 633 First Nations bands, representing 52 cultural groups and more than 50 languages (Assembly of First Nations, 2002). Other terms used include *Aboriginal*, *Native*, or *indigenous people*.

A primary source of information for Canadians, Health Canada conducts research projects and provides feedback on policy development. The ministry interacts with other nations about health-related issues and with the World Health Organization to keep Canadians up-to-date on health concerns around the world. In conjunction with WHO, Health Canada issues travel alerts and warnings for areas where health issues present cause for concern. The ministry also participates in producing and implementing national campaigns for health promotion and disease prevention, such as active lifestyle and anti-smoking campaigns.

HEALTH CANADA ORGANIZATION: MINISTRY LEVEL

The prime minister of Canada appoints an elected representative to head Health Canada as minister of health, a position that the prime minister can reassign at any time during the tenure of the party in power. The minister of health's responsibilities comprise "all matters over which Parliament has jurisdiction relating to the promotion and preservation of health for the people of Canada, not by law assigned to any other department, board or agency of the government of Canada" (House of Commons of Canada, 2001). These responsibilities include overseeing more than 20 health-related laws and associated regulations.

On occasion, the federal minister of health may also be responsible for other portfolios. For example, prior to his 2008 reassignment as minister of industry, the Honourable Tony Clement served as minister of health and minister for the federal economic development initiative in Northern Ontario in Stephen Harper's Conservative government. In the fall of 2008, Leona Aglukkaq became the first Inuk to hold a senior federal Cabinet position when she replaced Tony Clement as the minister of health.

Key responsibilities of the minister of health include overseeing the Public Health Agency of Canada, health promotion initiatives, and safety standards. The minister of health also supervises the collection and analysis of information carried out under the *Statistics Act*.

Perhaps one of the most important responsibilities of the federal minister of health is to work collaboratively with the provincial and territorial governments. The federal minister does not routinely become involved in internal matters within the provinces or territories; however, establishing a positive working relationship with the first ministers is essential for improving Canada's health care system across the country.

Rather than being an elected member of Parliament, the deputy minister of health is appointed from the civil service. The deputy minister works collaboratively with the minister of health, manages designated operations within the ministry, and may assume duties assigned to the minister of health if the minister is temporarily unavailable.

Several assistant deputy ministers of health and an associate deputy minister of health are also appointed from the civil service. Other agencies, such as the Departmental Secretariat and the chief public health officer, work collaboratively with the minister, deputy minister, and associate deputy minister. Their primary focus is to provide leadership to the Public Health Agency of Canada, whose principle mandate is to manage health promotion and health safety initiatives.

Thinking It Through

Officials of Health Canada are unelected employees that may work under the authority of many different governments. They are considered "apolitical" and remain in their positions even if a different party assumes power after an election.

1. Do you think having apolitical ministry employees is effective?
2. Would you rather see the deputy ministers of health be appointed from within the ranks of the party in power?

DEPARTMENTS OF HEALTH CANADA

The organizational makeup of Health Canada is complex and sometimes confusing, in part because it features both an internal arm (i.e., acts as a service provider for other groups under federal jurisdiction) and an external arm (i.e., provides leadership for health care in the provinces and territories). See Figure 4.1.

More than 20 **branches**, offices, and **bureaus** operate within Health Canada. Some, such as the Departmental Secretariat, oversee the financing, function, and organization of Health Canada. Other divisions are more directly aligned with public initiatives and health care. The Audit and Accountability Bureau, the Chief Financial Officer Branch, and the Corporate Services Branch are responsible for, and work with, a number of sub-units. The following sections summarize only the most relevant functions of some of the branches.

Branch
A division of a main office offering extended or supportive functions.

Bureau
Government department responsible for a specific entity or duty.

INTERNAL SERVICES
Departmental Secretariat
An executive office to which other departments report, the Departmental Secretariat acts as the link between the executive (appointed) and the political

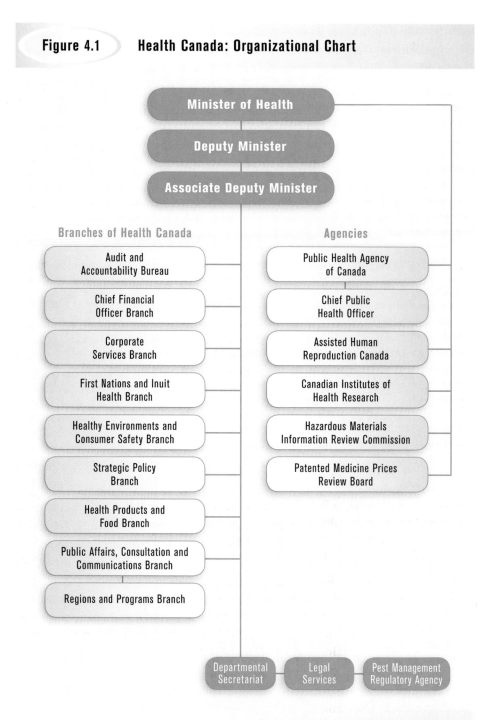

Figure 4.1   Health Canada: Organizational Chart

Minister of Health

Deputy Minister

Associate Deputy Minister

Branches of Health Canada

- Audit and Accountability Bureau
- Chief Financial Officer Branch
- Corporate Services Branch
- First Nations and Inuit Health Branch
- Healthy Environments and Consumer Safety Branch
- Strategic Policy Branch
- Health Products and Food Branch
- Public Affairs, Consultation and Communications Branch
- Regions and Programs Branch

Agencies

- Public Health Agency of Canada
- Chief Public Health Officer
- Assisted Human Reproduction Canada
- Canadian Institutes of Health Research
- Hazardous Materials Information Review Commission
- Patented Medicine Prices Review Board

Departmental Secretariat   Legal Services   Pest Management Regulatory Agency

Source: Health Canada. (2008). *About Health Canada. Branches and agencies.* Retrieved May 29, 2009, from http://www.hc-sc.gc.ca/ahc-asc/branch-dirgen/index-eng.php. Reproduced with the permission of the Minister of Public Works and Government Services Canada, 2009.

(elected) levels of Health Canada. Clients of the Departmental Secretariat include offices of the minister, deputy minister(s), and associate deputy minister.

The Departmental Secretariat receives communication from other divisions and either redirects that communication or responds to it appropriately and promptly. When ambiguous communication is received, this department attempts to clarify it before directing it to the proper program area. Examples of types of communication the Departmental Secretariat receives and redirects include briefing notes for members of Parliament and responses to letters. When possible, this department answers questions raised in the House of Commons and addresses requests that fall under the *Access to Information Act* and *Privacy Act*.

Audit and Accountability Bureau

The Audit and Accountability Bureau (AAB) is Health Canada's internal monitoring system. The bureau conducts internal audits and reports to the Departmental Audit and Evaluation Committee, chaired by the associate deputy minister. The AAB reviews different departments and bureaus to ensure that they are operating according to their mandate for performance and financial accountability. An audit might identify both operational strengths and areas for improvement.

Through audits, the AAB ensures taxpayer dollars are used effectively. It works with provincial and territorial departments to analyze the use of grant money and assesses the results of investments in programs and services. Such analyses and assessments make it possible to identify service gaps and to determine where improvements to overall management practices are necessary.

Chief Financial Officer Branch

The Chief Financial Officer Branch (CFOB) is made up of several organizational units, including the Departmental Performance Measurement and Evaluation Directorate, Departmental Resource Management Directorate, Financial Operations Directorate, Internal Control Division, Material and Assets Management Directorate, and Planning and Corporate Management Practices Directorate.

The CFOB oversees the use of Health Canada's departmental resources and ensures finances are spent wisely and efficiently to maximize results. This branch supports program management and operations by providing policies, systems, and **best practice** tools, all with the aim of promoting operational cost-effectiveness of each department or organization. It also ensures other departments and organizational units adhere to government policies and regulations; coordinates the management of risk; enhances performance measurement and reporting; and monitors the execution of the accountability framework.

Reporting to the deputy minister, the head of this branch, the chief financial officer (CFO), oversees the financial management of **central agencies**,

Best practice
The most current and effective methods of reaching a goal.

Central agency
An organization or department with the authority to direct or intervene in the activities of other departments. Central agencies aid with policy development and the coordination of activities.

including the Public Health Agency of Canada, the Privy Council, and the Treasury Board Secretariat. Monitoring trends and anticipating related needs, the CFO advises the minister, deputy minister, associate deputy minister, and departmental executives on financial matters and the competent management of resources.

Corporate Services Branch

Directorates within the Corporate Services Branch (CSB) include the Access to Information and Privacy Division, Facilities and Security Directorate, Human Resources Services Directorate, Information Management Services Directorate, and Planning and Operations Directorate.

The CSB provides support and services to Health Canada in such areas as human resources management; occupational health safety, emergency, and security management; access to information and privacy matters; and information technology. This department also supports the *Official Languages Act*, providing language training and support and managing related complaints (Box 4.1).

Box 4.1 **Canada's *Official Languages Act*, Section 2**

Section 2: "The purpose of the Act is to

(a) ensure respect for English and French as the official languages of Canada and ensure equality of status and equal rights and privileges as to their use in all federal institutions, in particular with respect to their use in parliamentary proceedings, in legislative and other instruments, in the administration of justice, in communicating with or providing services to the public and in carrying out the work of federal institutions;

(b) support the development of English and French linguistic minority communities and generally advance the equality of status and use of the English and French languages within Canadian society; and

(c) set out the powers, duties and functions of federal institutions with respect to the official languages of Canada."

Source: *Official Languages Act*, c. 31 (4th Supp.) (1985).

The CSB provides advice and guidance to the Human Resources Services Directorate on human resources management issues, as well as develops plans to recruit, train, and retain employees. It also collaboratively manages occupational health and safety alongside occupational health and safety committees.

Working with the Information Management Services Directorate, the CSB helps to ensure effective use of the information technology used to deliver Health

Canada's programs and services. The department also provides support for Health Canada infrastructure, including its computer systems, across the country.

Legal Services

Reporting to the Department of Justice, Legal Services employs lawyers to provide legal advice and other legal services to Health Canada. Through this unit, Health Canada can access specialized services provided by the Department of Justice, including advisory services relating to information privacy laws, administrative laws, and constitutional and criminal laws.

EXTERNAL SERVICES

Health Canada's external services consist of a variety of offices, directorates, branches, and other organizations. The structures, names, services, and related policies of these sub-departments change frequently. Several are discussed here. For current, more detailed information, see Web Resources at the end of this chapter for a link to Health Canada's Web site.

First Nations and Inuit Health Branch

The First Nations and Inuit Health Branch oversees the delivery of primary health care services to **Aboriginal peoples**, including public health and health promotion on First Nations reserves and within Inuit communities, as well as services provided to Aboriginal populations who do not live within Inuit communities or on reserves.

The branch also manages federal funding for health care services to these populations and works collaboratively with Aboriginal provincial and territorial councils to ensure high-quality health care. Providing adequate services remains a challenge, given Aboriginals' unique needs with respect to geography, demographics, population distribution, and other factors, such as lifestyle and mortality.

Strategic Policy Branch

The Strategic Policy Branch (SPB) develops and implements the federal government's and Health Canada's health care policies. Working collaboratively with both government and nongovernment groups as well as with provincial and territorial ministers of health, this department aims to improve health and health care delivery in Canada. The SPB also administers the *Canada Health Act* and creates health protection regulations and legislation, dealing with evolving problems on a priority basis and authorizing new agencies as required.

The SPB's programs are carried out by several offices and directorates, some of which are outlined below.

Health Care Policy Directorate

The Health Care Policy Directorate, an organization within the SPB, plays a key role in reshaping primary health care delivery with the objective of preserving the principles and conditions of the *Canada Health Act*. The directorate also assesses provinces' and territories' need for financial support for primary health care reform initiatives. The directorate monitors and analyzes the provision of community-based, continuing, and palliative care across Canada and gathers information that Health Canada uses to develop policies and initiatives that will assist the provinces and territories to improve health care in those areas.

Applied Research and Analysis Directorate

The Applied Research and Analysis Directorate assists Health Canada with the development and construction of its analytical foundation for policy decision making, performance measurement, and reporting. In addition, this directorate conducts economic analysis of health policy issues. Two or three times each year, it publishes *The Health Policy Research Bulletin*, which features health-related research developments and initiatives from Health Canada and its portfolio partners (see Web Resources at the end of this chapter).

Office of the Chief Scientist

The Office of the Chief Scientist helps to ensure that Health Canada has appropriate scientific information to make health-related decisions; provides leadership regarding decisions about potential health risks; and tracks the spread of diseases such as West Nile virus, SARS, mad cow disease (Creutzfeldt-Jakob disease), and the H1N1 virus.

Working with the Healthy Environments and Consumer Safety Branch and the Health Products and Food Branch, the Office of the Chief Scientist also helps to ensure that all products introduced to the Canadian market meet national standards of safety and abide by Canadian rules and regulations.

The office assists 50 research and diagnostic laboratories across Canada, which conduct research in a wide variety of areas, including fields as diverse as natural resources and medicine. One such laboratory, the National Research Council's Institute for Biodiagnostics in Winnipeg, assisted with the development of the first mobile MRI machine. Surgeons can use the mobile MRI during surgery to more accurately assess the status of a tumour.

A Health Canada scientist is currently researching how air pollution affects cardiopulmonary disease. Once the scientist has identified the specific toxic components that cause disease, the government can implement policies to restrict these components. Another Health Canada scientist is currently gathering information on factors that may influence the prevalence of cancer in certain regions.

Office of Nursing Policy

Created in 1999, the Office of Nursing Policy reflects the importance of nursing policy issues within health care. This office provides advice to Health Canada on select policy issues and programs from the nursing perspective and makes recommendations regarding the nursing workforce to help meet health care service needs. For example, it recommended hiring specially trained nurse practitioners to provide lower-cost comprehensive care in under-serviced areas. The Office of Nursing Policy also develops strategies to retain nurses by addressing issues such as burnout and frustration related to the occupational environment.

Health Products and Food Branch

The Health Products and Food Branch (HPFB) primarily reviews the health-related risks and benefits of drugs, vaccines, medical devices, natural health products, food, and veterinary drugs and ensures Canadians have the information necessary to make independent, informed choices. The many responsibilities and activities of the HPFB are carried out by several directorates and offices across the country, some of which are discussed below.

Office of Nutrition Policy and Promotion

The HPFB's Office of Nutrition Policy and Promotion develops the policies and standards for nutrition recommended in *Eating Well With Canada's Food Guide*. The food guide has evolved through years of research and collaboration with specialists from a variety of fields. A new guide adapted to the needs and lifestyles of First Nations, Inuit, and Métis populations has also been released (Box 4.2).

Box 4.2 **The First Ever Food Guide for First Nations, Inuit, and Métis**

In April 2007, the first ever national food guide for First Nations, Inuit, and Métis populations, *Eating Well With Canada's Food Guide—First Nations, Inuit and Métis*, was launched in Yellowknife. "This is the first time that Canada's Food Guide has been tailored nationally to reflect the unique values, traditions, and food choices of Aboriginal populations," said then minister of health, Tony Clement. "As a complement to the new 2007 version of Canada's Food Guide, this tailored food guide includes traditional food from the land and sea, and provides the best, most current information for eating well and living healthy."

Source: Health Canada. (2007, April 11). [News release 2007-44]. Retrieved May 29, 2009, from http://www.hc-sc.gc.ca/ahc-asc/media/nr-cp/_2007/2007_44-eng.php

Food Directorate

The Food Directorate regulates the safety and nutritional quality of food in Canada. The directorate monitors additives used in food products (e.g., aspartame, vitamins, and other nutrients); genetically modified products; and methods of processing and packaging foods.

Marketed Health Products Directorate

Through the Marketed Health Products Directorate (MHPD), Health Canada collects information about adverse reactions to foods and food products and ensures that the public is aware of any identified risks. Adverse reaction reports are currently collected by seven regional centres (British Columbia, Alberta, Saskatchewan, Manitoba, Ontario, Quebec, and Atlantic Canada), as well as by the national office in Ottawa. Through MedEffect, a program developed by the MHPD, Canadians can report adverse effects of, and obtain safety information on, health products and drugs (for online reporting, see Web Resources at the end of this chapter). The Canada Vigilance Program—which functions under MedEffect and is the point of contact for health care professionals and consumers (Health Canada, 2009)—collects and assesses all reports of suspected adverse reactions to health products marketed in Canada. This information allows Health Canada to continually gauge the safety of health products once they are available to consumers. And if, for example, a product's adverse affects outweigh its benefits, Health Canada will act to remove the product from the market either to reassess and modify it or to ban it completely.

Natural Health Products Directorate

In January 2004, the Natural Health Products Directorate developed Canada's first set of regulations directed at natural health products. These regulations cover all health products containing natural ingredients, including homeopathic medicines, vitamins and minerals, and traditional medicines. The regulations summarize and enforce licensing requirements for natural health products as well as stipulate packaging and labelling requirements—for example, product packaging must state health claims, ingredients, instructions for use, and potential side effects. Natural health product manufacturers must document and report any adverse reactions identified by consumers. Health Canada has the authority to request label changes and to remove any natural health product from the market at any time.

Despite these regulatory efforts, the use of natural products remains a concern to many health care professionals across Canada. The average consumer may not realize that a *natural* product may contain harmful ingredients or that it may interfere with prescription medications. For example, combining a prescription antidepressant with St. John's Wort (a herbal mood elevator) can cause nausea, vomiting, restlessness, dizziness, and headaches. St. John's Wort can also reduce the effectiveness of oral contraceptives. Ginseng, another popular herbal medication, can increase blood pressure so should not be taken by someone with hypertension or someone on antihypertensive medication. Even garlic, when taken with **hypoglycemic** medications (used by people with diabetes), can cause a drop in blood sugar and, possibly, a **hypoglycemic reaction**.

Hypoglycemic
Pertaining to low blood sugar.

Thinking It Through

A client tells you that she is taking a number of herbal medications, including synthetic estrogen preparations and metabolism boosters. She found on the Internet that these medications were recommended to combat fatigue and sluggishness. She believes it is unnecessary to tell her physician.

As an allied health professional, how would you respond?

Healthy Environments and Consumer Safety Branch

The Healthy Environments and Consumer Safety Branch (HECSB) develops and supports programs that promote a safe, healthy lifestyle and environment for Canadians. The HECSB provides information about the risks and benefits of various products and lifestyle habits with the goal of helping Canadians make constructive choices (e.g., an active lifestyle, healthy nutritional habits, and avoidance of self-imposed risks behaviours such as tobacco, drug, and alcohol use). The HECSB is also concerned with other matters, including drinking water quality, air quality, and the use of smoke detectors. A number of programs operate within the HECSB. Some are discussed below.

Hypoglycemic reaction
A response to a drop in blood sugar levels. The symptoms may include mild weakness or dizziness; headache; cold, clammy, or sweaty skin; problems concentrating; shakiness; uncoordinated movements or staggering; blurred vision; irritability; hunger; fainting; and loss of consciousness.

Safe Environments Program

The Safe Environments Program (SEP) identifies and assesses health risks to Canadians posed by environmental factors in an effort to promote healthy living, working, and recreational environments.

Drug Strategy and Controlled Substances Program

The Drug Strategy and Controlled Substances Program regulates the use and distribution of narcotics and other controlled drugs in Canada, primarily through the *Controlled Drugs and Substances Act* and narcotic control regulations. The program's responsibilities include licensing pharmaceutical companies that manufacture and distribute drugs and controlled substances and tracking the movement of drugs and controlled substances inside and outside the country. When individuals seek special permission to use specific controlled drugs for a health condition—for example, marihuana to control pain—the Drug Strategy and Controlled Substances Program manages these requests. The process for obtaining such permission is discussed in more depth in Chapter 8.

Tobacco Control Program

The Tobacco Control Program aims to reduce tobacco use in Canada by regulating the manufacture and sale of tobacco products, which has included implementing rules about the labelling of packages (e.g., the graphic anti-smoking warnings on cigarette packages). The program also works with provincial and territorial governments on anti-smoking media campaigns.

Some provinces have taken concrete steps to reduce smoking and to protect children from the effects of second-hand smoke (In the News: Legislation Versus Individual Rights).

In the **News**   Legislation Versus Individual Rights

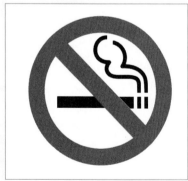

On June 16, 2008, Ontario joined Nova Scotia and Yukon in a bold, controversial move by banning smoking in cars that contain children. Under the law, any person (driver or passenger) smoking in a car while someone else under the age of 16 is present is committing an offence and will be fined $250. On April 7, 2009, British Columbia followed suit by attaching a fine of $109. Other provinces and territories may be considering similar legislation. Many people, although agreeing in principle with this legislation, feel it violates individual rights.

Sources: Ontario Ministry of Health Promotion. (2008, June 16). *New law bans smoking in motor vehicles* [News release]. Retrieved May 29, 2009, from http://www.mhp.gov.on.ca/english/news/2008/061608.asp; Fowlie, J. (2009, March 18). New B.C. law banning smoking in a vehicle with a child to take effect next month. *The Vancouver Sun*, Retrieved November 3, 2009, from http://www.vancouversun.com/health/banning+smoking+vehicle+with+child+take+effect+next+month/1402336/story.html

Photo credit: © iStockphoto.com/spxChrome.

Thinking It
Through

The federal, provincial, and territorial governments, in conjunction with anti-smoking campaigns, have tightened legislation regarding where individuals can smoke.

1. Do you think that the public education efforts made by governments are sufficient to help individuals understand the health risks of smoking and thus the rationale for increasing restrictions?

2. Do you believe that banning smoking inside one's own car (when children are present) goes too far in terms of infringing on individuals' rights?

Office of Sustainable Development

The Office of Sustainable Development's primary objective is to ensure sensitivity to environmental, social, and economic issues in the planning and implementation of Health Canada's programs and policies.

Product Safety Program

Before they reach the Canadian market, most products—products as diverse as children's toys and cosmetics—are researched and assessed by the Product Safety Program. Responsibilities of this unit also include researching and evaluating UV radiation, radiation-emitting devices (e.g., those used in some diagnostic tests), and workplace chemicals.

Regions and Programs Branch

The Regions and Programs Branch of Health Canada comprises the Regions, the Workplace Health and Public Safety Program, and the Programs Directorate.

Regions

Health Canada has divided Canada into eight regions: British Columbia, Alberta, Saskatchewan, Manitoba, Quebec, Ontario, the Atlantic Region, and the Northern Region. Each Health Canada region is headed by a regional director general, who reports to the assistant deputy minister of health. The regional director general ensures that services meet the needs of the region and are not duplicated. An important aspect of the regional director general's job is to maintain a positive working relationship with provincial or territorial groups.

Although the activities and programs (e.g., promotion of healthy environments and consumer safety; regulation of health products and food) launched by

Health Canada in the various regions bear similarities, each region faces diverse challenges related to demographics and geography. For example, some regions have a greater need for alcohol- and drug-abuse prevention programs, drug and dental coverage, vision plans, and transportation services to treatment centres. In many northern regions, water quality and other environmental issues present particular concern, so Health Canada employs environmental health officers to deal with these problems.

Workplace Health and Public Safety Program

The Workplace Health and Public Safety Program promotes a best practices philosophy in the workplace with the goal of encouraging physically safe and emotionally positive workplace environments. The program recommends that managers and administrators ensure employees are healthy and fit enough to handle jobs assigned to them and encourages the implementation of office ergonomics: a well-designed desk, chair, lighting, and computer workstation.

The Workplace Health and Public Safety Program also assumes responsibility for the health and safety of federal employees and for visiting dignitaries and politicians. To achieve this goal, the program collaborates with a number of departments, including the Emergency Preparedness and Response Unit, a group formed to respond to terrorist acts anywhere in Canada, be they biological, radiological, chemical, or nuclear.

Programs Directorate

Also under the umbrella of the Regions and Programs Branch, the Programs Directorate is responsible for a number of organizations, including the Canada Health Act Division, which provides policy advice related to the Act; monitors activities in the provinces and territories to assess their compliance with the principles and conditions of the *Canada Health Act*; and reports any incidents of noncompliance to the minister of health. Any province or territory may engage in activities that are not compliant with the *Canada Health Act* as long as these activities are authorized by the provincial or territorial government. However, the consequence of noncompliance may be restriction of federal funding. The Canada Health Act Division produces a year-end report that details each province's or territory's obedience to the principles and conditions of the Act (Health Canada, 2004).

Other divisions of the Programs Directorate are Drug Analysis Services, Office of Demand Reduction, Official Languages Community Development Bureau, Programs and Knowledge Exchange Division, and the Women's Health Bureau. Each of these sub-departments has unique responsibilities and services. For more information, refer to Health Canada's Web site.

Public Affairs, Consultation and Communications Branch

The Public Affairs, Consultation and Communications Branch (PACCB) performs a number of duties involving communication activities and responsibilities. Offices within this branch include Ethics and Internal Ombudsman Services and the Planning and Operations Division. Ethics and Internal Ombudsman Services acts as a confidential and unbiased resource for any employee within Health Canada, offering guidance and information about work-related concerns, regardless of occupation, title, or employment status. The Planning and Operations Division provides leadership to the PACCB with respect to human resources, contracts, finances, and strategic planning. Other offices of the branch are discussed below.

Public Affairs and Strategic Communications Directorate

The Public Affairs and Strategic Communications Directorate plays an important role in maintaining communication internally within Health Canada as well as externally—that is, with the public, the provinces and territories, nongovernment groups, and international associations and governments. In recent years, particularly since the release of the Romanow Report, Health Canada has reinforced its commitment to openness and accountability for its activities, policies, and programs. The Public Affairs and Strategic Communications Directorate handles much of the interaction between the ministry and the public regarding these matters, as well as managing emergency and risk communications when necessary.

Within this directorate, the Public Affairs Division, the ministry's first point of contact for the media, coaches and prepares Health Canada spokespersons to speak to the media. The Health Canada Web site provides a detailed list of telephone numbers and e-mail addresses to facilitate media contact with the organization.

Also within this directorate, the Horizontal Coordination Division manages communication across Health Canada; oversees external communication; and deals with issues related to access to information.

Marketing and Communications Services Directorate

The Marketing and Communications Services Directorate comprises the Web, Internal, and Corporate Communications Division; the Social Marketing Unit; and the Public Opinion Research and Evaluation Unit.

The Web, Internal, and Corporate Communications Division maintains the Health Canada Web site, which consists of more than 60,000 pages—an enormous task indeed. In 2005, the Web site was reorganized, with more than 100 sites being merged into one. (For a virtual introduction to the Web site, see the link in Web Resources at the end of the chapter.) This division also processes all public inquiries addressed to Health Canada.

The Social Marketing Unit manages all of Health Canada's advertising agencies. The unit is responsible for campaigns seeking to raise the public's awareness of certain disease risks and to encourage Canadians to develop healthy lifestyles.

Together with the Public Health Agency of Canada and Health Canada scientists, PACCB publishes a bulletin called *It's Your Health*, which delivers information and articles to the general public on a variety of health-related topics (see Web Resources at the end of this chapter).

The Public Opinion Research and Evaluation Unit conducts public opinion research, gathering information that is critical for helping Health Canada to understand Canadians' needs, perceptions, and expectations about health.

INDEPENDENT AGENCIES OF HEALTH CANADA

Several independent agencies report directly to the minister of health. The functions of some are described below.

CANADIAN INSTITUTES OF HEALTH RESEARCH

The Canadian Institutes of Health Research (CIHR) directs and funds research across Canada. CIHR distributes research funding based on priority and need, expanding research as required (e.g., in areas such as population health and health services research) and recruiting and training research scientists. CIHR is also responsible for ensuring that the research information gathered and analyzed is used properly—for example, to craft policies or to generate products and services for which a need has been determined.

CIHR operates 13 research institutes nationwide (Box 4.3) with a multi-million-dollar funding budget. More than 10,000 scientists and researchers in various hospitals, universities, and research institutes are involved with the agency. Targeted, ongoing, health-based research projects include those related to biomedical research, clinical science, and health care systems and services (Canadian Institutes of Health Research, 2007).

Box 4.3   CIHR Institutes Across Canada

Aboriginal Peoples' Health

Aging

Cancer Research

Circulatory and Respiratory Health

Gender and Health

Genetics

Health Services and Policy Research

Human Development, Child and Youth Health

Infection and Immunity

Musculoskeletal Health and Arthritis

Neurosciences, Mental Health, and Addiction

Nutrition, Metabolism, and Diabetes

Population and Public Health

Source: Canadian Institutes of Health Research. (2007). *CIHR institutes.* Retrieved from http://www.cihr-irsc.gc.ca/e/9466.html#a

HAZARDOUS MATERIALS INFORMATION REVIEW COMMISSION

The Hazardous Materials Information Review Commission (HMIRC) aims to protect workers in the province, while also protecting the industry's trade secrets. HMIRC is responsible for setting standards, policies, and rules for workplace safety.

The Workplace Hazardous Materials Information System (WHMIS), a combination of laws, regulations, and procedures, helps to reduce workplace injury and illness resulting from the use of hazardous chemicals. WHMIS represents a coordinated effort among the federal, provincial, and territorial governments to standardize workplace safety across the country. Through WHMIS, employers are obligated to supply employees with the training and knowledge to allow them to work safely with hazardous materials. Most individuals entering an occupational setting are required to take a WHMIS course and write a test before beginning employment.

PATENTED MEDICINE PRICES REVIEW BOARD

The Patented Medicine Prices Review Board (PMPRB), created in 1987, is a "watch" agency that monitors the prices of **patented drugs** to ensure fairness to both manufacturer and consumer. This board operates independently of other organizations within Health Canada that deal with product safety and inspection.

Patented drugs
Drugs that are legally protected from generic production for a period of 20 years from the date of filing.

Consumer price index (CPI)

A method of determining changes in the cost of goods and services through the monitoring of select items (e.g., food, rent, mortgages, gasoline) across Canada. Used to measure inflation, the CPI may affect such payments as social security, spousal support, and rent, which are periodically adjusted to reflect the CPI.

The board reviews the prices at which the manufacturer sells patented drugs to wholesalers, hospitals, and pharmacies. Pricing is determined in several ways:

- Pricing is subject to guidelines in the *Patent Act*.

- Drugs used to treat the same disease are generally priced similarly. Revolutionary drugs, which have no measures of comparison, are priced in line with similar products used in other countries.

- Using the **consumer price index (CPI)**, the PMPRB considers previous prices of similar drugs against the current price of those same drugs.

If a manufacturer is thought to be overcharging for a drug, the board will first offer the manufacturer an opportunity to voluntarily adjust its pricing. If the company refuses, a judicial hearing may take place, with a binding federal court decision resulting.

The PMPRB is not involved with the pricing of generic drugs, which are traditionally significantly less expensive than "brand-name" drugs.

In the **News**   Drug Price Rises by 800%

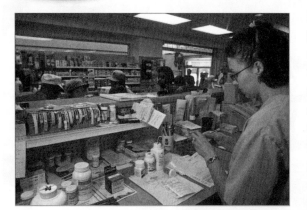

In May 2009, the media reported that the price of Premarin, a nonpatented hormone-replacement medication used to treat menopausal symptoms in women, rose by an astounding 800%. Effective April 1, 2009, a three-month supply of the drug cost more than $100 (before dispensing fee), up from $13. *The Globe and Mail* reported on June 4, 2009, that Wyeth Pharmaceuticals, the company that produces Premarin, claimed that the price adjustment was fair and that the drug was still priced below the national average prescription cost in Canada. The company cited higher costs for ingredients and a decrease in market use of the drug as criteria for the price increase.

Source: Alphonso, C. (2009, June 4). Jump in cost of HRT drugs shocks users. *The Globe and Mail*, Retrieved July 8, 2009, from http://www.theglobeandmail.com/life/jump-in-cost-of-hrt-drugs-shocks-users/article1168071

Photo credit: © Jim West/Alamy.

Thinking It
Through

Billions of dollars are spent annually on research, development, and clinical trials to test the safety and effectiveness of new drugs. Patent protection allows pharmaceutical firms 20 years to make a profit on drugs they have brought to market. Companies that produce generic drugs, however, are pushing for a reduction in patent protection time so they can bring cheaper, generic brands of patented drugs to market earlier.

1. Do you think that the patent protection time frame should be reduced?
2. Bearing in mind the tremendous cost of bringing the original drug to market, should pharmaceutical firms receive compensation for the money lost to them if generic drugs are brought to market earlier?

OTHER PERTINENT AGENCIES

PUBLIC HEALTH AGENCY OF CANADA

Created in 2004 and headed by Canada's chief public health officer, the Public Health Agency of Canada (PHAC) has a mandate to promote health and prevent diseases, including chronic infirmities such as cardio-respiratory conditions and cancer. PHAC also aims to reduce accidents, prevent injuries, and respond to other public health issues such as health emergencies and infectious disease outbreaks.

PHAC promotes strategies for healthy pregnancies, campaigns for active lifestyles, and initiatives to combat childhood obesity and diabetes. In Canada, most Web-based data regarding health issues is organized and posted by PHAC (a function formerly carried out by the Canadian Health Network, a national Internet-based health information service funded by PHAC).

In terms of "health watch" activities, PHAC tracks outbreaks of seasonal flu, tuberculosis, measles, and other illnesses and recommends corrective and preventive measures. Worth special mention is a branch called the Centre for Infectious Disease Prevention and Control (CIDPC), which has several departments, including the Blood Safety Surveillance and Health Care Acquired Infections Division and the Community Acquired Infections Division. CIDPC works closely with other agencies, such as the Centers for Disease Control and Prevention (CDC) in the United States.

Assisted Human Reproduction Canada

Established in March 2004, Assisted Human Reproduction Canada (AHRC) is a federal regulatory agency that examines the ethical principles of human reproduction technology and related matters. The members of AHRC's board of directors are selected from different backgrounds and professions to bring diverse representation and viewpoints to reproductive issues and debates.

The *Assisted Human Reproduction Act* guides the introduction and application of human reproductive technologies with the goal of protecting both the mother and the child or children resulting from the use of these technologies (*Assisted Human Reproduction Act*, 2004).

Canadian Institute for Health Information

An independent organization, the Canadian Institute for Health Information (CIHI) works closely with CIHR and Statistics Canada (see Chapter 2) to gather and assimilate information from numerous sources, including surveys, hospitals, clinics, and other health care centres. Funded by the federal, provincial, and territorial governments, CIHI reports to an independent board of directors that represents government health departments, regional health authorities, hospitals, and health-sector leaders across the country.

The data collected, organized, and distributed by this agency provide valuable, comprehensive information for organizations and individuals within and outside of Health Canada—the general public, government bodies, hospitals, professional organizations, educational facilities, researchers, and organizations at the municipal level (e.g., regional health authorities). The information helps in planning, organizing, and implementing policies and strategies.

CIHI maps the pattern of health care in Canada by working with 20 national and provincial information systems to gather data about the costing and delivery of health care services and the supply and distribution of health care professionals. The organization produces an annual report of general information as well as a number of specific reports, such as *Women's Health*; *Supply, Distribution and Migration of Canadian Physicians*; and *Health Indicators*.

Pest Management Regulatory Agency

Pesticides are used in various forms all across Canada—for example, to control species of mosquitoes that carry the West Nile virus, to protect agricultural crops from disease and infestation, and to keep lawns free from weeds, destructive insects, and other pests. Many pesticides, however, are harmful to the environment, wildlife, and humans.

The Pest Management Regulatory Agency (PMRA) tests pesticides to ensure they meet human health and environmental safety standards. Pesticides already in use are re-evaluated as standards and regulations change. PMRA works with other departments, such as Environment Canada, the Canadian Food Inspection Agency, and Agriculture and Agri-Food Canada, providing them with information on the effects of potentially harmful substances and responding to identified environmental concerns.

In April 2007, the minister of health announced new regulations regarding pesticide use in Canada. Now, pesticide companies must report to Health Canada all adverse effects of their products and submit all sales information to Health Canada annually. Because environmental safety is a concern, promoting eco-friendly pesticide use has become a priority.

INTERNATIONAL HEALTH AGENCIES WORKING WITH HEALTH CANADA

Health Canada collaborates with international health agencies and governments by sharing current information about new technologies and medications, identifying and tracking health risks, and helping to contain outbreaks of potentially damaging diseases.

WORLD HEALTH ORGANIZATION

The United Nations' authority on health issues, the World Health Organization (WHO), provides leadership in health matters on a global level. The organization spearheads global research, provides technical support to members, monitors and assesses health trends, and sets standards within the fields of health and medicine. WHO recommends policies and actions regarding population health initiatives to countries around the world. It is also instrumental in gathering information and producing statistics on health matters at an international level.

A total of 193 countries compose the membership of WHO. Each member country of the United Nations may become a member of WHO by accepting its constitution. Countries outside the United Nations may be admitted as members if their applications are approved by a majority vote of the World Health Assembly. Jurisdictions without responsibility for their international affairs (regions within a country, for example) may become associate members if approved.

To respond to an increasingly complex world, WHO has developed a six-point agenda (Box 4.4).

Box 4.4   The World Health Organization: The Six-Point Agenda

1. *Promoting health development.* Giving priority to those countries and regions affected by poverty and socioeconomic inequities and other disadvantaged and vulnerable groups.

2. *Fostering health security.* Tracking and responding to outbreaks of epidemic-prone diseases and implementing measures to control and perhaps eliminate these threats.

3. *Strengthening health systems.* Working to extend health services to all those in need, implementing strategies to reduce poverty and to diminish those elements identified by population health initiatives that contribute to poor health.

4. *Harnessing research, information, and evidence.* Gathering and distributing relevant health information and using this information to set priorities, shape approaches and plans, and target outcomes.

5. *Enhancing partnerships.* Working collaboratively with organizations, including UN agencies, international organizations, and the private sector, to launch health initiatives and programs within countries; making the best use of available resources and facilities.

6. *Improving performance.* Working to continually improve each organization's effectiveness in meeting its goals and its many responsibilities.

Source: World Health Organization. (2008). *The WHO agenda 2008.* Retrieved May 29, 2009, from http://www.who.int/about/agenda/en/

International Coding Systems

The international statistical classification of diseases and related health problems (ICD) is a system of codes developed to classify things such as clinical signs, diseases, and causes of injury and death. Primarily used for research purposes, the coding system can assign a code up to six characters in length to every health condition. Published by the World Health Organization, this classification system tracks international morbidity and mortality statistics. The ICD-9 system (i.e., the system's ninth edition), adopted by Canada in 1979, allows international organizations to standardize the information they collect for research and statistical purposes.

The ICD-10 system, the most recent edition, came into use in WHO member states in 1994. ICD-10 is more comprehensive than earlier editions and more relevant for use outside of the hospital setting (e.g., in clinics or physicians' offices). It contains codes for a broader range of problems, including, for example, the following:

- Z56.3: represents a stressful work schedule
- Z63.0: indicates problems with a partner or a spouse

- Z72.3: refers to lack of exercise

- Z59.1: represents inadequate housing

- Z72.4: indicates inappropriate diet and eating habits

The Canadian Institute for Health Information received permission from WHO to modify the ICD-10 coding system to make it more relevant to the Canadian health care system. This "Canadian enhancement," dubbed ICD-10-CA, includes an additional 3000 codes. As a member state of WHO, however, Canada must use the international standard, ICD-10 coding, for the reporting of illness and death. The next version of ICD, ICD-11, is projected to launch in 2015.

Canada also uses a system published by the United States to more accurately describe the condition and clinical health status of clients, called the ICD-9-CM coding system (*CM* stands for *clinical modification*). We have a unique coding system for provincial and territorial billing called the Canadian Classification of Health Interventions (CCI), which replaced the Canadian Classification of Diagnostic, Therapeutic, and Surgical Procedures (CCP) and the intervention portion of ICD-9-CM in Canada. This system, regarded as a companion to the next version, the ICD-10-CM system, is used to code surgical and nonsurgical interventions and diagnostic services. It would be used, for example, in a doctor's office to code a biopsy, an electrocardiogram, or a stress test.

Pandemic Alerts

WHO has created an alert system consisting of six phases (Figure 4.2) to help countries prepare for and respond to a **pandemic**. The alert system defines the stages of a pandemic, outlines the role of WHO, and makes recommendations for national measures before, during, and after the pandemic (Box 4.5).

Pandemic
A sustained, worldwide human-to-human transmission of disease.

| Figure 4.2 | The World Health Organization: Pandemic Influenza Phases |

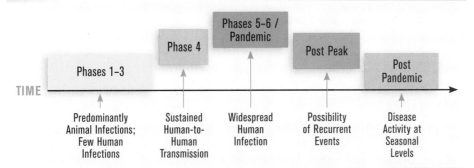

Source: World Health Organization. (2009). *Current WHO phase of pandemic alert*. Retrieved May 29, 2009, from http://www.who.int/csr/disease/avian_influenza/phase/en/index.html. Reproduced by permission.

> ### Box 4.5   The World Health Organization: Pandemic Influenza Phase Guidelines
>
> ### Interpandemic Period
>
> **Phase 1**: No new influenza virus subtypes have been detected in humans. An influenza virus subtype that has caused human infection may be present in animals. If present in animals, the risk of human infection or disease is considered to be low.
>
> **Phase 2**: No new influenza virus subtypes have been detected in humans. However, a circulating animal influenza virus subtype poses a substantial risk of human disease.
>
> ### Pandemic Alert Period
>
> **Phase 3**: Human infection(s) with a new subtype but no human-to-human spread, or at most rare instances of spread to a close contact.
>
> **Phase 4**: Small cluster(s) with limited human-to-human transmission but spread is highly localized, suggesting that the virus is not well adapted to humans.
>
> **Phase 5**: Larger cluster(s) but human-to-human spread still localized, suggesting that the virus is becoming increasingly better adapted to humans but may not yet be fully transmissible (substantial pandemic risk).
>
> ### Pandemic Period
>
> **Phase 6**: Pandemic: increased and sustained transmission in general population.
>
> Notes: The distinction between *phases 1* and *2* is based on the risk of human infection or disease resulting from circulating strains in animals. The distinction is based on various factors and their relative importance according to current scientific knowledge. Factors may include pathogenicity in animals and humans, occurrence in domesticated animals and livestock or only in wildlife, whether the virus is enzootic or epizootic, geographically localized or widespread, and other scientific parameters.
> The distinction among *phases 3*, *4*, and *5* is based on an assessment of the risk of a pandemic. Various factors and their relative importance according to current scientific knowledge may be considered. Factors may include rate of transmission, geographic location and spread, severity of illness, presence of genes from human strains (if derived from an animal strain), and other scientific parameters.
>
> Source: Centers for Disease Control and Prevention. (2005). *Stages of a pandemic*. Retrieved May 29, 2009, from http://www.cdc.gov/flu/pandemic/phases.htm

SARS, WHO, and Canada

WHO warnings first affected Canada in a significant and direct way during the SARS crisis of 2003. This event has had a prolonged and profound effect on emergency preparedness in Canada, as well as in other countries.

Estimates state that SARS killed 44 Canadians (Ontario Ministry of Health and Long-Term Care, 2004), caused serious illness for thousands of others, and brought Ontario and much of Canada economically to its knees when WHO issued an alert warning people against travel to Canada. Canada clearly was not ready to effectively handle this calamity. With many questions unanswered regarding Canada's response to, containment of, and management of the crisis, Mr. Justice Archie Campbell was charged with investigating the country's response to the SARS crisis. His final report was released on January 9, 2007. He concluded that the handling (or mishandling) of the situation fell on the shoulders of many individuals, as well as on departments and agencies across the health care system. He concluded that the SARS crisis was further worsened by inadequate, ineffective policies and procedures—in effect, the health care system itself—which led to errors in judgement, treatment, and containment (through isolation) and inadequate protection for health care workers, especially nurses (SARS Commission, 2006).

The Ministry of Health and Long-Term Care in Ontario claims to have learned lessons from the outbreak—along with the rest of the country. Hospitals and other health care agencies and organizations have committed to more open communication and improved policies and procedures for dealing with such outbreaks. Most jurisdictions across Canada have Web sites detailing the signs of SARS and steps for individuals to take if they suspect they have encountered the disease or any other potentially disastrous virus.

Lessons Learned

Health Emergency Preparedness

Individual Canadians faced with any health-related emergency are initially responsible for their own protection. Depending on the complexity and seriousness of the threat, however, various levels of government become involved as resources, and more expertise becomes necessary to deal with the event. Under 1985's *Emergency Preparedness Act (EPA)*, each federal department must have an emergency response plan relating to its areas of responsibility. Such plans include the National Counter-Terrorism Plan and the Canadian Pandemic Influenza Plan. Each province and territory has its own legislation to deal with emergencies within its boundaries. However, in the event of a national emergency, federal plans under the *EPA* would take priority and be implemented collaboratively with each jurisdiction. The SARS crisis emphasized the importance of all levels of government working together to effectively deal with such an event.

To address national emergencies such as SARS, the Canadian government has taken steps to ensure rapid, effective responses and, in 2004, created two organizations for this purpose—Public Safety Canada and the Public Health Agency of Canada (PHAC). As well, the federal government developed the National Security Policy and National Emergency Response System (NERS). The establishment of these organizations and policies addresses a wide variety of emergencies and concerns that Canadians may encounter. PHAC, in particular, is charged with both recognizing and responding to public health threats.

PHAC's key goals are public awareness, ongoing surveillance, early detection, prompt action to contain viruses, effective communication across the health care system, and collaboration among health care professionals, organizations, and agencies at all levels of government. The government has created a Web site for the Centre of Emergency Preparedness and Response to provide access to resources in every province and territory (see Web Resources at the end of this chapter).

With the outbreak of the H1N1 virus, Canada and most other developed nations appear more prepared to respond, in terms of surveillance, testing, containment, and treatment.

The H1N1 Virus

In April 2009, an outbreak of a flu-type virus appeared to originate in Mexico. Clinical specimens of the virus were sent to Canada's National Microbiology Laboratory in Winnipeg, Manitoba, for analysis. The lab confirmed the virus as a human swine influenza—new but related to others such as the AH1N1 human swine virus. The virus causes a respiratory illness with symptoms similar to those of seasonal flu. The virus was deadly, killing an estimated 80 Mexicans within the first few days of its appearance and affecting young, healthy individuals. Reporting of this outbreak was prompt, and the response was swift. Within days, Mexican officials closed schools, museums, and libraries in Mexico City and cancelled any activities involving crowds. Canada and other countries immediately implemented measures to monitor individuals returning from Mexico.

Initially, WHO called the swine flu outbreak in Mexico and the United States a "public health emergency of international concern" and asked countries around the world to step up their reporting and surveillance of influenza. WHO uses six phases to categorize the risks of such an outbreak and to determine its pandemic alert level (see Box 4.5 and Figure 4.2). Within a week of the outbreak, WHO placed the alert level at phase 3, since human-to-human transmission was very limited. By June 11, 2009, however, with nearly 30,000 confirmed cases reported in 74 countries, WHO raised the pandemic alert level to phase 6—placing the world at the start of an influenza pandemic.

Phase 6 is a full pandemic alert (World Health Organization, 2005). To declare a pandemic, WHO considers the following factors:

- *Is the virus new?* The Centers for Disease Control and Prevention said the H1N1 strain of swine flu included genetic material from four sources: North American swine influenza viruses, North American avian influenza viruses, human influenza virus, and swine influenza viruses found in Asia and

Europe—a new combination that had not been identified anywhere in the world before.

- *Does it cause severe disease?* The vast majority of individuals who have contracted the H1N1 virus do not become seriously ill. In centres in which large outbreaks have occurred, most cases have appeared in people under the age of 25. Alarmingly, whereas the majority of deaths from seasonal flu typically occur in older adults and those with chronic diseases or compromised immune systems, nearly half of the fatal H1N1 infections have occurred in middle-aged adults in good health.

- *Does it move easily between people?* Even countries with effective tracking and testing systems are seeing the virus spread easily. Countries without effective systems cannot monitor the spread of disease well, which, in turn, promotes its spread. WHO has estimated that the H1N1 virus may well infect as many as 2 billion people by 2011—about one of every three people in the world.

With the development of an H1N1 vaccine, it is hoped that the spread of the virus can be controlled. Since the SARS outbreak, pharmaceutical companies have invested more money into producing flu vaccines and are better prepared to respond to market needs. As well, governments are more willing to provide additional funding to companies that invest in developing and producing the vaccine. Pharmaceutical companies will, of course, endeavour to meet demands; however, if vaccines are in short supply, decisions must be made as to who will receive them. Front-line health professionals and those most vulnerable will likely be first in line.

In the **News**   **Health Canada Responds to Melamine Found in Milk in China**

In 2008, milk and other dairy products from China were found to be contaminated with melamine, a synthetic material used in such items as household cleaning products, plastics, and fertilizer that is dangerous to humans if ingested in sufficient amounts. A number of infant deaths in China resulted from product consumption. The Chinese government notified the Canadian Embassy on September 12, 2008.

As a result of the contaminated milk, WHO produced a report outlining what it considered to be safe and acceptable standards of melamine exposure. Canada adopted those standards in December 2008. As well, the Canadian Food

Continued on next page

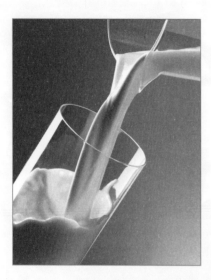

Inspection Agency (CFIA) implemented a number of measures to monitor and test high-risk products from China, such as infant formula and infant foods containing milk and milk-based ingredients. On November 14, 2008, the chief public health officer of Canada announced that no known cases of illness resulted from melamine ingestion in Canada. Nonetheless, after the WHO alert, some products were recalled.

In March 2009, the *New England Journal of Medicine* found evidence that infants who drank melamine-contaminated formula had a higher incidence of kidney stones. Although Canada may not have experienced imminent danger to the same degree as China, Health Canada's response almost certainly minimized any related potential health problems.

Sources: Health Canada. (2008). *Health Canada's human health risk assessment supporting standard development for melamine in foods.* Retrieved May 29, 2009, from http://www.hc-sc.gc. ca/fn-an/pubs/melamine_hra-ers-eng.php; Guan, N., Fan, Q., Ding, J., Zhao, Y., Lu, J., Ai, Y., et al. (2009). Melamine-contaminated powdered formula and urolithiasis in young children. *New England Journal of Medicine, 360,* 1067–1074. Retrieved May 29, 2009, from http://content.nejm. org/cgi/content/abstract/360/11/1067

Photo credit: © iStockphoto.com/Elhenyo.

World Health Assembly

The World Health Assembly is the policymaking body for WHO. The assembly's executive board comprises 34 members, all with qualifications in the health care field, who are elected for a three-year term. Each year, in Geneva, the assembly meets with representatives from member nations to discuss policies of WHO and to approve a budget for proposed programs for the upcoming year. The executive board tables reports that require further action, study, or investigation, as well as ensures that planned activities for the upcoming year are implemented.

PAN-AMERICAN HEALTH ORGANIZATION

The Pan-American Health Organization (PAHO) aims to improve health and living standards in the Americas. Among other activities, this international public health agency serves as the Regional Office for the Americas of WHO and functions as part of the United Nations. Member countries include the 35 nations that comprise the Americas. Because many member states lack basic health care, clean drinking water, and adequate sanitation, one of PAHO's main priorities is to promote current, effective, and community-based primary health care strategies.

ORGANISATION FOR ECONOMIC CO-OPERATION AND DEVELOPMENT

The Organisation for Economic Co-operation and Development (OECD) consists of 30 member countries (including Canada) that adhere to the principles of democracy and a free market economy. Through the organization, governments compare policy experiences and seek answers to common problems. The organization, among other things, measures the quality of medical care in member countries and rates health outcomes. For example, a report released in November 2007 called *Health at a Glance* provided valuable information on different aspects of health care performance in member countries. It also identified variations in indicators of health status and health risks and compared these to standards of practice in related health care systems (Organisation for Economic Co-operation and Development, 2007).

SUMMARY

❖ The federal government plays a significant leadership role in health care. Through its complex and frequently changing hierarchical structure, Health Canada works to fulfill its mission to make Canadians among the healthiest populations in the world.

❖ Contrary to the belief of many Canadians, the federal government has little legal power over health care in the provinces and territories. Health Canada plays an authoritarian role in enforcing compliance with the *Canada Health Act*. However, the federal government's only real power over the provinces and territories is financial—it therefore withholds federal-to-provincial transfers of funds when a province or territory breaches the principles and conditions of the Act.

❖ Health Canada is led by the minister of health, who is supported by a deputy minister, assistant deputy ministers, an associate deputy minister, a chief public health officer, and the Departmental Secretariat. The minister of health is appointed by Parliament; deputies and assistant deputies are not.

❖ The many branches, offices, bureaus, and agencies that make up Health Canada work both independently and collaboratively within and outside of the organization. The Audit and Accountability Bureau, the Chief Financial Officer Branch, the Corporate Services Branch, and Legal Services have primary responsibilities supporting the internal workings of Health Canada. They all ensure that the departments function in an organized, collaborative, effective, and financially accountable manner.

❖ Other sections, such as the First Nations and Inuit Health Branch, the Health Products and Food Branch, the Healthy Environments and Consumer Safety Branch, and the Public Affairs, Consultation and Communications Branch, are responsible for activities more directly aligned with the public's health and safety.

❖ The Public Health Agency of Canada plays a significant role in health promotion and disease prevention initiatives; tracks outbreaks of seasonal flu, tuberculosis, measles, and other illnesses; and recommends corrective and preventive measures.

❖ Health Canada is active on an international level, working with a number of organizations to improve health at both a national and international level. The World Health Organization, a key player in such initiatives, provides leadership on health matters globally. WHO recognizes health threats such as the H1N1 virus and initializes pandemic alerts in response to information gathered.

REVIEW QUESTIONS

1. State the primary role of the federal government in health care.

2. In terms of health care, which population groups is the federal government responsible for?

3. Explain the primary responsibilities of the deputy minister of health.

4. What function does the Audit and Accountability Bureau of Health Canada perform?

5. What branch of Health Ca[...] the safety and regulation of [...]

6. What is meant by patent protection for a n[...] drug, and which Health Canada department is responsible for patent regulation?

7. Explain the functions of the World Health Organization, the Pan-American Health Organization, and the Organisation for Economic Co-operation and Development.

DISCUSSION QUESTIONS

1. Select a Health Canada branch or agency and research the key issues it currently faces. How is the branch or agency addressing these issues?

2. Research the occurrence of SARS in Canada and the measures the federal government has taken to ensure preparedness if a similar outbreak occurs. Include what preparations hospitals and other facilities in your geographic area have made. Present your findings in class.

3. Assume that you work in a busy health clinic. What current threats and travel advisories issued by WHO would you share with clients?

4. Research the etiology of the H1N1 virus, how it is spread, and what precautions and measures Canada has taken to deal with it. Track the spread of the virus to its current level. What threats does it now pose? How effective does the vaccine appear to be?

WEB RESOURCES

About Health Canada: About Missions, Values, Activities
http://www.hc-sc.gc.ca/ahc-asc/activit/about-apropos/index-eng.php

Health Canada is the federal department responsible for helping Canadians maintain and improve their health. The department partners with other agencies and health care organizations to ensure that its efforts meet the needs of all Canadians. This link provides information on Health Canada's mission, values, and activities.

Health Canada: Branches and Agencies
http://www.hc-sc.gc.ca/ahc-asc/branch-dirgen/index-eng.php

This Web link directs you to current information about Health Canada's sub-departments.

Canadian Food Inspection Agency
http://www.inspection.gc.ca

The Canadian Food Inspection Agency (CFIA) is mandated to safeguard Canada's food supply. The agency's plans and priorities link directly to the Government of Canada's priorities for bolstering economic prosperity, strengthening security at the border, and ensuring the safety of the food supply.

Public Health Agency of Canada
http://www.phac-aspc.gc.ca

The Public Health Agency of Canada provides research, information, and statistics on a wide variety of health-related issues, including diseases and conditions, healthy travel abroad, maternal health, and health and safety for all stages of life.

EB RESOURCES

Centre for Emergency Preparedness and Response
http://www.phac-aspc.gc.ca/cepr-cmiu/

A division of the Public Health Agency of Canada, the Centre for Emergency Preparedness and Response creates and executes plans to deal with any type of emergency, including pandemics, natural disasters, accidents, and terrorist acts.

World Health Organization
http://www.who.int/en/

The World Health Organization is the authority for health within the United Nations system. All United Nations member countries may become members of WHO by accepting its constitution. Non-UN member countries may be admitted as members by a majority vote of the World Health Assembly. WHO currently has 193 member states.

Canadian Institute for Health Information
http://www.cihi.ca

An independent, nonprofit organization, the Canadian Institute for Health Information (CIHI) provides essential data and analyses on Canada's health care system and the health of Canadians, with a focus on services, spending, and human resources in health care and on population health.

Swine Flu Outbreak International "Public Health Emergency": WHO
http://www.cbc.ca/world/story/2009/04/25/flu-mexico-090425.html

This article discusses the outbreak of the "swine flu" in April 2009 and provides the early figures and estimates as well as an overview of the early impact on Canada. It supplies information about the virus itself and explains the WHO rationale in declaring the outbreak a public health emergency.

Canadian Surveillance of H1N1 Virus
http://www.phac-aspc.gc.ca/alert-alerte/h1n1/surveillance-eng.php

The Public Health Agency of Canada maintains this site to keep Canadians informed about the impact of the H1N1 virus in Canada. It includes updated information about deaths reported due to the virus.

Reporting Adverse Reactions
https://www6.hc-sc.gc.ca/medeffect/intro.do?method=intro&applanguage=en_CA

This Web page provides a path to an online form intended for the reporting of suspected adverse reactions to pharmaceuticals, biologics, natural health products, and radiopharmaceuticals.

Health Policy Research Bulletins
http://www.hc-sc.gc.ca/sr-sr/pubs/hpr-rpms/index-eng.php

This Web page provides a path to a collection of Health Canada's policy research bulletins and policy research working papers.

Introduction to the Health Canada Web Site
http://www.hc-sc.gc.ca/home-accueil/tour/index_e.html

Health Canada is the federal department responsible for helping Canadians maintain and improve their health. It partners with other agencies and health care organizations to ensure its efforts meet the needs of all Canadians.

Canada Becomes First Country to Adopt New World Health Organization Recommendations Regarding Melamine in Food
http://www.hc-sc.gc.ca/ahc-asc/media/nr-cp/_2008/2008_181-eng.php

This news release reports that Canada adopted the WHO recommendations regarding melamine levels in food on December 12, 2008.

The Government of Canada Responds to Melamine in Food Products
http://www.hc-sc.gc.ca/fn-an/securit/chem-chim/melamine/index-eng.php

This article discusses the steps taken by the Government of Canada in addressing the issue of melamine in food products.

WEB RESOURCES

Statement From Canada's Chief Public Health Officer Regarding Melamine
http://www.phac-aspc.gc.ca/media/
cpho-acsp/080928-eng.php

This link provides the official statement regarding melamine found in food products from China, issued by Dr. David Butler-Jones, chief public health officer of Canada. The statement provides information on the recall and recommends steps to be taken by people who had recently adopted a baby from China or who find baby formula from China in a store.

Health Canada First Nations and Inuit Health Branch
http://www.hc-sc.gc.ca/fniah-spnia/index-eng.php

In recognition of the unique needs of First Nations and Inuit peoples in Canada, the federal government established the First Nations and Inuit Health Branch (FNIHB) within Health Canada. The branch works closely with First Nations and Inuit organizations and communities to carry out initiatives aimed at helping people keep healthy and at preventing chronic and infectious diseases.

It's Your Health
http://www.hc-sc.gc.ca/hl-vs/iyh-vsv/index-eng.php

Written in consultation with Health Canada's and PHAC's scientists and experts, "It's Your Health" is a series of articles that cover a wide range of health issues. The articles also provide Internet links and references to further information.

WHO Extends Its SARS-Related Travel Advice to Beijing and Shanxi Province in China and to Toronto, Canada
http://www.who.int/csr/sarsarchive/2003_04_23/
en/

This Web page provides a WHO situation update on SARS from April 23, 2003, recommending, as a measure of precaution, that persons planning to travel to Beijing or Shanxi Province, China, or to Toronto, Canada, consider postponing all but essential travel.

Government of Canada: Is Your Family Prepared?
http://getprepared.ca/

This site provides emergency management organization (EMO) information for each province and territory, including tips on determining risks, creating an emergency plan, and preparing an emergency kit.

REFERENCES

Assembly of First Nations. (2002). *Top misconceptions about Aboriginal peoples*. Fact sheet. Retrieved May 29, 2009, from http://www.afn.ca/cmslib/general/FS-TM-e.pdf

Assisted Human Reproduction Act, S.C., c. 2 (2004).

Canadian Institutes of Health Research. (2007). *About CIHR*. Retrieved May 29, 2009, from http://www.cihr-irsc.gc.ca/e/37792.html

Health Canada. (2004). *Canada Health Act provincial submissions: 2005–2006*. Retrieved May 29, 2009, from http://www.hc-sc.gc.ca/hcs-sss/pubs/cha-lcs/2005-cha-lcs-ar-ra/nu_e.html

Health Canada. (2007). *About Health Canada*. Retrieved May 29, 2009, from http://www.hc-sc.gc.ca/ahc-asc/activit/about-apropos/index-eng.php

Health Canada. (2009). *Canada Vigilance Program*. Retrieved May 29, 2009, from http://www.hc-sc.gc.ca/dhp-mps/medeff/vigilance-eng.php

House of Commons of Canada. (2001). Bill C-95. An act to establish the Department of Health and to amend and repeal certain acts. Retrieved May 29, 2009, from http://www2.parl.gc.ca/HousePublications/Publication.aspx?DocId=2328421&Language=e&Mode=1&File=34

REFERENCES

Ontario Ministry of Health and Long-Term Care. (2004). *SARS: Severe acute respiratory syndrome.* Health update. Retrieved May 29, 2009, from http://www.health.gov.on.ca/english/public/updates/archives/hu_03/hu_sars.html

Organisation for Economic Co-operation and Development. (2007). *Health at a glance 2007.* Retrieved May 29, 2009, from http://www.oecd.org/health/healthataglance

SARS Commission. (2006). *Spring of fear: The SARS Commission final report.* Toronto: Author.

World Health Organization. (2005). *WHO global influenza preparedness plan.* Retrieved May 29, 2009, from http://www.who.int/csr/resources/publications/influenza/GIP_2005_5Eweb.pdf

CHAPTER FIVE

Provincial and Territorial Governments

Learning Outcomes

1. Discuss the common structural elements among the provincial and territorial governments.

2. Describe the purpose and general structure of regionalization initiatives.

3. Explain how provincial and territorial health care is financed.

4. Summarize eligibility criteria for health care coverage.

5. Outline the health care services covered under the provincial and territorial plans.

6. Describe in general terms how health care is delivered in the provinces and territories.

7. Describe the roles of private health care and private health insurance in Canada.

KEY TERMS

Co-payment, p. 173

Deductible, p. 177

Dispensing fee, p. 178

Drug identification
number (DIN), p. 179

Enhanced services, p. 170

Formulary list, p. 178

Inpatient, p. 171

Medically necessary, p. 151

Methicillin-resistant *Staphylococcus
aureus* (MRSA), p. 179

Nonprofit, p. 157

Vancomycin-resistant *Enterococcus*
(VRE), p. 179

Vancomycin-resistant *Staphylococcus
aureus* (VRSA), p. 179

This chapter provides an overview of the structure of the provincial and territorial health care systems, emphasizing the common elements among them and outlining their differences. While not every detail can be covered, the chapter will help you to develop a general understanding of the 13 health care systems across the country and how they operate. To better understand specific details about your own province or territory, answer the Review Questions at the end of the chapter and visit the Web site of your provincial or territorial department of health (see Web Resources at the end of this chapter).

This chapter follows two families who are new to Canada as they navigate their way through their respective provincial health care systems. You will learn how the Jaeger family in British Columbia (Case Example 5.1) and the Wongs in Nova Scotia (Case Example 5.2) become eligible for health care and what services are available to them.

Case Example 5.1

On January 1, 40-year-old Joseph Jaeger and his family arrive in Toronto from Germany and are en route to British Columbia. Joseph and his wife, Helga, 36, have three children: Anna, 16; Luca, 10; and Alois, 3. Although delighted to be in Canada, the family has little general information about their new country and even fewer details about an area of real concern to them—their health care. Anna is 3 months pregnant, Luca has asthma, and Alois requires updated immunizations. Joseph, who is overweight and on medication for high blood pressure, is a bricklayer and was told that, due to a shortage of skilled tradespeople in Canada, finding a job would be easy.

Case Example 5.2

Quang Wong, 36, and his wife, Ling, 35, arrive in Sydney, Nova Scotia, on January 15 with their two children: a son, Huan, aged 10, and a daughter Niu, aged 6. Quang, a doctor, plans to certify in Sydney; Ling is an architect. The family has no outstanding health problems.

PROVINCIAL AND TERRITORIAL HEALTH CARE PLANS

DIVISION OF POWERS

Both Canadians and non-Canadians often ask, "Does Canada have a national health insurance plan?" The answer is *no*, Canada does not have a national health insurance plan. Rather, Canada has 13 separate insurance programs run by 10 provinces and three territories, loosely bound together by federal agreements and the *Canada Health Act*. As mentioned in Chapter 3, these programs are frequently referred to collectively as *Medicare*.

Although the federal government works in partnership with the provinces and territories to deliver health care, the provinces and territories maintain the bulk of the responsibility for health care. Under the *Constitution Act* (Box 5.1), provincial and territorial governments oversee matters relating to the personal health of their populations—promoting good health, preventive care, health maintenance, and the diagnosis and treatment of health problems. To receive continued federal funding for health care, however, provinces and territories must abide by the principles and conditions of the *Canada Health Act*, which obliges them to operate a health insurance plan that covers hospital care and **medically necessary** treatment for eligible residents. The Act is not concerned with the specifics of public or private health care delivery and does not address coverage of diagnostic services such as positron emission tomography (PET scans), magnetic resonance imaging (MRIs), and computed axial tomography (CT scans). Each province and territory controls which services are covered and how they are delivered.

Box 5.1   The *Constitution Act*: A Clarification

The original *British North America Act* of 1867 became the *Constitution Act* in 1982, when Britain surrendered the power to make Canada's laws, including the Constitution. Among other things, the *Constitution Act* outlines the division of health care responsibilities.

STRUCTURE OF THE HEALTH PLANS: AN OVERVIEW

Within each provincial and territorial government is a ministry assigned to managing health care (Box 5.2). Some jurisdictions combine the health ministry with the ministry for social services, a combination reflected in the ministries' names. Several ministries' names suggest multiple focuses. For example, Alberta's ministry responsible for health care is called the Ministry of Health and Wellness, emphasizing its attention to health promotion and disease prevention. Likewise, Manitoba highlights healthy living in its title. In Ontario, the Ministry of Health and Long-Term Care stresses the province's focus on long-term care.

The health ministries or departments oversee a variety of sub-divisions, branches, agencies, and programs that assume responsibilities for various matters and types of health care. Ministries also work with other service partners in the community—some government-funded, others private.

Each ministry is headed by an elected member of Parliament appointed by the premier to the position of minister of health (MOH). Typically, a government also appoints a deputy minister of health (sometimes more than one), who is not an elected member of Parliament. One or more associate deputy ministers and a management committee may also be assigned. Ultimately responsible for the health care system in the province or territory, the MOH has numerous organi-

---

Box 5.2   Ministries Responsible for Health Care Across Canada

Province/Territory	Ministry Title
Alberta	Alberta Health and Wellness
British Columbia	Ministry of Health Services
Manitoba	Manitoba Healthy Living
New Brunswick	Department of Health
Newfoundland and Labrador	Health and Community Services
Northwest Territories	Department of Health and Social Services
Nova Scotia	Department of Health
Nunavut	Department of Health and Social Services
Ontario	Ministry of Health and Long-Term Care
Prince Edward Island	Department of Health
Quebec	Santé et Services sociaux
Saskatchewan	Saskatchewan Health
Yukon	Yukon Health and Social Services

zations within the ministry reporting to him or her. These organizations provide leadership, direction, and support to service delivery partners such as regional health authorities, physicians, and other health care professionals.

One of the ministries' greatest responsibilities is implementing and regulating the provincial or territorial health insurance plan—that is, overseeing hospital and medical care. In some jurisdictions, this responsibility belongs to a single authority. In others, two administrative bodies share the duty—one handles hospitals and other health care facilities; the other, medical care. For example, in British Columbia, the Medical Services Commission administers the medical care plan, and the government, through the Ministry of Health Services, administers hospital services under the *Hospital Insurance Act*, reimbursing facilities for the medically necessary services they provide. But in Prince Edward Island, both the hospital and medical services plans are administered by the Department of Health.

The provincial and territorial ministries must also negotiate salaries and other policies with physicians' professional associations. Committees are typically created to manage these negotiations.

All provinces and territories provide three general categories of health care—primary, secondary, and tertiary—which are discussed below. The interaction between these categories is illustrated in Figure 5.1.

Figure 5.1	**Access to Primary, Secondary, and Tertiary Health Care**

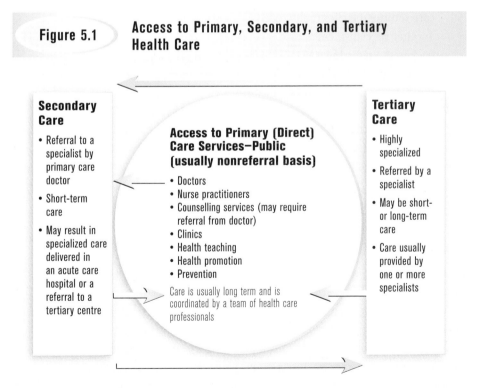

Secondary Care

- Referral to a specialist by primary care doctor
- Short-term care
- May result in specialized care delivered in an acute care hospital or a referral to a tertiary centre

Access to Primary (Direct) Care Services—Public (usually nonreferral basis)

- Doctors
- Nurse practitioners
- Counselling services (may require referral from doctor)
- Clinics
- Health teaching
- Health promotion
- Prevention

Care is usually long term and is coordinated by a team of health care professionals

Tertiary Care

- Highly specialized
- Referred by a specialist
- May be short- or long-term care
- Care usually provided by one or more specialists

1. *Primary care* refers to "first contact" services to which the public has direct access, including family doctors, nurse practitioners, counselling services, clinics, emergency care services, and telephone helplines for health care advice. Primary care professionals diagnose and treat health concerns, make referrals to secondary health care services when required, and provide preventive care, health promotion, and health education. Although typically long term and comprehensive in nature, primary care does not usually include hospitalization. *Primary care* should not be confused with the concept of *primary health care*, which encompasses essential medical and curative care received at the primary, secondary, or tertiary levels.

2. A client must obtain a physician referral to access *secondary care*, including consultation with a specialist, such as a dermatologist, urologist, internist, or orthopedic surgeon. A specialist assists the primary care physician to diagnose a client's problem and to provide specialized treatment, but the specialist's involvement is usually short term. Secondary care may involve admission to a general hospital or referral to a highly specialized facility, which provides tertiary care.

3. Highly specialized, *tertiary care* also requires a referral. A cancer centre or cardiology centre, for example, would provide tertiary care. In a tertiary care setting, the client may receive care from the referring specialist or from another specialist. Once care is considered complete, the client may be sent back to the referring specialist, who will then discharge the client back to his or her family doctor. Alternatively, the tertiary care centre itself may refer the client back to the family doctor.

Although ultimately accountable for all aspects of health care, the provincial or territorial ministry or department of health assigns responsibilities to various departments. The most common method of delivering primary, secondary, and tertiary care is under a regional model using organizations commonly called *regional health authorities* (RHAs).

Regionalization: Why and When

In the early 1990s, because of the rising cost of health care and the increasing demand for services in a variety of settings, governments conducted public forums, reviews, and other studies to determine a way to improve health care delivery. The conclusion: to decentralize decisions about health care issues through regionalization (Box 5.3), a concept of assessing the need for specific types of care and delivering that care within a given jurisdiction. The regional approach was based on the belief that involving the community in decisions regarding health care needs would both increase public participation in health care initiatives and enable the ministry to address the unique needs of each community in a more streamlined, cost-effective manner.

Box 5.3   Regional Health Authorities: A Definition

Regional health authorities (RHAs) are autonomous health care organizations responsible for health care administration in a defined geographic region within a province or territory. Through appointed or elected boards of governance, RHAs manage the funding and delivery of community and institutional health care services within their regions.

Source: Ferrell, B., & Coyle, N. (2006). *Textbook of palliative nursing.* New York: Oxford University Press.

Regionalization took different forms across the country, but every province and territory eventually became involved, with Ontario the last to regionalize care, in 2006. Each regional health authority is run by a board; in some regions, the provincial government appoints the board members; in others, board members comprise a mix of elected and appointed officials. The RHAs across Canada differ in terms of size, structure, responsibility, and name.

In most provinces and territories, although RHAs have the authority to disperse funds and direct services, they ultimately answer to the ministry and must provide financial statements and performance reports regarding services they have funded. RHAs oversee long-term care, residential and acute care services, and, in some regions, public and mental health, addiction, and health promotion programs.

Over the past 15 years, most provinces and territories have altered the original structures of their health care delivery systems, merging or eliminating some RHAs and shifting some responsibilities among the ministry, other departments, and the RHAs.

PROVINCIAL AND TERRITORIAL REGIONAL HEALTH AUTHORITIES

British Columbia

Prior to 2001, health care in British Columbia was delivered through 52 health authorities. In 2001, restructuring gave rise to a new governance and management structure, resulting in six RHAs, five of which develop and manage regional services for 16 designated areas. The sixth, called the Provincial Health Services Authority, coordinates specialized services, such as cardiac and cancer care. Each

RHA has an appointed board and is managed by an executive team, which participates in decision making at the operational level. The RHAs also manage community health centres (CHCs), which offer a variety of services throughout the province, including primary care clinics, health promotion, addictions services, home care, community mental health services, and specialized services, such as assistance for new immigrants, support for new mothers, and youth health drop-in centres. The range of services each CHC offers reflects the needs of the community it serves.

Alberta

In 2008, Alberta's nine RHAs, the Alberta Mental Health Board, Alberta Cancer Board, and Alberta Alcohol and Drug Abuse Commission were all replaced by one provincial governance organization, the Alberta Health Services Board. Reporting to the minister of health and wellness, this board is responsible for health care delivery for the entire province.

This new governance model aims to strengthen Alberta's approach to managing health care services, including surgical access, long-term care, chronic disease management, addiction and mental health services, and primary care access.

Three advisory councils have been created to advise and guide the Alberta Health Services Board on issues such as cancer research and addiction and mental health services.

Saskatchewan

In Saskatchewan, 12 RHAs provide the bulk of health care to the province's residents. The RHAs oversee hospitals, emergency response and ambulance services, long-term care and home care programs, community health services (including public health), and mental health and rehabilitation services.

The Saskatchewan Cancer Agency plans and implements cancer services in the province. The agency's duties include evaluating and developing guidelines for standards of care, treatment, and health promotion initiatives.

The Athabasca Health Authority, established under the *Non-Profit Corporations Act*, has a funding arrangement with Saskatchewan Health for providing care for those living in the Athabasca Basin.

Manitoba

Under Manitoba's *Regional Health Authorities Act*, the province developed 11 RHAs in 1997. The Act outlines the conditions under which the RHAs are incorporated and defines the scope of practice of the RHAs as a whole. Reporting to the minister of health, these 11 authorities assess and prioritize community needs and deliver hospital care, long-term care, home care, public health services, rehabilitative services, ambulance services, and laboratory services. Manitoba also delivers health care services (e.g., medical care, counselling, health education) through community health centres, divisions of the RHAs run by local community boards.

The largest RHA, the Winnipeg Regional Health Authority, divided its region into 12 parts, established six community health advisory councils, and made each council responsible for two geographic divisions.

Ontario

In Ontario, 14 local health integration networks (LHINs) regionalize and distribute funding for the areas they serve—again, responding to the region's specific health care needs. LHINs are responsible for hospitals, community care access centres, community support service organizations, mental health and addiction agencies, CHCs, and long-term care homes.

While the Ministry of Health and Long-Term Care retains responsibility for such things as the provincial health plan, ambulance services, provincial drug programs, and public health, LHINs have control over two-thirds of the Ontario health care budget and must submit an annual financial report to the ministry. Each LHIN operates within the scope of agreements made with the ministry and must report on its performance, including its status toward reaching designated goals, meeting standards, and using allotted finances. These agreements are redefined annually.

More than 50 CHCs exist across the province. Ten Aboriginal health care centres serve families both on and off reserves. Two other health care centres, located in Timmins and Toronto, also provide services for local Aboriginals. (Although Aboriginals can access any health care centre, these ones provide culturally based health care.) As well, the province introduced family health teams in 2004, primarily to address wait times and a shortage of family doctors. The responsibility of LHINs, family health teams are **nonprofit**, community-governed teams of health care professionals who deliver a wide range of services based on community need.

Nonprofit
Not seeking or producing a profit.

Quebec

Quebec has practised regionalization since 1997, longer than it has been in practice in any other province or territory. Quebec's 18 RHAs bear the responsibility for hospitals, long-term care, home care, public health, mental health, rehabilitation, social services, and laboratory and ambulance services—a more comprehensive list of responsibilities than those of most other jurisdictions.

In 2004, 95 local service networks were established across the province to work under their respective regional health authorities. These networks provide comprehensive, accessible health care services to the populations in their region. At the heart of these local networks lie health and social services centres, created by merging local community health centres, residential and long-term care centres, and general and specialized hospital centres. By constructing service agreements with partners and stakeholders within the local services networks (e.g., rehabilitation centres, physician groups, medical clinics, youth protection centres, mental health organizations, university hospital centres), these centres ensure seamless access to primary, secondary, and tertiary care and adequate follow-up for the populations they serve.

New Brunswick

In 2002, eight RHAs were established in New Brunswick. The minister of health approves financing for each RHA, depending on the needs of its region as outlined in its business plan. Each RHA must have a professional advisory committee, which is responsible for quality control issues, health criteria for admission and discharge from facilities, and the overall clinical care of clients under medical and hospital care. Other responsibilities of the province's RHAs include home care and local ambulance and laboratory services.

Nova Scotia

Nine district health authorities (as RHAs are called in Nova Scotia) and the Izaak Walton Killam (IWK) Health Centre, an independent women's and children's tertiary care hospital, provide the bulk of Nova Scotia's health care services.

Four medical officers of health oversee the regions within the district health authorities. District health authorities are responsible for hospitals, public health, mental health, rehabilitation, and laboratory services. The district health authorities receive funding from the Department of Health; in return, they prepare financial statements and service summaries for the ministry at designated intervals.

Nova Scotia's medical insurance plan is administered by Medavie Blue Cross (formerly Blue Cross), an agency that reports to the Department of Health. Medavie Blue Cross has the authority to receive money from the province to pay physicians, to determine the eligibility of health care professionals who bill the provincial plan, and to provide educational seminars for physicians about their entitlements and responsibilities under the medical insurance plan.

Prince Edward Island

In 2005, Prince Edward Island replaced its Health and Social Services Department with the Department of Health and the Department of Social Services and Seniors. These departments are led by the minister and deputy minister of health and supported by eight senior directors and a departmental management committee.

The Department of Health manages the delivery of health care services. Under the restructured model, five community hospital authorities replaced five RHAs. Governed by a board that answers to the minister of health, each of the community hospital authorities has a mandate to deliver the programs and services offered through community hospitals.

The Department of Health retains responsibility for public health, primary and acute care, community hospital care, and continuing care services for the island population.

Newfoundland and Labrador

In 2005–6, the government of Newfoundland and Labrador restructured the delivery of health care to increase both the financial accountability and health care accountability to the government and the populations served. Fourteen health boards were reorganized to form four integrated RHAs, responsible for a wide range of services, including public health and community services and acute and long-term care. The government has established boards of trustees and a senior executive team to oversee the RHAs' implementation of services.

Northern Regions

The spread-out populations and great distances between centres in the northern regions of Canada present unique and complex challenges in the delivery of health care. Technological advances (e.g., electronic health records, Telehealth, video links to large health centres) have contributed to significant improvements in the quality and accessibility of health care over the past four or five years; however, care in the North remains woefully inadequate. This vast area comprises the Northwest Territories, Nunavut, Yukon, and the northern regions of other provinces, particularly British Columbia, Alberta, Saskatchewan, Manitoba, Ontario, and Quebec.

The federal government funds much of the health care for northern Inuit, Innu, and First Nations populations. These isolated populations endure higher incidences of diseases such as diabetes, tuberculosis, and depression, and more commonly face issues such as substance abuse, family violence, and suicide. Inadequate housing, unemployment, tainted drinking water, and isolation itself contribute to the frequency of these problems. The Inuit, Innu, and First Nations are, to a large extent, peoples caught between their traditions and a modern world. Many struggle with identity and respect issues as they strive to maintain their unique way of life in the larger society.

In the **News**   **Government Intervention in Preventive Care**

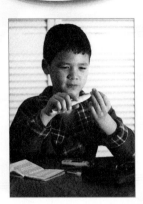

In November 2008, in support of World Diabetes Day, the Government of Canada announced that more funding will be devoted to the Aboriginal Diabetes Initiative, a program first developed in 1999 to address the rising epidemic of diabetes among Aboriginal peoples. In 1999, the government allocated $58 million over five years for this initiative. Another $190 million is being invested until 2010. Diabetes rates among Aboriginal peoples are three to five times higher than the national average.

Source: Public Health Agency of Canada. (2008). *Canada's government recognizes World Diabetes Day*. Retrieved May 29, 2009, from http://www.phac-aspc.gc.ca/media/nr-rp/2008/2008_14-eng.php

Photo credit: Stuart Nimmo/GetStock.com.

Northwest Territories

The Northwest Territories health and social services system consists of the Department of Health and Social Services, under which eight RHAs operate. Nongovernment organizations and private groups, agencies, and health care professionals also provide services through agreements with the department and authorities. Physicians and specialists from larger centres in more southern regions routinely visit the communities of the Northwest Territories.

Community health programs in the territory include daily drop-in clinics, public health clinics, home care, school health programs, and educational programs. As well as offering the community health programs, the department provides social service programs, including early intervention and support to families and children, child protection services, adoption services, family violence prevention, mental health and addiction services, and corrections services.

Yukon

The vast territory of Yukon consists of fewer people than most mid-size towns elsewhere in Canada, with between 25,000 and 32,000 residents who are eligible for government-funded health care. The Department of Health and Social Services manages and delivers all components of health care in the territory. Its initiatives include a children's drug and optical program (including prescription eyeglasses) for low-income families and youth under the age of 19; a chronic disease program, which offers benefits for prescription drugs, health care supplies and equipment, and food supplements; a pharmacare program for seniors; and an extended health plan to cover essential medical and health care supplies (e.g., hearing aids, dental care, eye care) for seniors. Yukon health insurance does not cover nursing home services.

Nunavut

Named a territory in 1999, Nunavut spans one-fifth of Canada's land mass and has communities spread across three regions—Baffin, Kivilliq, and Kitikmeot. Approximately 85% of the territory's population of roughly 30,000 people is Inuit. The territory has one regional hospital, in the capital, Iqaluit.

In 2000, the restructuring of the Department of Health and Social Services resulted in the closing of three regional boards and the incorporation of their staff and responsibilities into the new department. Under the authority of a minister and deputy minister of health, three regional offices (one in each region) now manage care in the jurisdiction. Primary care is delivered through 22 CHCs.

Health care funding is centrally managed and distributed, with the bulk of expenses going toward medical travel and out-of-territory treatments. Some of the Northwest Territories' health-related legislation has been adopted pending Nunavut's development of its own legislation to better meet the needs of its population.

HEALTH CARE: WHO PAYS FOR IT?

Each province and territory has a method (e.g., premiums, payroll tax, general revenues) of financing health care services not covered by federal funding. Private and volunteer organizations provide significant revenue for specific services or hospitals. For example, when a community hospital builds a new wing, a government grant usually covers part of the expense, and volunteer groups and the municipal government frequently make up the balance. A formal building campaign, often launched by the hospital undergoing the expansion, provides a conduit for donations.

HEALTH CARE PREMIUMS

Only two provinces—British Columbia and Ontario—currently charge premiums for health care services (Albertans stopped paying health care premiums as of January 1, 2009). British Columbia and Ontario residents cannot use premium payments as income tax deductions.

British Columbia

British Columbia charges a health care premium of approximately $54 per month for a single person, $96 per month for a family of two, and $108 per month for a family of three or more, at which point the premium payment is capped.

Those who have been residents of Canada for the previous 12 consecutive months may qualify for financial assistance (Health Canada, 2004). The province offers two premium-assistance packages to those in need. Regular premium assistance covers from 20% to 100% of the premium cost, depending on the individual's or family's income, less certain deductions. For example, a person or couple earning less than $20,000 per year would receive 100% coverage of their premiums through this plan. The temporary premium-assistance program offers total premium coverage on a short-term basis for families or individuals undergoing unexpected financial difficulties.

Ontario

Dalton McGuinty's Liberal government introduced health premiums to Ontario in 2004. Individuals who have an annual taxable income below $20,000 pay no premium; those with higher incomes pay graduated amounts to a maximum of $900 per individual per year (Public Works and Government Services Canada, 2008). This premium, introduced despite election promises to the contrary, generated resentment and anger among Ontario residents. The government promised that the money raised would be invested in health care.

Payroll Tax

Manitoba, Newfoundland and Labrador, Ontario, Quebec, Nunavut, and the Northwest Territories levy a payroll tax (HRinfodesk, 2009), a tax collected from employers that specifically raises funds for health care, education, and social services. Employers with a payroll below a certain amount may be exempt; others may pay a reduced amount based on their salary or wage payout. Note that in Ontario, this tax is in addition to health care premiums paid by residents (discussed above).

The payroll tax in Manitoba—known as the health and postsecondary education tax levy—is an obligatory tax on employee wages paid by all employers with permanent residency in the province. The tax amount the employer pays depends on the total payroll. In 2008, the government of Manitoba exempted employers with an annual payroll of less than $1.25 million. Those with payrolls between $1.5 and $2.5 million pay 4.3% on the amount in excess of $2.5 million, and those with payrolls over $2.5 million pay 2.15% of the total payroll (i.e., the $1.25 million deduction is not considered).

In Newfoundland and Labrador, employers pay a health and postsecondary education tax. Employers whose annual payroll exceeds a predetermined exemption threshold must pay a tax of 2%. In 2008, the exemption threshold was increased to $1 million (Government of Newfoundland and Labrador, 2008).

In Ontario, premiums are collected from the employer and the employee for employment insurance and the Canada Pension Plan. These funds support employees who lose their jobs, take parental leave, or retire. The rates of taxation change slightly each year but are based on a percentage of wages paid to employees.

In Quebec, employer contributions to health care services are paid at a rate of 2.7% of the payroll for payrolls under $1 million. Those with payrolls between $1 million and $4.999 million pay a rate ranging from 2.7% to 4.26% of the total wages paid. For employers with payrolls of $5 million and greater, the tax rate is 4.26%.

The Northwest Territories and Nunavut require that all employers with one or more employees pay a 2% payroll tax on employees' wages. The tax also applies to employers who do not live in the territories but who pay employees for services performed there (Northwest Territories Finance, 2009).

OTHER SOURCES OF FUNDS

Provincial, territorial, and municipal governments provide some funds for services such as preventive health measures, medical- and hospital-based services (both inpatient and outpatient), the treatment of chronic diseases, community-based rehabilitation care, and care for nursing home residents.

Provincial and territorial health ministries fund and regulate hospitals. They may also contribute financially to community health organizations, services delivered by certain health care professionals (other than physicians), and teaching and research institutions.

DISTRIBUTION OF FUNDS

Precisely how finances are organized and administered varies among the provinces and territories. In some provinces, for example, the ministry responsible for health care may directly manage hospital and medical insurance and cardiology and cancer care. Other provinces or territories may establish separate public organizations to oversee and finance these services. Currently, most provincial and territorial governments provide funding—at least in part—to RHAs, which, in turn, finance hospitals and health care services within their regions depending on each area's particular needs. For example, an RHA responsible for hiring community nurses would contract with private nursing agencies to provide care in a certain region. Managing its own funds, each nursing agency would then hire the nurses and deliver the care.

In some jurisdictions, other ministries provide funds for additional health-care-related services. For example, the Ministry of Labour might oversee occupational health matters, and the Ministry of Community and Social Services might provide services for those with specific health issues such as learning and physical disabilities (e.g., counselling, group homes, special education).

The provinces and territories also allocate funds to supplementary benefits (e.g., medical supplies such as surgical dressings and syringes; prescription drugs; hearing aids). These funds, most commonly distributed through the RHAs, finance regional facilities and services.

Thinking It Through

Some provinces charge premiums for health care; others do not.

1. Do you think that charging premiums is a fair way to offset the cost of health care?

2. Would you be in favour of your province or territory charging a tax that goes directly toward covering the cost of health care?

HEALTH INSURANCE

Health insurance coverage is provided by provincial and territorial plans and by private insurance companies.

Third-party health insurance plays a significant role in offsetting the costs of services not covered by provincial and territorial health services. Approximately 60% of Canadians carry private health insurance, either provided through group employment benefits or purchased personally (Drug Coverage, 2007). Usually including coverage for employees' families and dependants, employee plans provide benefits for health care services not covered by provincial or territorial plans, such as vision and dental care, private nursing services, assistive devices, and enhanced medical services (e.g., semi-private hospital room).

PROVINCIAL INSURANCE PLANS

Eligibility

All of the following criteria must be met for a person to be eligible for provincial or territorial health insurance:

- Canadian citizenship or permanent resident status
- Resident of the province or territory in which he or she is seeking health coverage

- Physically in that jurisdiction for at least six months of the year (this criterion varies slightly among jurisdictions—see Chapter 3) (babies born in a given province or territory are insured from birth in most circumstances)

People with study or work permits, issued under the federal *Immigration and Refugee Protection Act*, may be considered residents. Terms and conditions for insuring other population groups can be obtained from the provincial or territorial health Web sites. No Canadian can be denied medically necessary hospital or physician care under any circumstances.

Application for Coverage

In each province and territory, newcomers must apply to the ministry or department of health for health insurance coverage. The application process and documentation required can vary. Specific instructions for applying for health care coverage can be found on the Web sites of the provincial and territorial health departments. The application processes of Nova Scotia and British Columbia are illustrated as our two families, the Jaegers (Case Example 5.3) and the Wongs (Case Example 5.4), apply for provincial health coverage.

Case Example 5.3

In British Columbia, the Jaegers have several means of obtaining application forms:

- Forms can be downloaded from the Medical Services Plan, filled out, and mailed in or completed and sent electronically.

- Paper forms can be obtained from the Medical Services Plan or through the province's access centres. The Jaegers can call a toll-free number to be connected to the nearest Service B.C. Centre.

- A forms-by-fax service is available from the provincial government 24 hours a day, 7 days a week.

If Mr. Jaeger were employed, his employer would likely complete a group insurance form for him so that he could receive supplementary benefits.

Documents required for provincial or territorial health insurance applications vary. Usually a citizen of Canada must present proof of that citizenship, proof of residency in a particular province or territory, and further (or supporting) proof of personal identification (all original documents). To prove

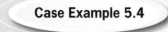

Case Example 5.4

To apply for health insurance in Nova Scotia, the Wongs can call the Medical Service Insurance plan's registration department. The Wongs will receive application forms, which they must complete and submit with the required documentation—a copy of their landed immigrant papers and a copy of their permanent resident cards. Upon approval, each member of the Wong family will be issued a health card, which will expire every four years. When their health cards expire, the Wongs will call the same number to get a renewal form.

citizenship, a birth certificate, passport, citizenship card, or similar documentation is acceptable. To show residency, an income tax assessment, a child tax benefit statement, or a utility or property tax bill is acceptable. Proof of personal identification includes a credit card, an employee ID card, or a driver's licence.

Under the *Canada Health Act*, the waiting period is not to exceed three months, so in most provinces and territories, health coverage begins within three months of moving to that jurisdiction. The following case examples show variations for the Jaegers (Case Example 5.5) and the Wongs (Case Example 5.6).

Under the reciprocal agreement (Box 5.4), health card holders qualify for health care services anywhere in Canada (other than Quebec), barring some exceptions; for example, people may not seek elective surgery in another province or seek a service that is uninsured in their province or territory of origin.

Case Example 5.5

In British Columbia, new residents are eligible for coverage after a waiting period that consists of the balance of the arrival month plus two months. If the Jaeger family arrives in British Columbia on January 5, they will be covered as of April 1. However, if Mr. Jaeger arrives January 5, and Mrs. Jaeger and the children follow on February 5, family coverage will not begin until May 1. Note that when Anna Jaeger delivers her baby, the baby will be insured from birth.

When one family member arrives at a later date, it is the latest arrival that determines when coverage for the whole family will start. The family will need supplementary health insurance until their three-month wait ends.

Case Example 5.6

The Nova Scotia health insurance plan covers the Wong family as soon as their applications are approved. In Nova Scotia, the family will not have to pay premiums for their health care coverage.

Box 5.4   Reciprocal Agreement

The reciprocal agreement supports the principle of health insurance portability (see Chapter 3) among the provinces and territories. Through the agreement, a person's province of origin will pay for required health services in another province or territory at the rates imposed by the host province. This interprovincial agreement is not mandatory. For example, Quebec has not signed it.

As a result of this agreement, Canadians, for the most part, will not face point-of-service charges for medically required hospital and physician services when they travel within Canada. In most cases, a person can receive care in a host province by simply presenting his or her health card, and the client's province of origin will pay the host province for services delivery.

Source: Health Canada. (2007). *Health care system—Canada Health Act*. Retrieved May 29, 2009, from http://www.hc-sc.gc.ca/hcs-sss/medi-assur/cha-lcs/administration-eng.php

Thinking It Through

You are considering immigrating to Canada. You find out that some provinces and territories have no wait time before you qualify for health care coverage, and others do, and that some provinces charge you health care premiums, and others do not.

If you have a choice of where you will settle, would these factors sway your decision?

Health Cards

Once an application is approved, the ministry or department of health issues the applicant a health card, identified by a number, for the province or territory in which he or she resides. Some jurisdictions assign a number to a whole family and then, when the children reach a certain age, issue the children an individual health number. Other jurisdictions issue a personal health number to each person. In Ontario, for example, babies are issued an individual health number at birth.

Increasingly, health care facilities require individuals to present their health cards at the point of service. (Note, however, that only providers of provincially or territorially funded health care can ask a person to produce a health card.) The card may be validated at that time. If an "invalid" message appears (e.g., if the card has expired or was reported lost, or if an address change has since occurred), the cardholder will have to pay for the service he or she is seeking. After finding his or her health card or renewing an invalid one, the person can submit the receipt to the ministry for reimbursement.

Health card fraud has become a significant problem across Canada, resulting in an enormous cost—in the millions of dollars—to the provinces and territories. It is virtually impossible to detect fraudulent use on older health cards that have no special security features or photo identification (e.g., Ontario's old "red and white" cards). Most jurisdictions now have photo identification health cards (for those over a certain age—usually 15 or 16) and increased security measures, such as a holographic topcoat and hidden ultraviolet ink printing that can be viewed only under UV light, to protect the information on the cards. These cards must be renewed at designated intervals, unlike the older-style cards, which never expired. Some cards also require signatures. A magnetic strip on the health card contains coded information, such as the holder's name and address. It is a serious offence in all provinces and territories to knowingly facilitate the illegal use of a health card. Health care professionals are encouraged to watch for and to report anything suspicious—for example, a client unable to provide his or her address or a person who looks decidedly different from the picture on the health card. Many jurisdictions have a hotline for health care professionals or the public to call if they suspect fraudulent use.

Lost cards must be reported immediately, as must changes of address or name. All provinces and territories have a protocol to follow for lost or misplaced health cards. As soon as a card is reported lost or missing, it is invalidated and the user is issued a new card with a new number or other variation, such as a version code.

Insured and Uninsured Services

Provincial and territorial governments are responsible for administering the health care insurance plan in their jurisdictions (Health Canada, 2009). They must decide on the need for different types of hospital beds (e.g., acute care, rehabilitation, long-term care), the mix of professional health care staff, and the structure of the system that will best serve various regions within the province or territory. In addition, the governments approve hospital budgets and negotiate physicians' fees with medical associations.

Under the *Canada Health Act*, medically necessary hospital and medical services are insured everywhere in Canada. The *Canada Health Act* also requires the provinces and territories to insure extended health care services, which include "intermediate care in nursing homes, adult residential care service, home care service and ambulatory health care services" (*Canada Health Act*, 1985).

Some provinces and territories may choose to provide supplementary benefits and services outside of the *Canada Health Act*. The governments will then determine eligibility guidelines for specific services, funding formulas, and the length of time these services will be insured. Supplementary benefits are health care services, such as optometric, dental, and chiropractic services, that are insured by the province or territory but not mandated by the *Canada Health Act*.

All provinces and territories provide specific services (e.g., eye care, dental care, drug benefits) to certain population groups, such as those receiving income assistance or guaranteed income supplements, older adults (i.e., those over 65), and disabled persons. Many jurisdictions also provide some of these services to children of low-income families.

As noted in Chapter 4, the federal government, rather than the provincial and territorial governments, provides health insurance to First Nations, Inuit, and Innu populations living on reserves. Some supplementary services (e.g., prescription drugs, eyeglasses, dental work, medical supplies, diabetic supplies) for these population groups are provided through the federal Noninsured Health Benefits Program (Box 5.5).

Box 5.5   Noninsured Health Benefits Program

Like all Canadians, First Nations people, Innu, and Inuit are insured for select health care services by their provincial and territorial governments. A number of services, however, are not insured. To help Aboriginal populations reach a health status comparable to that of other Canadians, Health Canada's Noninsured Health Benefits Program provides coverage for a limited range of these services, including drugs; dental care; vision care; medical supplies and equipment; short-term, crisis-intervention mental health counselling; and medical transportation.

Source: Health Canada. (2008). *First Nations, Inuit and Aboriginal health: Non-insured health benefits for First Nations and Inuit.* Retrieved May 29, 2009, from http://www.hc-sc.gc.ca/fniah-spnia/nihb-ssna/index-eng.php

Other groups for whom the federal government bears responsibility (e.g., federal public service employees) receive coverage under plans separate from the provincial and territorial ones.

Contrary to what many Canadians believe, private health care has existed in some form or another since before the inception of the *Canada Health Act*. Despite some private clinics in Canada being perceived as illegal under the principles of the *Canada Health Act*, several such clinics exist across the country. They circumvent the legal principles of the Act largely by offering services not technically considered medically necessary, since they cannot charge for medically necessary procedures that are covered by the public health plan. For example, private clinics may provide 3-D imaging of fetuses for pregnant women or provide MRIs that are not medically necessary for individuals wanting them. The emergence of these private clinics raises many concerns (Box 5.6).

Box 5.6   Private Clinics: Concerns

Significant concerns exist across Canada about private clinics. At the forefront lies the worry that the availability of private clinics will lengthen wait times for those using the public system because private clinics use the services of physicians and other health care professionals who also work in the public system. The prevailing thought is that doctors' time in the public system will be lessened. Those making cases against this belief argue that physicians working in the private sector do so on their own time, thus not interfering with services offered in the public system. For example, an orthopedic surgeon may have only two days of operating room time available to him or her, leaving three days a week during which he or she cannot perform surgical procedures. On such days, the surgeon can see clients in a private clinic, perhaps doing knee or hip replacements, and, conversely, shorten the line in the public system.

Another concern is that clients paying for private services or **enhanced services** will unfairly move to the top of wait lists because of the additional revenue for the clinic. In many jurisdictions, in the public system, a client requiring a hip replacement will receive offers of "upgrades" (e.g., titanium), which generate revenue for the hospital. Some claim that cases exist in the public system in which people purchasing such upgrades move up the list.

Bundled services, some claim, provide another method by which individuals can jump the queue. For example, a clinic performing cataract surgery can "bundle" an uninsured laser surgery with the insured cataract surgery. The client paying for the laser portion of the procedure could be bumped up the list, while someone wanting cataract surgery only continues to wait.

Enhanced services
Allows patients to pay for enhanced or optional health services such as, choice in hospital rooms, enhanced medical goods and services, and the ability to purchase services not covered by a province's public health insurance system.

Private clinics charge substantial fees to individuals using their services for non–medically necessary procedures. A growing trend, particularly within the past five years, has seen physicians and specialists pooling their services to offer routine and specialized care via "health packages." Such groups (e.g., the Copeman Healthcare Centres in Vancouver, Calgary, and Edmonton) charge an enrolment fee and an annual membership fee. In return for fairly steep fees ($29,000 per year for the "elite" program at Copeman), clients receive the guarantee of prompt access to an impressive team of health care professionals, including family doctors, dietitians, psychologists, and specialists, along with an array of other services. Fees are generally tax deductible, and many of the services are covered by third-party insurance. Critics of this type of private health care point out that the fees are well out of reach of the average Canadian family.

To what extent a two-tier system will continue to develop in Canada is anyone's guess. The availability of private clinics and services suggests that, in one form or another, a two-tiered system will continue to exist.

Hospital Services

In the hospital setting, insured services for **inpatients** include standard hospital accommodation, meals, certain medications (in some regions, clients are asked to bring their own medications), operating room and delivery room services, anaesthetic facilities, diagnostic and laboratory services, routine medical and surgical supplies used for hospitalized clients, routine nursing care, and certain rehabilitative services (e.g., physiotherapy). Provincial and territorial plans do not cover private nursing care unless a doctor orders it, at which point it becomes medically necessary and is covered. Note that the cost of a private room may be covered by the provincial or territorial plan under some circumstances (e.g., for infection control, isolation purposes, or compassionate reasons).

Inpatient
A person admitted to, and staying in, a hospital for one or more nights.

Insured outpatient hospital services include emergency treatment, day surgery, and diagnostic and radiological procedures at a hospital or specialized clinic (e.g., outpatient cancer centre, orthopedic clinic). As well, most jurisdictions insure physiotherapy, occupational therapy, and respiratory therapy services for a limited period if deemed medically necessary.

Medical Services

Under the *Canada Health Act*, medically necessary care provided by a medical doctor (i.e., family doctor or specialist) is an insured service, with some conditions. In Ontario, for example, a person can claim coverage for only one visit to a medical doctor per day unless the physician submits the claim for special review.

Rules also govern insured services provided by a specialist. For instance, in most provinces and territories, a doctor must refer a client to a specialist; the client may see the specialist again for the same problem within a calendar year. After that, or for a new symptom or complaint, the family doctor must provide another referral. In most jurisdictions, when a client requests the opinion of a second specialist, the provincial or territorial plan will pay for that visit if the family doctor provides another referral request. After receiving a second opinion, however, the client would usually have to pay for further consultations even if referred by his or her family doctor.

Each province and territory generates its own list of insured services, which is reviewed periodically by the ministry or department of health and the province's or territory's medical association. At this time, some services may be delisted, and others added. Since "medically necessary" is subjective, these services vary from one jurisdiction to another. For example, having wax removed from one's ear is insured in British Columbia, but not in Nova Scotia (although it is covered for children). Ontario's provincial plan covers an annual checkup, but British Columbia's does not. In several provinces, a complete checkup is performed only in response to a symptom or complaint.

Doctors may choose to offer services that are not deemed medically necessary by their provincial or territorial health care plan. For these services, physicians may bill clients directly, or they may bill a third party—an insurance company, the Workplace Safety Insurance Board (WSIB), or an employer or other payer.

The amount a doctor charges for uninsured services depends on guidelines set out by his or her provincial or territorial medical association (Box 5.7). Since physicians are legally bound to inform clients about charges for uninsured services, price lists for such services are often posted in doctors' offices. As an alternative to charging clients each time an uninsured service is performed, some doctors use *block payments* or an *uninsured services plan*. Essentially, they charge the client or family an annual fee for any and all uninsured services that might be rendered during the year.

Box 5.7   Uninsured Chargeable Physician Services

- Telephone prescription renewal
- Travel advice
- Missed appointments
- Form completion (e.g., passport, driver or pilot fitness test)

- Back-to-work or back-to-school note

- Faxing or transfer of medical records

- Nonmedical TB skin testing

- Cosmetic procedures

- Uninsured vaccinations

- Telephone advice (dependent on practice guidelines)

Thinking It Through

Physicians are required to inform clients of the price of any procedure, assessment, or treatment not covered by their provincial or territorial plan before carrying out any such procedure. Some doctors use what is called a *block payment plan*, whereby clients pay a lump sum annually that covers any uninsured procedure the physician performs during the course of the year, including third-party or camp medicals and return-to-school or -work notes.

1. If you had undergone an uninsured treatment provided by a doctor but did not learn until after the treatment was completed that you were required to pay for it, what would you do?

2. Would you be more likely to opt for a block payment plan or a pay-as-you-go plan for uninsured services?

Ambulance Services

In most jurisdictions, either land and air ambulance services are under regional management and costs are shared with the provincial or territorial government, or these services are delivered privately through performance-based contracts. Because ambulance services are not addressed in the *Canada Health Act*, provinces and territories can establish their own guidelines, including fee schedules, for these services.

People using an ambulance even for medically necessary reasons may be responsible for a **co-payment** (Case Example 5.7). However, fees are not usually charged for transportation between hospitals—whether the destination hospital is within a short distance, in another part of the province, in another province altogether, or outside of the country—as long as the transfer is for

Co-payment
A predetermined dollar amount or percentage of the cost of a health care service or medication that an individual must pay.

medically necessary reasons (Case Example 5.8). Interfacility transfers (e.g., from one nursing home to another) usually require a co-payment. Most jurisdictions either reduce or eliminate the co-payment for low-income individuals and families.

In Ontario, the cost of using an ambulance is approximately $240, with the client's portion set at $45 (Ontario Ministry of Health and Long-Term Care, 2008). Nova Scotia's ambulance fees increased in April 2009 to approximately $135 for provincial residents; $672 for out-of-province Canadians; and $1009 for non-Canadians. Nova Scotia does not charge for interhospital transfer (Canadian Legal Information Institute, 2002). Newfoundland provides ambulance services for its residents at no charge. Yukon residents are eligible for ambulance or air medevac services only within the territory.

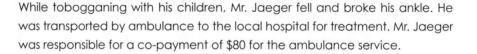

Case Example 5.7

While tobogganing with his children, Mr. Jaeger fell and broke his ankle. He was transported by ambulance to the local hospital for treatment. Mr. Jaeger was responsible for a co-payment of $80 for the ambulance service.

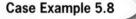

Case Example 5.8

When Anna Jaeger went into labour eight weeks before her due date, her parents brought her to Vancouver General Hospital. Anna was carrying twins, who would require intensive care accommodation once they were born. No neonatal ICU beds were available in British Columbia, but Ontario had space. Anna was transported by air ambulance to Women's College Hospital in Toronto, where she delivered two healthy baby girls. Two weeks later, Anna and her babies were returned to Vancouver General Hospital. The British Columbia medical services plan covered the entire cost of the round trip air ambulance because the province was unable to meet Anna's medical needs at home.

British Columbia recently changed ambulance co-payment fees to a flat rate ($80) regardless of distance travelled or means of travel (ground or air); the province also adjusts rates downward for low-income individuals. A person without insurance coverage in British Columbia would have to pay a staggering $2746/hour for an air ambulance (British Columbia Ministry of Health, 2007).

Insured Health Care Professionals Other Than Physicians

Some provinces and territories provide residents with limited insurance coverage for the services of health care professionals other than doctors. A monetary limit may be imposed per calendar year, or coverage may be provided only for lower-income households (Box 5.8). For example, Manitoba's residents receive partial coverage for up to 12 chiropractic adjustments per year. The covered portion increases for individuals living north of the fifty-third parallel (Manitoba Chiropractors' Association, n.d.). Saskatchewan and Alberta also partially insure chiropractic care. The British Columbia Medical Services Plan will pay $23 per visit for a total of 10 visits per year for chiropractic care, massage therapy, naturopathy, physical therapy, and nonsurgical podiatry care for eligible residents (i.e., those on premium assistance) (British Columbia Ministry of Housing and Social Development, 2008).

Box 5.8   **Coverage of Supplementary Services**

The provinces and territories provide varying degrees of coverage for optometric care. Ontario covers one eye examination yearly for individuals under 20 or over 65 years of age. Ontario residents with medical conditions requiring medically necessary eye examinations (e.g., diabetic retinopathy, macular degeneration) are insured for at least one assessment per year. In British Columbia, individuals under 18 and over 65 years of age are insured for routine (annual) eye examinations. Manitoba provides no coverage for routine eye exams. In Nova Scotia, children younger than 10 years of age and adults over 65 are eligible for eye examinations every two years. Newfoundland and Labrador covers those under 19 years of age or over 65 for an eye examination every 12 months. Those receiving social assistance who have a medical condition deemed to require close surveillance (e.g., diabetic retinopathy) may qualify for more extensive coverage.

Most provincial plans partially cover problems related to hearing loss. In most cases, the diagnosis of hearing loss is made by a specialist and is, therefore, covered by provincial and territorial health plans. Diagnostic testing done by independent audiologists, however, may not be covered by the provincial or territorial plan, although it may be covered by supplementary insurance. Some hearing aid providers will cover the cost of a hearing test if the client purchases a hearing aid from them. All jurisdictions have plans that cover (in part or full) the cost of designated hearing devices for those who cannot afford to purchase them.

Private carriers insure most dental care across Canada. Only dental surgical procedures performed in the hospital are insured under the provincial or territorial health plan. As previously noted, some jurisdictions will provide limited coverage for children of low-income families (e.g., the Healthy Kids program in British Columbia).

Extended Health Care Services

Long-term care homes offer 24-hour nursing care and support to individuals no longer able to live on their own. The terms *long-term care facility* and *old-age home* are often used interchangeably, but, in some provinces and territories, subtle differences may exist. For the most part, these facilities offer residents more intensive care than retirement homes provide. They may be owned and operated by private corporations (either profit or nonprofit), municipal councils, churches, or ethnic, cultural, or community groups. In most provinces and territories, these facilities are overseen by one or more pieces of legislation. In Nova Scotia, for example, nursing homes are under the governance of the *Homes for Special Care Act*. In Ontario, three acts—the *Aged and Rest Homes Act*, the *Nursing Home Act*, and the *Charitable Institutions Act*—were replaced by the *Long-Term Care Homes Act* in 2007.

The province or territory sets standards of care in long-term care facilities and performs regular inspections to ensure these standards are met. Long-term care facilities are encouraged to seek accreditation through Accreditation Canada (formerly known as the Canadian Council on Health Services Accreditation), an organization that conducts reviews on a three-year cycle. The Qmentum accreditation program introduced in 2008 has revised some assessment standards and added new ones, such as an improved survey process and more effective tools for measuring compliance. Assessments include reviews of client care, staff management, information management, administrative management, and partnerships. Accreditation reflects a level of transparency and shows the public that the facility meets national standards of care and operation. More details about Accreditation Canada can be found in the Web Resources at the end of this chapter.

Provincial and territorial governments design their own funding formulas for funding long-term care facilities. The funding of long-term care facilities is covered in more detail in Chapter 6.

Most provinces and territories offer a variety of other services:

- *Home care* helps individuals with basic personal care, meals, and household maintenance, allowing them to remain at home even once they find it difficult to care for themselves.

- *Adult day care programs* provide community day-activities as well as respite care and in-home support to individuals with disabilities.

- *Respite care*, which allows nonprofessional caregivers some relief from caring for disabled family members, is often offered in long-term care facilities or the equivalent for a designated time frame.

- *Assisted living accommodation* helps to keep a person in his or her home by providing individualized support and care as required.

- *Group homes* allow persons with disabilities to live in an environment that provides supervision and assistance.

- *Hospice care* is provided in a home-like setting for those unable or unwilling to die at home. Individuals receive nursing and medical care, pain management, counselling, and other supportive care needed while dying.

- *Palliative care* provides care, medication, and some medical supplies for individuals dying at home.

Assistive Devices and Medical Products

Those in need of but unable to afford health care products and assistive devices—mobility devices (e.g., wheelchairs, walkers, motorized carts), prosthetic devices (e.g., post-mastectomy products, artificial limbs), bathing and toileting aids, and home care beds and accessories—can receive supplemental coverage; however, the coverage for such items varies across jurisdictions.

Alberta offers two income-based programs: the Alberta Aids to Daily Living (AADL) and the Dental Assistance for Seniors programs. The AADL offers eligible Albertans with a long-term disability, chronic illness, or terminal illness financial support for the purchase of medical equipment and supplies. The dental assistance program provides required dental care to low- and moderate-income seniors to a maximum of $5000 for eligible services every five years. Other supplementary services, including audiology, physiotherapy, occupational therapy, and speech therapy, are delivered through RHAs, which assess eligibility and prioritize referrals based on service availability within each community.

In British Columbia, the Pharmacare Program, run by the province's RHAs, covers medical devices and equipment for designated population groups. A physician must make a referral, outlining the client's medical eligibility criteria for the program.

Manitoba offers similar assistance with medical supplies and assistive devices, also delivered through RHAs.

DRUG PLANS

Medications consume a huge portion of the health care dollars spent across Canada, second only to hospital spending. The enormity of this expenditure stems, in part, from the use of newer, more expensive drugs and an aging population with multiple health problems who are prescribed an astonishing array of medications.

As is the case with dental care, the majority of Canadians have private or employer-sponsored insurance plans with drug benefits. Both types of plans may insure only certain medications. Publicly funded drug benefit packages (discussed below), unlike private insurance plans, have co-payments or **deductibles**

Deductible
The amount of money that an individual or family is required to pay toward health care costs before an insurance plan will take over.

(usually percentage-based) that beneficiaries pay, depending on their income and drug costs.

Private insurance plans require beneficiaries to pay **dispensing fees** themselves. For individuals on a public drug plan, the dispensing fee is either calculated as a percentage of the prescription cost or set at a flat rate, depending on the plan.

To qualify for provincial or territorial drug benefits, an individual must first apply for assistance. For example, residents in Nova Scotia, British Columbia, Manitoba, and Yukon apply to Pharmacare; in Ontario, to the Ontario Drug Benefit Program or the Trillium Drug Program; and in Saskatchewan, to the Drug Plan and Extended Benefits Branch of Saskatchewan Health. The organization would then assess the applicant's annual income, considering how many people that income supports, and calculate how much coverage the family should get for eligible prescription drugs.

Most jurisdictions require the family or individual to pay a predetermined deductible for prescription drugs. Once the deductible is reached, the public plan will pay a percentage of the beneficiary's eligible drug costs. Some jurisdictions also set a maximum amount or a "cap" that the family or person must pay, after which point, the plan will cover 100% of the drug costs.

Some plans (both private and public) will cover only drugs prescribed from a **formulary list**. Formulary lists, although they include hundreds of drugs, are limited, containing, for the most part, cheaper, generic versions of common drugs. Some brand-name drugs may be covered, but only if there is not a less expensive alternative. Many combination drugs, time-release drugs, and so-called "lifestyle" drugs (e.g., sildenafil [Viagra], used for erectile dysfunction; orlistat [Xenical, Alli], used to treat obesity) are not available on most formularies. However, most plans will cover a nonformulary drug if the generic drug does not produce the desired therapeutic effect or causes adverse side effects (Case Example 5.9). Doctors may also seek approval to prescribe (and have covered) a nonformulary drug. Many private insurance plans offer an "open access" plan that will insure all prescription medications approved by Health Canada that are prescribed on an outpatient basis.

Dispensing fee
A service fee charged by a pharmacy for dispensing a prescription medication (i.e., reading the prescription and preparing the medication for the client).

Formulary list
A list of prescription medications (often generic brands) selected for coverage by a public or private health insurance plan.

Case Example 5.9

Quang Wong is receiving assistance through Pharmacare because he does not yet have a job. He has developed an irregular heartbeat, and his doctor put him on aspirin for its anticoagulant effects (i.e., ability to prevent blood clots). Within days, Quang developed a pain in his stomach and other gastrointestinal (GI) symptoms. The doctor decides that the aspirin is causing the GI upset and wants to switch Quang to clopidogrel bisulfate (Plavix)—another drug to prevent clots. This drug is not on the Nova Scotia drug formulary list. The doctor fills out a special request form so that Pharmacare will cover the drug. He must note the **drug identification number (DIN)** and explain the situation.

Each formulary includes a "limited use" list (LU), which lists drugs deemed unsuitable or too expensive to be on the formulary list. These drugs may, however, have therapeutic benefits in special circumstances—for example, an antibiotic that can treat resistant bacteria such as **vancomycin-resistant** *Staphylococcus aureus* **(VRSA)**, **vancomycin-resistant** *Enterococcus* **(VRE)**, and **methicillin-resistant** *Staphylococcus aureus* **(MRSA)**.

Some drugs are not on either the formulary or the LU list. The physician must seek special permission to have these drugs covered by a publicly funded drug benefit plan. Recently, Ontario implemented an Exceptional Access Program, which aims to provide easier and faster access to drugs that are not on the formulary.

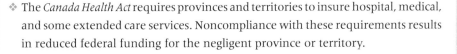

SUMMARY

❖ The *Canada Health Act* requires provinces and territories to insure hospital, medical, and some extended care services. Noncompliance with these requirements results in reduced federal funding for the negligent province or territory.

❖ Supplementary services are offered at the discretion of the province or territory. All jurisdictions provide some form of benefits for drugs, assistive devices, medical supplies, home care, ambulance services, and access to select nonphysician health care professionals. Provincial and territorial governments make many of these services available at no charge, or with fees adjusted to the family's or individual's income, to seniors, low-income families, and select population groups.

❖ Third-party and private insurance plays a significant role in covering supplemental benefits for most Canadians. Many people receive insurance through employment benefit packages.

Drug identification number (DIN)
A unique number assigned to each medication approved by Health Canada for use in Canada.

Vancomycin-resistant *Staphylococcus aureus* **(VRSA)**
A strain of *Staphylococcus aureus* that has become resistant to the antibiotic vancomycin.

Vancomycin-resistant *Enterococcus* **(VRE)**
A form of the bacteria *Enterococcus* that has become resistant to many antibiotics, including vancomycin—one of the most effective antibiotics to treat enterococcal infections.

Methicillin-resistant *Staphylococcus aureus* **(MRSA)**
A strain of *Staphylococcus aureus* that has become resistant to the antibiotic methicillin.

REVIEW QUESTIONS

1. What health care services are offered under the *Canada Health Act*?

2. What body or bodies administer the provincial or territorial health care plan in your province or territory?

3. What is meant by *regionalization of health care services*?

4. How can a drug formulary list reduce the cost of insured drugs for a province or territory?

5. Which provinces and territories charge health care premiums?

6. Which provinces require a three-month wait before a newcomer to the province is covered by health insurance?

7. Explain the *reciprocal agreement*.

DISCUSSION QUESTIONS

1. Explain the differences among primary, secondary, and tertiary health care. Describe these services in your province or territory.

2. Review the organizational structure of the ministry or department of health in your province or territory. If an organizational plan is available, use it as a guide. Briefly explain the function of each department.

3. Review Case Examples 5.3 and 5.4. What process would the Jaegers or the Wongs have to follow to apply for a health card in your province or territory? How long will they have to wait before they are eligible for provincial or territorial coverage?

4. What do you pay for health premiums in your province or territory? If your jurisdiction charges no premiums, explain how health care is funded.

5. Describe the structure and function of regional health authorities or the equivalent in your province or territory.

6. Should Canadians have the right to spend their own money to jump the queue and have medical or surgical services performed in their home province in a timely manner? After all, they can quite legally go abroad to access these services. Defend your stand on this issue.

WEB RESOURCES

Accreditation Canada

http://www.accreditation-canada.ca

Accreditation Canada, formerly known as the Canadian Council on Health Services Accreditation, is an independent, national, nonprofit organization that assesses long-term care facilities. Its accreditation process consists of a self-assessment, an on-site survey, and follow-up action for improvements. Accreditation Canada has developed a set of standards it calls "Patient

Safety Goals and Required Organizational Practices," which have been an integral part of the accreditation program since January 2006.

Health Canada First Nations and Inuit Health Branch

http://www.hc-sc.gc.ca/fniah-spnia/index-eng.php

In recognition of the unique status and needs of First Nations and Inuit peoples in Canada, the federal government established the First Nations and Inuit Health

WEB RESOURCES

Branch (FNIHB) within Health Canada. The branch works closely with First Nations and Inuit organizations and communities to carry out initiatives aimed at helping people keep healthy and at preventing chronic and infectious diseases.

Health Canada
http://www.hc-sc.gc.ca

Health Canada is the federal department responsible for helping Canadians maintain and improve their health. It partners with other agencies and health care organizations to ensure its efforts meet the needs of all Canadians.

Health Council of Canada
http://www.healthcouncilcanada.ca

Canada's first ministers established the Health Council of Canada in their 2003 Accord on Health Care Renewal. It is funded by the Government of Canada, reports to the Canadian public, and operates as a nonprofit agency that informs Canadians on health care matters while promoting accountability and transparency.

Provincial and Territorial Health Departments
In Canada, the administration and delivery of health care services is the responsibility of each province or territory, guided by the provisions of the *Canada Health Act*. The provinces and territories fund their health care services with assistance from the federal government.

- Alberta Health and Wellness
  http://www.health.alberta.ca/

- British Columbia Ministry of Health Services
  http://www.gov.bc.ca/health/

- Manitoba Healthy Living
  http://www.gov.mb.ca/healthyliving/

- Newfoundland and Labrador Health and Community Services http://www.health.gov.nl.ca/health/

- New Brunswick Department of Health
  http://www.gnb.ca/0051/index-e.asp

- Northwest Territories Department of Health and Social Services http://www.hlthss.gov.nt.ca/

- Nova Scotia Department of Health
  http://www.gov.ns.ca/health/

- Nunavut Department of Health and Social Services
  http://www.gov.nu.ca/health/

- Ontario Ministry of Health and Long-Term Care
  http://www.health.gov.on.ca/

- Prince Edward Island Department of Health
  http://www.gov.pe.ca/health/index.php3

- Quebec Santé et Services sociaux
  http://www.msss.gouv.qc.ca/en

- Saskatchewan Health http://www.health.gov.sk.ca/

- Yukon Health and Social Services
  http://www.hss.gov.yk.ca/

REFERENCES

British Columbia Ministry of Health. (2007). *Flat rate benefits patients travelling longer distances*. Retrieved May 29, 2009, from http://www.bcas.ca/assets/News/PDFs/2007/0912-nr-flat-rate-benefits-patients.pdf?zoom_highlight=fees+changed#search=%22fees%20changed%22

British Columbia Ministry of Housing and Social Development. (2008). *Ministry of Housing and Social Development BC employment and assistance rate tables: Health supplements and programs*. Retrieved May 29, 2009, from http://www.hsd.gov.bc.ca/mhr/hsp.htm

Canada Health Act. R.S.C., c. C-6 (1985).

Canadian Legal Information Institute. (2002). *Ambulance Fee Regulations*, N.S. Reg. 133/2002. Retrieved May 29, 2009, from http://www.canlii.org/ns/laws/regu/2002r.133/20080215/whole.html

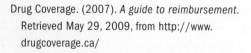

REFERENCES

Drug Coverage. (2007). *A guide to reimbursement.* Retrieved May 29, 2009, from http://www.drugcoverage.ca/

Government of Newfoundland and Labrador. (2008). *Department of Finance backgrounder: Budget 2008 tax and fee measures.* Retrieved May 29, 2009, from http://www.releases.gov.nl.ca/releases/2008/fin/0429n03bk1.htm

Health Canada. (2004). *British Columbia: Provincial submission to the Canada Health Act annual report 2005–2006.* Retrieved May 29, 2009, from http://www.hc-sc.gc.ca/hcs-sss/medi-assur/cha-lcs/pt-plans-bc-eng.php

Health Canada. (2009). *Health care system. Page 1– Canada Health Act annual report 2007–2008.* Retrieved May 29, 2009, from http://www.hc-sc.gc.ca/hcs-sss/pubs/cha-lcs/2008-cha-lcs-ar-ra/page1-eng.php

HRinfodesk. (2009). *Payroll rates—Quick reference, Table 11.* Retrieved May 29, 2009, from http://www.hrinfodesk.com/preview.asp?article=8453#tableofcontent

Manitoba Chiropractors' Association. (n.d.) *Chiropractic health care coverage.* Retrieved May 29, 2009, from http://www.mbchiro.org/about_chiro/coverage.html

Northwest Territories Finance. (2009). *Payroll tax/information for employers.* Retrieved May 29, 2009, from http://www.fin.gov.nt.ca/taxation/payroll/index.htm

Ontario Ministry of Health and Long-Term Care. (2008). *OHIP: Ambulance services billing.* Retrieved May 29, 2009, from http://www.health.gov.on.ca/english/public/pub/ohip/amb.html

Public Works and Government Services Canada. (2008). *Information notice to employees: Tax changes—Effective July 1, 2004.* Retrieved May 29, 2009, from http://www.tpsgc-pwgsc.gc.ca/remuneration-compensation/dr-cd/dr-cd-2004-008-avis-notice-eng.html

The Dollars and "Sense" of Health Care Funding

KEY TERMS

Accord, p. 189

Active ingredients, p. 206

Capitation-based funding, p. 210

Electronic health
record (EHR), p. 215

Empirical studies, p. 202

Laparoscopic surgery, p. 199

Nursing home, p. 212

Organisation for Economic
Co-operation and Development
(OECD), p. 209

Renal dialysis, p. 197

Thinking It Through

Before you begin reading this chapter, write down—even if it is just a guess—what you think Canada spends on health care in one year and how much you think a visit to your family doctor for an intermediate assessment (for example, for an earache, a sore throat, or a cold) might cost. Next, write down how much you think a knee replacement, a hip replacement, and an appendectomy might cost. Keep these numbers handy to compare with figures you will see later in this chapter, and see the "Conclusion" section at the end of the chapter for the true costs of these services.

Can you imagine going to the doctor for an ear infection and having the administrative assistant ask for cash or a credit card to pay for the visit? Or a parent or aunt or uncle having cardiac bypass surgery or a hip replacement and being sent an invoice? Remember that, in addition to these procedures, the client would need a preoperative physical examination, blood work, and perhaps an X-ray, an MRI, an arteriogram, or a CT scan. He or she would have to pay for the hospital stay, tests, nursing care, and supportive care (e.g., physiotherapy, respiratory therapy)—and would even be charged for the tray and equipment used to remove the sutures and the bandages used on the wound. What would you do if you needed such a procedure and knew it would cost you thousands of dollars?

Health care is free, right? A common and dangerous belief, this idea contributes to the overuse of the health care system and sends the cost of health care soaring. Canadians value their health care system highly. It gives them a sense of pride and security despite the cutbacks, the shortages of family doctors and hospital beds, and the long waits for specialists and surgeries. When they are sick, they seek care, present their health card, and, although they may have to wait, they ultimately receive the medical attention they need. No money comes out of their pockets. Unfortunately, many Canadians believe that because they do not have to shell out money at the point of service or pay a bill at the end of the month, health care is free.

The reality is that health care costs taxpayers billions of dollars each year. In fact, in 2008, it set us back an estimated $172 billion—an average of $5200 for each Canadian. This chapter examines the actual cost of health care and how health care is funded. Remember that the numerous statistics and dollar values presented are approximate because costs change yearly, monthly, sometimes even daily.

This chapter also looks at the cost of health care in a general sense, considering different types of service. It examines hospital expenses relative to the services offered and steps that hospitals have taken to reduce costs. The chapter also considers the cost of other sectors within the health care industry (e.g., doctors, community-based services, private health care).

LEVELS OF HEALTH CARE FUNDING

Health care in Canada is funded, for the most part, by the federal, provincial, territorial, and municipal governments through a blend of personal and corporate taxes, and by Workers' Compensation Boards. Some provinces also use revenue from sales taxes and lotteries for health care. Although not mandated by the *Canada Health Act*, British Columbia and Ontario require eligible residents to pay health care premiums (see Chapter 5). At the community level, many volunteer organizations (e.g., hospital auxiliaries, Rotary Clubs, Kinsmen, and Rebecca Lodges) also raise money for local hospitals to support such initiatives as expansion, updating facilities, and purchasing equipment. Often the provincial, territorial, or municipal government will match funds raised or a portion thereof. The Canadian Institute for Health Information (2008e) estimates health care spending to be a 30/70 mix, with 30% coming out of consumers' pockets and through private insurance. That leaves 70% of the cost of health care to come from public health plans.

According to Dr. Albert Schumacher, former president of the Canadian Medical Association, an estimated 75% of the health care services funded publicly are delivered privately (Canadian Broadcasting Company [CBC], 2006), including many home care services, ambulance costs (with some exceptions), and uninsured hospital services, such as preferred accommodation with television, several lab tests and vaccinations, and services delivered by many family doctors. Recognizing which services are privately delivered but publicly funded can be difficult but is important. When you go to see your family doctor for a health complaint, to a lab for blood work, or to a radiology clinic for a bone scan, you are, much of the time, using privately owned services operating on a for-profit basis. Family doctors, unless salaried, operate a private business even though their services are paid for by your provincial or territorial plan. Dr. Schumacher's 75% figure also includes a percentage of dental services, drugs, and much of the cost of the country's long-term care.

The provincial and territorial governments will probably never agree with the federal government about how much money it contributes to the cost of health care—the amount the provinces and territories claim to receive is invariably less than what the federal government claims to give them. Currently, the provinces and territories claim that the federal government contributes approximately 16 cents on the dollar, compared with 50 cents on the dollar four decades ago. The federal government, however, denies this calculation and presents different figures using its own accounting system (Health Canada, 2004).

The exact dollar figure that the federal government transfers to the provinces and territories remains a mystery. The federal government cannot dictate specifically how this money is spent, although most federal transfers must remain within the realm of health care services. For example, Saskatchewan may choose to fund a certain portion of a drug plan, while New Brunswick may have different formulas or fund a drug plan differently. The province or territory will usually base its funding on the needs of its population.

The amount of money spent on health care at the provincial and territorial level is also difficult to determine because of the complexity of the federal government's transfer payments, which are made in the form of both cash and tax points. Tax points replace actual cash transfers of money. The federal government may reduce the amount of income tax charged to a province or territory, which, in turn, increases the province's or territory's income tax base by the same amount. The federal government calls this "tax room." The tax points thereby surrendered by the federal government can be applied to personal or corporate income tax by the province or territory. The total taxation amount does not change; the only difference is which level of government levies the tax and collects the revenue.

Federal health transfer payment amounts are calculated using a complex formula and distributed through the following five main transfer models:

1. **The Territorial Financing Formula**. The federal government uses the Territorial Financing Formula to calculate money given to the territorial governments for public services. This money—allotted to these jurisdictions because of their unique geography, population distribution, and related high cost of delivering health care and other public services—constitutes over

60% of the total monetary resources in Yukon and the Northwest Territories and over 85% in Nunavut.

2. **Equalization Payments**. Some provinces and territories have more money than others and thus can provide more public services to their residents. Provinces and territories with less money receive equalization payments from the federal government to allow them to offer their residents services similar to those available in richer jurisdictions (Table 6.1). A needy jurisdiction will receive the difference between its *fiscal capacity* (i.e., its ability to generate income) and the *10-province standard* (i.e., the national average). Without equalization payments, these provinces and territories would have to raise their taxes significantly to generate revenue.

In 2009–10, Ontario received its first equalization payment since the program formally began in 1957. In total, the province will get an estimated $347 million, distributed as 12 payments over the fiscal year. Exempt in 2009–10 are British Columbia, Alberta, Saskatchewan, and Newfoundland and Labrador.

Table 6.1	Equalization Payments to the Provinces

Receiving Provinces ($ millions)

Year	Prince Edward Island	Nova Scotia*	New Brunswick	Quebec	Ontario	Manitoba
2008–9	322	1571	1584	8028	0	2063
2009–10	340	1571	1689	8355	347	2063

* Includes both equalizations and offsets.

Source: Department of Finance Canada. (2008). *Canada's finance ministers meet to discuss global financial crisis.* Retrieved May 29, 2009, from http://www.fin.gc.ca/news08/08-085e.html

In the **News**	**A Shift in the Balance of Equalization Payments**

In 2008, federal Finance Minister Jim Flaherty announced a groundbreaking change to the list of provinces that would be receiving equalization payments (the so-called have-not provinces). For the first time in the 51-year history of the equalization program, Ontario would receive an equalization payment. A weakened economy due, in large part, to a struggling manufacturing sector

Continued on next page

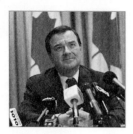

was to blame. Newfoundland and Labrador, on the other hand, would, for the first time, *not* be receiving an equalization payment thanks to an economy strengthened by healthy oil revenues. "Newfoundland and Labrador is now a have province. That's a momentous day for the people of this province," said Premier Danny Williams.

Sources: Canadian Broadcasting Corporation. (2008, November 3). Ontario to receive $347M in equalization: Flaherty. *CBC News*. Retrieved May 29, 2009, from http://www.cbc.ca/canada/story/2008/11/03/flaherty-ministers.html#socialcomments; Canadian Broadcasting Corporation. (2008, November 3). Have-not is no more: NL off equalization. *CBC News*. Retrieved May 29, 2009, from http://www.cbc.ca/canada/newfoundland-labrador/story/2008/11/03/have-not.html

Photo credit: Tara Walton/GetStock.com.

A new version of equalization payments was established in the Constitution in 1982 (Box 6.1). The provinces and territories are free to determine how they will spend their equalization payments; many use this money, at least in part, for health care (Department of Finance Canada, 2009b).

Box 6.1   Equalization Payments Embedded in the Canadian Constitution

"Parliament and the Government of Canada are committed to the principle of making equalization payments to ensure that provincial governments have sufficient revenues to provide reasonably comparable levels of public services at reasonably comparable levels of taxation."

Source: Department of Justice Canada. (1982). *Constitution Act, 1982*. Subsection 36(2). Retrieved May 29, 2009, from http://lois.justice.gc.ca/en/const/annex_e.html

---

3. **The Canada Health Transfer**. The Canada Health Transfer (from the federal to the provincial and territorial governments) consists of tax points and cash. Unlike equalization payments, this money must be used on health care. The 2004 Health Accord provided legislation that determined the cash amounts to be transferred to each of the provinces and territories until 2014. Alberta and Ontario receive the least amounts because of their higher tax bases.

4. **The Canada Social Transfer**. The Canada Social Transfer provides funding to the provinces and territories, through cash and tax points, for social programs, child care and early childhood development and learning programs, and postsecondary education. The money must be applied to

these designated areas. Money transferred through the Canada Social Transfer will increase by 3% annually (referred to by the government as an "automatic escalator") until 2014, at which time the legislation will be renewed (Department of Finance Canada, 2009a).

5. **The Health Reform Transfer**. The Health Reform Transfer, implemented in 2003, provides additional funds for primary health care reform, home care services, and the catastrophic drug cost coverage recommended by the Romanow Report (see Chapter 3). The funds used for drug coverage are meant to help Canadians without insurance coverage pay for costly medications.

Prior to April 2004, the Canada Social Transfer and the Canada Health Transfer together composed the Canada Health and Social Transfer, a single transfer payment that paid for both health and education. The transfer was separated into two transfers to provide greater transparency regarding the allocation of funds.

NEGOTIATING FUNDS: HEALTH ACCORDS

Bargaining for health care funding is ongoing among the provinces, territories, and federal government. Needs are studied and analyzed, proposals are made, and agreements, often referred to as **accords**, are signed.

One of the more recent and most productive of these first ministers' bargaining meetings occurred in September 2000 and resulted in the expenditure of $800 million over six years, ending in 2006, to improve the delivery of primary care services, to reduce wait times, and to ease the volume of clients in and demands on emergency rooms. At the same time, the federal government vowed to pay out an additional $2.3 billion more over five years, with $500 million earmarked for developing health care information technology across Canada, and $1 billion, used over a two-year period, to update and buy costly medical equipment (Table 6.2).

In 2004, the first ministers reached an agreement to introduce $41.3 billion in federal funding to the provinces and territories over 10 years, beginning in the 2004–5 fiscal year (Department of Finance Canada, 2008). This money was promised, in part, to address the following recommendations from the Romanow Report:

- Improve health care services in rural and remote communities
- Shorten wait times for diagnostic services
- Improve home care services (e.g., nursing care, physiotherapy, home support)

Accord
An agreement between two or more parties.

Table 6.2	Approximate Cost of Select Diagnostic Equipment in Canada

Equipment	Cost
MRI machine	$3 million
CT scanner	$1.7 million
Single-plane cardiac catheterization lab (to view blocked vessels to the heart)	$1.3 million
Linear accelerator (used for cancer treatment)	$3.5 million

Source: Canadian Institute for Health Information. (2008). *Medical imaging in Canada, 2007*. Retrieved May 29, 2009, from http://secure.cihi.ca/cihiweb/products/MIT_2007_e.pdf

- Initiate primary health care reform (e.g., family health groups)
- Implement an electronic medical records system

FEDERAL GOVERNMENT COSTS FOR DIRECT HEALTH CARE

As discussed in Chapters 3 and 4, under the Canadian Constitution, the federal government is responsible for direct health care services for certain groups: First Nations living on reserves, Inuit and Innu populations, veterans, inmates of federal penitentiaries, members of the Royal Canadian Mounted Police (RCMP) and the Canadian Armed Forces, and refugee claimants. Refugee claimants are citizens of other countries who arrive in Canada claiming refugee status because they need protection from a threat or danger in their country of origin. Until a refugee claim is settled, the federal government retains responsibility for the claimant's health care needs.

The federal government spends over $5.6 billion annually on direct health care services—and this amount increases every year (CIHI, 2008e).

PROVINCIAL AND TERRITORIAL COSTS FOR DIRECT HEALTH CARE

Canada's total health care spending was projected to reach $171.9 billion in 2008, a $10.3 billion, or 6.4%, increase over 2007. Spending on health care in recent years has grown faster than the Canadian economy, and 2008 marked the twelfth year that health care spending outpaced inflation and population growth. In fact, in 2008, health care spending was projected to reach 10.7% of gross domestic product (GDP), the highest percentage ever reached (CIHI, 2008e).

Health expenditures per capita (i.e., per person) vary across the provinces and territories (Table 6.3). This variation can be explained by several factors, including differences in services offered. For example, chiropractic care is covered only in Alberta, Manitoba, and Saskatchewan, and British Columbia covers acupuncture as a supplementary benefit. Expenditures also depend on which services each province or territory considers medically necessary. For instance, male babies may be circumcised under provincial or territorial insurance in one jurisdiction but not in another, and some laboratory tests may be covered in some provinces or territories but not others.

Table 6.3	Provincial and Territorial Spending per Capita: 2008 (Projected)		
Province/Territory	**Amount**	**Province/Territory**	**Amount**
Alberta	$5730	Ontario	$5229
British Columbia	$5093	Prince Edward Island	$5182
Manitoba	$5555	Quebec	$4653
New Brunswick	$5280	Saskatchewan	$5393
Newfoundland and Labrador	$5395	Northwest Territories	$9652
		Nunavut	$11,379
Nova Scotia	$5451	Yukon	$7837

Source: Canadian Institute for Health Information. (2008). *National health expenditure trends, 1975–2008.* Ottawa: Author.

Other factors, such as population distribution, geography, and the age and health of a population, affect spending, as well. Delivering health care to sparsely populated regions can be more expensive than to urban settings.

In 2007, the provinces and territories spent, on average, 39.2% of their total program expenditures on health care (CIHI, 2008e). That is, over one-third of the money available for all provincial and territorial spending went toward health care—and yet the prevailing thought is that Canada needs to spend more money on health care.

INDIRECT COSTS OF POOR HEALTH

Unsurprisingly, governments at all levels want to find ways to reduce costs, while still providing high-quality health care. The burden of poor health on the Canadian economy includes not only the direct costs of treating sick people but also the indirect costs associated with loss of productivity and earnings while a person is incapacitated. This economic loss costs Canada billions of dollars annually.

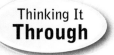

Thinking It
Through

Health care expenditures rise each year in order to meet demands.

Using the latest statistics available, calculate the annual expenditure for health care in your jurisdiction and determine the change from the previous statistics available. Do you think the change makes sense?

MAJOR AREAS OF HEALTH CARE EXPENDITURE

Hospitals, drugs, and physicians represent the three top health care expenditures. The total health care budget is broken down in Figure 6.1.

HOSPITALS

More health care dollars are spent in the hospital sector than in any other sector. In 2007, hospital spending amounted to nearly 28.4% of the combined federal

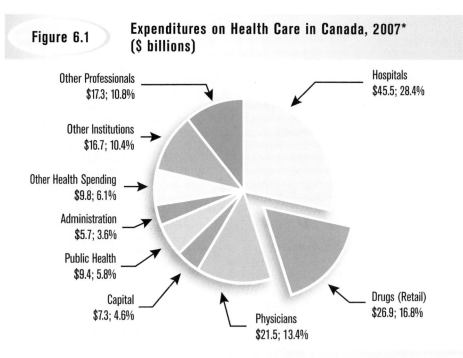

Figure 6.1   **Expenditures on Health Care in Canada, 2007***
($ billions)

Other Professionals $17.3; 10.8%
Other Institutions $16.7; 10.4%
Other Health Spending $9.8; 6.1%
Administration $5.7; 3.6%
Public Health $9.4; 5.8%
Capital $7.3; 4.6%
Physicians $21.5; 13.4%
Hospitals $45.5; 28.4%
Drugs (Retail) $26.9; 16.8%

*Forecast.
Source: Canadian Institute for Health Information. (2008). *Drug expenditure in Canada, 1985 to 2007.* Ottawa: Author, p. 5. Retrieved May 29, 2009, from http://secure.cihi.ca/cihiweb/products/Drug_Expenditure_in_Canada_1985_2007_e.pdf

and provincial health care budget. Nevertheless, this is a drop of nearly 15% from what was spent on hospitals in the mid-1970s (CIHI, 2008e).

Provincial and territorial government expenditures account for 90% of hospital income. In other words, hospitals receive most of their money from government. Direct payments from the private sector and from insurance companies account for the remaining 10%. Hospital income from individuals and insurance companies constitutes about 3.5% of revenue; the remaining 6.5% comes from nonclient sources, such as food services, parking, rentals (e.g., office space rented to doctors), and donations from volunteer and community organizations (CIHI, 2008e).

A number of different types of health care facilities exist, including general and acute care facilities, nursing homes, chronic care facilities, rehabilitation centres, and psychiatric hospitals. All are publicly funded, in part or in whole. Some hospitals treat certain conditions (e.g., Princess Margaret Hospital in Toronto specializes in cancer treatment) or specific age groups (e.g., Vancouver's B.C. Children's Hospital and Sunny Hill Health Centre for Children). Other hospitals (e.g., long-term care facilities) may be covered only in part by provincial or territorial insurance, in which case, clients pay a portion of the services they use. Psychiatric hospitals, as well as the services of psychiatrists, however, are fully covered in all provinces.

Problems facing hospitals, communities, and individuals include cuts to services, reductions in hospital beds, closures or merging of hospitals, rationalization (i.e., improving efficiency) of services, insufficient and demoralized staff, and long wait lists for surgery, related tests, and admission to hospitals. The following sections will examine how hospitals are funded, how they operate, why operational costs are high, and what is being done to lower costs.

Hospital Funding Mechanisms

The provincial or territorial ministry or department of health provides funds to hospitals to deliver services to the community. The hospital is then expected to operate as a business, ending the fiscal year with a balanced budget.

The terms under which this money is given vary, depending on the funding model the hospital functions under. Currently, hospitals in several provinces and territories are working closely with regional health authorities to revise funding models to increase efficiencies.

In the case of *block funding*, popular since the 1970s, a hospital's funding amount is determined by its previous year's expenditures.

In the case of *line-by-line funding*, still popular in British Columbia and New Brunswick, the costs of specific services and equipment within a hospital, referred to as *line items* or *inputs,* are itemized, and the hospital receives the sum needed for each service.

Service-based funding (also called the *case-mix approach*) is gaining popularity (Ontario hospitals are reviewing this model). The types of cases treated and the volume of clients seen provide the foundation for an analysis of expenditure needs. Clients who suffer similar types of medical problems and undergo similar treatments are grouped using a formula; the cost of their treatments and services is estimated; and the amount of funding the hospital receives relates to how many clients it treats requiring each combination of services. The funding is then provided in the form of a global budget (i.e., an annual lump sum of money). Many hospitals adopting this funding approach also use line-by-line funding. For example, a hospital would receive money to complete a designated number of hip or knee replacements.

The *population-based funding model,* used by Alberta and Saskatchewan for several years, grants hospitals money based on demographics (e.g., clients' ages, gender, socioeconomic status). In all, more than 100 different individual prototypes exist based on these criteria, with varying amounts awarded depending on location and on how many clients fall into certain categories. For example, a hospital in an area with a large population of older adults may receive more money than one with a mainly younger clientele, and since lower socioeconomic groups require more health care services, hospitals catering to clients in that category receive more funding. The hospital's size and location, as well as the services it offers are also factored into the budget.

After completing its budget, the hospital assesses its financial needs, prepares documentation, and negotiates with the minister of health for appropriate funding. To facilitate these activities, the hospital must track the expenses of all departments and services.

You may have heard or read media reports about whether a hospital is in the black (i.e., posting a surplus) or in the red (i.e., posting a deficit) at the end of the fiscal year. A hospital in the red must look for ways to reduce costs. It must critically examine the services it offers, the cost of each, and determine where cuts can be made. A hospital may have to reduce services and staff, close beds, decrease operating time, or do all of these things to keep within its budget. Under certain circumstances, the ministry or department of health may grant extra money to hospitals with budget shortfalls.

The Cost of Hospital Care

Hospitals offer diagnostic tests, treatment, and client care for a variety of illnesses and diseases. More than half of hospital expenditures in 2005–6 were incurred to diagnose and treat—in order of expense—cardiovascular disease, gastrointestinal

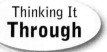

Thinking It Through

Many Canadians believe health care is free, not realizing that they pay for health care services with their tax dollars.

1. If people were given a receipt showing the cost of each doctor's visit, hospital stay, and services received, do you think they might use health care services more prudently?

2. Do you think that being unaware of the costs of services contributes to the attitude that health care is free?

disorders, respiratory illnesses, musculoskeletal issues, connective tissue disorders, and pregnancy and childbirth (CIHI, 2007a).

On a per client basis, however, this cost ranking changes. In the same time period, cardiovascular diseases (e.g., congestive heart failure, stroke) ranked first among hospital expenditures, with an average cost of $16,100 per client, followed by burns, at an average cost of $14,100, and musculoskeletal disorders, at an average cost of $6400 (CIHI, 2007a). Pregnancy and childbirth, the leading cause of hospital admissions for women of childbearing age, costs $2300 per person on average, although the cost varies with the nature of delivery. An uncomplicated vaginal delivery costs just under $2000, while a Caesarean section costs just over $4000 (CIHI, 2007a).

Many Canadians remain unaware of how much the government pays for various procedures. Table 6.4 provides a list of the costs of some of the more common procedures and conditions for which individuals are admitted to hospital.

The Cost of Hospital Services

The staff and infrastructure needed to provide hospital care incur significant costs. Nursing for inpatient services imposes the greatest cost, at 37% of a hospital's entire budget in 2005–6. Diagnostic and therapeutic services are next, composing 21% of a hospital's budget in 2005–6 (CIHI, 2008a). You might think that medical staff—doctors, residents, interns—would represent the highest costs, but most of these individuals operate independently of the hospital, although some medical staff members may be on contract or in salaried positions.

Administration and Support Services

Every hospital has administrative expenses, such as human resources (e.g., clinical secretaries, admission clerks), information technology (e.g.,

Table 6.4 — Average Cost of Different Procedures and Conditions for Inpatients, 2004–2005

Procedure/Condition	Average Cost per Hospitalization ($)
Normal newborn singleton delivered vaginally	610
Oral cavity/pharynx intervention	1615
Symptom of digestive system	2097
Poisoning/toxic effect of drug	2413
Fever	2487
Seizure disorder	2495
Chemotherapy/radiotherapy session neoplasm	2830
Laparoscopic cholecystectomy (gallbladder removal)	2946
Lower urinary tract infection	3503
Cellulitis	3626
Diabetes	3661
Hysterectomy (no diagnosis of cancer)	3767
Non-extensive burn	4724
Chronic obstructive pulmonary disease	4810
Depressive episode without electroconvulsive therapy	5043
Heart failure without cardiac catheter	5049
Unilateral knee replacement	7652

Source: Canadian Institute for Health Information. (2007). *Health care in Canada 2007*. Ottawa: Author, p. 12. Retrieved May 29, 2009, from http://secure.cihi.ca/cihiweb/products/hcic2007_e.pdf

communication, systems support), and finance. Support services include materials management, volunteer services, health records, registration, food services, laundry, and security.

Nursing Services

Registered nurses, practical nurses (called *registered practical nurses* in Ontario and *licensed practical nurses* in all other provinces and territories), nurses' aides, and personal support workers make up the nursing staff within health care facilities. The particular mix of regulated and nonregulated health care professionals used will vary with each facility. Typically, acute care hospitals rely on regulated professionals to deliver nursing care, but, again, the mix may vary among facilities, depending on the level of care required. Nursing staff work in most departments that interact with either inpatient or outpatient clients. In analyzing their costs, most hospitals separate out the cost of nursing services for inpatient care. Expenditures for other nursing staff may be accounted for in the costs of specialized departments (e.g., outpatient clinic, **renal dialysis**, cancer day treatments).

Medical Staff

Depending on its size and scope of services, the hospital may have physicians on salary or on contract. Other physicians may assume teaching responsibilities for interns and residents. Doctors who admit and visit inpatients are usually not paid by the hospital. Rather, they bill their provincial plan for services or receive payment in other ways.

The Operating Room and Labour and Delivery Units

The operating room has specific expenses, including costs for its actual use; supplies, instruments, and other equipment (e.g., devices implanted into a client, such as an artificial hip); and staff with specialized skills (e.g., nurses with specialized training). Labour and delivery units also have specific costs for specialized equipment and perhaps staff.

Ambulatory Care and Outpatient Services

Clinics within hospitals have specialized diagnostic and other equipment based on their particular needs. The services of health care professionals working in clinics, who typically also provide care in other areas of the hospital (e.g., laboratory services, physiotherapy, respiratory therapy), would not be charged specifically to a clinic.

Emergency Room

Many hospitals employ physicians to work in the emergency room (ER). These physicians are usually paid by the hour. In some cases, however, a physician seeing clients in the ER will bill the provincial or territorial plan on a fee-for-service basis (see pages 209–210), although this practice is no longer common. ER services include assessment, diagnosis, and treatment.

Diagnostic and Therapeutic Services

The diagnostic and therapeutic services department supplies services related to diagnosis for inpatients, outpatients, and the community at large. In most jurisdictions, anyone can go to the hospital lab for tests ordered by a physician, although many communities also have privately run, publicly funded labs that offer the same or similar services. Highly technical tests, however, are more likely to be available in hospital facilities.

Renal dialysis
A mechanical process to remove unwanted elements normally taken from the blood by the kidneys. This process becomes necessary when a person's kidneys are not functioning.

Community and Social Services

Community and social services departments offer care to individuals within the community, such as discharged clients or outpatients. This department is assuming a greater role (and thus incurring a greater expense) as the move toward community-based care broadens. While adding to a hospital's expenses, these services result in a decrease in admissions and hospital stays, thereby offsetting their cost.

Pharmacy and Medications

All hospitals have pharmacies. Pharmacy expenses include staff (e.g., pharmacists, pharmacology assistants, technicians) and the cost of drugs for inpatients.

Cost Reduction Strategies

To reduce costs, hospitals have tried to decrease clients' length of stay and to rationalize services. These strategies are discussed in detail below.

Length of Stay

Decreasing the length of hospital stays is an important way to reduce costs and to make beds available for those who need them. Over the past 10 years, great strides have been made toward this goal.

The province or territory determines the cost of an insured bed to a hospital (paid for out of its budget) by estimating the services required by the person occupying the bed. For example, a client in an acute care bed recovering from hip surgery would be deemed more expensive than one recovering from an appendectomy. A long-term care bed typically costs the hospital less than beds in other wards because the person occupying the bed usually requires less care. Interestingly, the use of semi-private and private rooms generates income for a hospital (Case Example 6.1).

Case Example 6.1

Mary, a 65-year-old woman who will be admitted to hospital for knee replacement next week, is wondering whether she can afford private accommodation. A semi-private room (i.e., a room containing two beds) would cost approximately $220 more per person per day than would a ward or standard bed, and a private room, a further $220 per person per day above that. So, if Mary had regular provincial or territorial health insurance and wanted a private room, she would pay $440 per day out of her own pocket. However, if she had semi-private coverage through a private insurance or group benefits plan and wanted to have a private room, she would pay $220 per day out of her own pocket.

The following strategies have helped to reduce the length of stays in hospitals across Canada.

Same-Day Admissions

In the past, individuals scheduled for major surgery were admitted one or two days prior to their operation for tests and what was called "preop" preparation, which consisted of a medical history, a physical, bowel cleansing, shave if needed, preoperative instruction, and nighttime sedation to ensure a sound sleep.

Today, for many surgeries, this preparation is done on an outpatient basis. The family doctor typically performs the physical and takes a preoperative history a week or so prior. Tests, such as blood work and an electrocardiogram, are done several days before the surgery. Pre- and postoperative instruction is given on an outpatient basis: The client makes an appointment at the hospital, watches a video, and has an opportunity to have questions answered, usually by a surgical nurse or nurse educator. Any necessary preparation (e.g., not eating or drinking for eight hours before the operation) is done at home by the client (shave preps are frequently omitted). On the morning of the surgery, the individual is admitted, preoperative information not already obtained is gathered, and the preoperative sedation, if any, is administered. Considering the large number of surgeries that take place within each province or territory each day, omitting one night in hospital for every client results in a significant savings.

Technology and Day Surgery

Because of technological advances in many fields, particularly in **laparoscopic surgery**, many surgeries are now done on an outpatient basis. For example, the routine removal of the gallbladder (called a *cholecystectomy*) once required a large abdominal incision but now requires only a small incision using a laparoscope. The client, admitted as an outpatient, goes home the same day. When the surgery required a larger incision, the client would stay in hospital for seven days or more. However, even when larger incisions are done today, the client seldom remains in hospital longer than two or three days.

Services Within the Community

Gaining support in all jurisdictions, community-based care offers clients a variety of services delivered within their own community or at home. Often accessed through a central body, such as Community Care Access Centres in Ontario (CCAC), these services support clients through illness, providing medical care, supportive and rehabilitative care as necessary, long-term support, and palliative care. A significant number of people with health problems now

Laparoscopic surgery
A type of surgical procedure in which a small incision is made in the body, through which a viewing tube (laparoscope) is inserted. A small camera in the laparoscope allows the doctor to examine internal organs. Other small incisions may be made to insert instruments to perform surgery.

receive care at home instead of in the hospital. Clients are first accepted into a home care program, their health and care needs are assessed, and care is provided.

Community-based care reduces both hospital admissions and the length of stay for individuals who do become hospitalized. Canadian Home Care Association, the Victorian Order of Nurses, and Meals on Wheels are just three organizations that offer community-based care services. Home care services are not always fully covered by provincial or territorial insurance plans, but these organizations themselves often provide coverage in whole or in part; any residual uninsured costs remain the responsibility of users. Various levels of government, regional health authorities, insurance companies, or private corporations may hire an organization to provide a specific service.

Timely Discharge

Hospitals endeavour to discharge inpatients by 10:00 or 11:00. Depending on the policies of the jurisdiction, the province or territory will charge the hospital for an additional 24-hour period if a client is not discharged by a certain time, often noon. If a discharged client cannot arrange to go home (or to another destination) before the discharge time, the nurses will, if possible, have the client vacate his or her bed and perhaps wait in a lounge so that the room can be cleaned and readied for an admission. Individuals undergoing day procedures such as surgery are likewise kept only until they are deemed stable, and then they are discharged.

Discharge of Postoperative Clients

Even those undergoing major surgeries may receive early discharge. Several years ago, a person having a hip replacement would be in an acute care hospital bed for up to 10 days and then moved to a rehabilitation bed for several weeks. Today, hip replacement clients are often discharged within a week; a visiting nurse will follow up with them at home to assess their progress, to dress the incision, and to provide any other necessary medical care. Afterward, a physiotherapist will make home visits to help the client become mobile again.

Palliative Care Clients

Palliative care is care provided to individuals with terminal illnesses. In the past, when people became too ill to be cared for at home, they were admitted to hospital to die. Many still are, especially if their need for pain control cannot be met at home or if family members simply cannot emotionally or physically manage without the intervention of community services. However, many terminally ill people prefer to spend their remaining time at home. A visiting nurse and other community support services then provide the necessary care, supporting both the family and the client.

Other Conditions Managed at Home

Many other medical conditions, including cancer, can now be managed on an outpatient basis. Previously, a client receiving chemotherapy following cancer surgery would have been admitted to hospital for a day or more to receive treatment. Today, oncology outpatient clinics provide this treatment. The client comes in at a designated time, receives his or her treatment, and goes home. Outpatient cancer treatments are made possible, in part, because of improved chemotherapy drugs. Whereas, in the past, many chemotherapy drugs caused severe nausea and vomiting, today's have fewer side effects. Antinauseant medications (e.g., Gravol) also make a difference.

A variety of other medical problems can also be managed at home. Clients receiving fluids through an intravenous needle (IV) used to be hospitalized. However, advances in IV equipment and monitoring mean IVs can be used safely at home. A visiting nurse comes several times a day, if needed, to assess the infusion (called *parenteral therapy*) and to provide IV antibiotics or other medications as necessary. Individuals needing parenteral pain management may also use "pain pumps" (electronic infusion pumps that deliver a prescribed amount of painkillers intravenously), which come in a variety of types.

People with multiple chronic diseases may also remain at home and manage their illnesses with support from organizations or individuals, such as family doctors, outpatient clinics, community nurses, and community health centres.

Community Health Centres

Fairly similar in structure across the country, community health centres (CHCs) offer the services of a health care team that includes doctors, nurse practitioners, counsellors, community workers, and dietitians. CHCs offer support, treatment, and preventive services to Canadians who have difficulty accessing health care because of language and cultural barriers, disabilities, poverty, or homelessness. These nonprofit centres also are pivotal in keeping individuals out of hospital by supporting them within the community setting.

Rationalization and Mergers

Governments have also cut costs by rationalizing hospital services (e.g., restructuring, downsizing, decentralizing, closing) in an effort to prevent the duplication of services, to provide care at the necessary level within a community, and to better use resources. For example, in Kitchener, Ontario, cardiac and cancer services are centralized—St. Mary's Hospital has become the cardiac centre, and Grand River Hospital, the cancer centre. Government funds were invested in both hospitals to update, upgrade, and expand services in these specialty areas. Obstetrical services are offered only at Grand River Hospital, although both hospitals maintain a viable emergency department. Eliminating the duplication of services saves money, and, ultimately, a higher level of care results because more sophisticated and technologically advanced equipment can be purchased and operated by highly skilled health care professionals.

Rationalization also involves delivering the right kind of care at the right level to the right person. Adopting regional health authorities and similar organizations across the country has contributed to supplying appropriate health care for individual communities.

Since 1984–85, the number of approved hospital beds has continued to drop with the simultaneous rise in hospital day programs (e.g., outpatient clinics, day surgery). Mental health beds have also decreased since care for the mentally ill has shifted to the community (CIHI, 2005; Statistics Canada, 1997).

Hospital mergers occur in two main ways:

1. The horizontal model merges several hospitals under one administration—one board, one CEO, one budget—but maintains several sites.

2. The vertical model merges specific programs within a single organization; however, the administration of various programs may remain independent of one another, thus not be under the direction of one board.

The advantages to merging are broad: reduced duplication of services, higher levels of efficiency, lower administration and management costs, and the ability to offer more services with better results for client care and recovery. Larger institutions are also believed to attract more staff. However, studies have shown some negative outcomes when larger hospitals merge, one of the greatest being the effects on staff. Mergers often result in a disruption in a hospital's culture, lost seniority, and displacement of staff members, either through a reorganization of positions or layoffs. Mergers of smaller hospitals appear to be more successful because the resulting facility broadens its service base while retaining staff and improving care.

Empirical studies
Studies based on observation and experience.

A few **empirical studies** on the effectiveness of mergers have been undertaken. Despite claims by one such study that Canadian hospitals overall have saved 4% of operating costs by merging, little concrete evidence exists to support this claim. For example, although managers of a hospital in Victoria, British Columbia, reported a hefty savings in staffing by merging, no comparison study of hospitals of a similar size that did not merge exists. In other cases, some hospital mergers have shown reduced expenditures, while others have not. For instance, Chedoke and McMaster hospitals in Hamilton, Ontario, claimed savings after merging, while a hypothetical merger (a plan created in a virtual situation) of two hospitals in Peterborough, Ontario, showed that no increase in savings would result (Canadian Health Services Research Foundation, 2002).

Some reports claim that mergers negatively affect the quality of client care because hospital management and staff get immersed in the process of merging, and client care suffers, which, in the long run, can increase costs. The merging of hospitals may also result in some people having to travel farther for some services. Evidence shows that those in lower socioeconomic groups are less able, and thus less likely, to seek certain treatments and services. This is especially true in rural settings.

Another contradiction results from the claim that mergers improve staffing and staff retention. Each hospital has its own culture. Staff members who are moved to a new location and expected to adopt different philosophies and styles of care delivery can end up resentful. Some health care professionals in these situations lose seniority or a position they enjoyed. Moreover, morale and trust in the new institution can plummet, creating a climate of discontent and disharmony. Managers who oversee more than one facility may also be less supportive, as their time and attentions are divided, thus affecting client care, interprofessional relationships, staff attendance, and job stability—and then costs in the human resources sector increase.

DRUGS

Next to hospital services, drugs represent the second largest health care expense. Total drug expenditures in Canada reached $29.8 billion, or $897 per Canadian, in 2008, compared with $25.3 billion in 2006 and $26.9 billion in 2007, showing an annual growth rate of approximately 8.3%—an increase exceeding that in other major spending categories, including hospitals and physicians. Spending on drugs in 2008 accounted for 17.4% of total health care spending, with costs of prescribed drugs swallowing up 84% of the total drug budget. This expenditure is expected to continue to grow.

Expenditures by the private sector accounted for more than 79.5% of total spending for prescribed drugs in 1975. This share decreased to 52.3% by 1992. In 2008, it was projected to be 55.5% (Figure 6.2) (CIHI, 2008b, 2008e). In March or April of each year, the Canadian Institute for Health Information releases new figures, which can be accessed from the organization's Web site (see Web Resources at the end of this chapter).

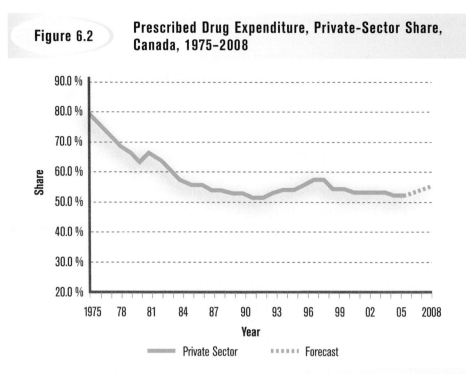

Figure 6.2   Prescribed Drug Expenditure, Private-Sector Share, Canada, 1975–2008

Source: Canadian Institute for Health Information. (2008). *National health expenditure trends, 1975 to 2008*. Ottawa: Author, p. 21. Retrieved May 29, 2009, from http://secure.cihi.ca/cihiweb/products/nhex_2008_en.pdf

Currently, thousands upon thousands of pharmaceutical products are available to Canadians. These products are used to treat, palliate, alleviate, and prevent illness and disease. Broadly speaking, several factors drive drug expenditure in Canada, including increased usage (i.e., more people using prescription drugs), increased costs, an aging population, health care system factors (e.g., variations in drug subsidies among jurisdictions), and the introduction of new drugs (which tend to be more expensive than older ones) (CIHI, 2009).

Drug Insurance

All provinces and territories provide some kind of drug insurance to certain groups, such as older adults and people who cannot afford necessary medications, although the jurisdictions do charge some type of co-payment and deductible to most of these insured groups (see Chapter 5). Some pharmacies will waive deductibles and co-payments in certain circumstances. Most provinces and territories will assume the cost of very expensive drugs for specific health conditions when the family is unable to cover the expense. This coverage stems from the Romanow Report recommendation that catastrophic drug costs (see

Chapter 3) be paid by the government to ensure no Canadian resident goes without necessary drugs.

A drug's accessibility and coverage through an insurance plan are determined by its category: Over-the-counter (OTC) medications can be purchased without a prescription and are rarely covered by public or private health plans; prescription medications can be purchased only with a prescription from a health care professional (e.g., family doctor or specialist; in some jurisdictions, nurse practitioner or midwife) and may be covered in part or in full by insurance.

Occasionally, a province or territory will "delist," or remove, a drug from the list of drugs that may be obtained only with a prescription. On one hand, delisting makes the drug more available to the general public, but on the other hand, that drug is no longer likely to be covered by any type of insurance—which saves money for insurance companies and provincial and territorial plans, but costs consumers more.

The cost of drug insurance to governments has risen for a number of reasons:

- More people are taking more drugs for more reasons. Many conditions that in previous years could not be treated (e.g., high cholesterol, hypertension, heart disease, depression) are now controlled with effective medications.

- Consumers demand drugs. Antibiotics, painkillers, tranquillizers, sleeping pills, and antidepressants top the list of requested drugs. Physicians besieged by irate and insistent clients often buckle to their demands.

- Newer and more effective drugs (e.g., treatments for HIV/AIDS, new chemotherapy drugs) are expensive.

- People are living longer, although often with multiple conditions requiring several different medications. On average, nine out of every 10 older adults not living in long-term care facilities take three different types of medications. Older women tend to take a wider variety of medications than their male counterparts—more than 27% of women aged 65 or older take at least five types of medication, compared with only 16% of men in the same age group (Statistics Canada, 2006).

- Pharmaceutical companies have begun advertising drugs, and information about them is available on the Internet. Consumers then demand these drugs from their health care professionals, who may comply, thereby contributing to overprescribing.

- Many new drugs on the market are under patent protection, making them more expensive (see page 206), yet doctors and clients alike want to try the new drug. In reality, many of these newer drugs are no more effective than older ones available as generic drugs, which, on average, cost 50% less than brand-name drugs. Estimates suggest that the use of generic drugs saves our health care system over $1 billion annually (Canadian Health Services Research Foundation, 2007; National Center for Policy Analysis 2007).

- A 2004 study found that Canadian physicians are generally oblivious to drug prices and often prescribe an expensive pharmaceutical when a cheaper one would do (Allan & Innes, 2004). Soaring drug bills in Canada could be decreased if doctors considered the cost of the medications they prescribe.

Nationally, an average of 47.9% of total health care expenditures went toward prescription drugs in 2007. This national average was exceeded by Quebec (52.2%), Manitoba (52.7%), Saskatchewan (51.5%), Alberta (50.2%), Yukon (68.7%), the Northwest Territories (55.4%), and Nunavut (70.6%) (CIHI, 2008c).

Brand–Name and Generic Drugs

Brand-name drugs—those that are owned and sold by the company that developed them—cost more than generic drugs. They are protected under a piece of legislation called the *Patent Act*. Currently, patents last 20 years from the time the pharmaceutical company applies to the board for approval to sell the drug in Canada. Once a patent expires, any drug company can produce the drug (these are called *generic drugs*) and sell it at a lower cost. Note that brand-name drug names are always capitalized; generic drug names are not (e.g., *ibuprofen* is a generic drug; *Advil* is a brand-name drug).

Active ingredients
Those ingredients in a drug that have therapeutic value meant to cure, palliate, or otherwise treat a health problem.

Because they do not have to spend money on research and development, companies producing generic drugs can do so at a greatly reduced cost. Generic drugs contain the same **active ingredients**, although the other ingredients (called *nonmedicinal ingredients*) vary. All generic drugs go through an approval process and analysis similar to those of brand-name drugs. One method of testing, called *comparative bioavailability*, is conducted on human volunteers to ensure that the generic drug's effectiveness equals that of the brand-name drug it replaces. Despite this testing, some people claim that brand-name drugs are of a higher quality and that different nonmedicinal ingredients can alter the action of the drug. Unless a doctor specifically indicates on a prescription "no substitution," pharmacists often substitute a generic drug for a brand-name one.

Discussion about how long patent protections should last is ongoing in Canada. Generic drug companies, of course, lead this debate. When a patent expires, the production of the drug in question is fair game, and once a drug can be produced generically, the public pays less—one of the defining arguments for shortening patent protection time. However, the drug companies who spend the money to research and develop the drug—and by doing so, stand at the forefront of pharmaceutical research—would then have less time to recoup their costs and less incentive to continue researching new drugs.

Controlling the Cost of Patented Drugs

An independent government agency, the Patented Medicines Prices Review Board (PMPRB), regulates the price at which patentees sell their patented medicines in Canada to wholesalers, hospitals, pharmacies, and others (e.g., clinics), called the factory-gate price. Although the PMPRB can ensure that drug companies do not charge excessive prices, the board does not have jurisdiction over retail prices (i.e., the prices pharmacies charge their customers) or pharmacists' professional fees. For the duration of the patent, the PMPRB regulates the prices of all patented and generic drug products, including those available only through prescription, those sold over the counter, and those available through Health Canada's Special Access Program (a program that provides physicians access to existing drugs not currently on the market that might prove effective for treating serious or life-threatening conditions when mainstream medications have proven ineffective, are not readily available, or cannot be tolerated by the client). Importantly, the PMPRB has no authority to regulate the prices of nonpatented drug products (i.e., drug products that were never patented or for which the patent has expired). Finally, also outside the purview of the PMPRB are matters such as distribution, prescribing, and whether the cost of a medicine is reimbursed by public drug plans (S. Dupont, personal communication, March 15, 2009).

What Is the Answer to Rising Drug Costs?

A large number of Canadians have insufficient or no drug coverage at all (CBC, 2008; Health Canada, 2006), and as the cost of medications continues to rise, many worry about being unable to afford the medications they need (Case Examples 6.2 and 6.3).

Case Example 6.2

George, 24, suffers from asthma, but he cannot afford the cost of inhalers, so he often has difficulties breathing. George does not qualify for welfare or provincial drug relief, and his parents are not in a position to help him. Ultimately, George's family doctor supplies him with a temporary supply of the appropriate medications from samples a pharmaceutical representative left. (Pharmaceutical sales representatives provide physicians with sample

Continued on next page

medications, which the physicians give to clients in certain circumstances at their discretion. George's case is an example of when this would be appropriate. However, pharmaceutical samples are not a resource for supplying clients with medications long term.) George's options are limited: appealing to the province for help or otherwise finding funds with which to purchase his medications. This case illustrates a challenge many Canadians face. No easy answer exists—many Canadians simply go without.

Case Example 6.3

At 35 years old, Jim is a brittle diabetic (one whose diabetes is poorly controlled even if the sufferer consistently adheres to his or her dietetic regime). Jim's best option, an insulin pump, is not covered by either private or public insurance in his province. Although he cannot afford the pump, he does not qualify for provincial assistance. In the present economy, Jim has lost his manufacturing job and now works for a moving company. Jim struggles to balance this very physical occupation with his insulin needs and diet. Jim ends up in the ER in insulin shock and nearly dies.

To address the concern of drug costs, both the Kirby and Romanow reports (see Chapter 3) suggested a universal Pharmacare plan that would cap costs to ensure all Canadians get the medications they need on a uniform basis. The implementation of such a plan is particularly important as the Canadian population ages and relies on a multitude of medications to stay productive and healthy.

HUMAN HEALTH RESOURCES

The term *human health resources* refers to all people who work in the health care field. Health care professionals include doctors, nurses (both registered and practical nurses), chiropractors, physiotherapists, and midwives. In recent years, several new related professions have been introduced, such as those of physician assistants, nurse endoscopists, clinical specialist radiation therapists, and anaesthesia assistants.

Despite popular belief, the number of doctors and nurses in Canada has actually expanded in recent years. Between 1997 and 2006, the number of physicians grew by 12.9%; between 2003 and 2006, the number of nurses grew by 4.6% (CIHI, 2008c). These numbers, however, are still insufficient to meet the needs of an aging population and to replace the large number of health care professionals retiring or leaving their occupations.

Estimates suggest that more than one and a half million people work in the health care field in Canada (CIHI, 2008c). The largest of these regulated professions is nursing, followed by medicine (i.e., physicians). Currently, postsecondary institutions offer more than 150 different health care programs across the country, with more emerging.

Compared with other countries in the **Organisation for Economic Co-operation and Development (OECD)**, Canada spends significantly more on health care. Despite this, Canada has fewer physicians and nurses than do other countries. In 2006, Canada had 2.1 practising physicians/1000 population (the average among OECD countries at that time was 3.1) and 8.8 qualified nurses/1000 people (again, lower than the OECD average of 9.7) (Organisation for Economic Co-operation and Development [OECD], 2008). While the number of physicians per capita between 1990 and 2006 remained relatively stable, the number of nurses decreased, causing significant concern for federal, provincial, and territorial governments. All are taking steps to rectify this nursing shortage (see Chapter 5) (CIHI, 2007b, 2007c; OECD, 2008).

Organisation for Economic Co-operation and Development (OECD) Established in 1961 and now representing 30 countries, the OECD provides a setting in which member governments compare policy experiences, seek answers to common problems, identify best practices, and coordinate domestic and international policies.

How Physicians Are Paid: Billing Options

In 2006, physicians accounted for 13% of total health care expenditures in Canada, the third-largest category of expenditure. This category was forecast to have grown by 6.2% in 2008 over 2007, to a total cost of $23.1 billion (CIHI, 2008e).

Most physicians are paid through the fee-for-service method, although alternative billing options exist and, as part of primary health care reform, are under review to determine the most effective option.

The following sections summarize the most common payment options for physicians in Canada.

Fee for Service

Fee for service (FFS) is the oldest and most widely accepted method of physician payment in Canada. Using this method, doctors charge the provincial or territorial plan for every service they perform. Each province or territory has slightly different parameters for FFS billing. Invariably, though, the amount the doctor bills relates to the complexity of the client visit and the length of time it takes.

Within the FFS model, doctors can also bill for things other than the actual office visit. For example, doctors who make house calls can charge more to ensure they are compensated for travel, for seeing a client away from the office, for the time of day or night the house call is made, and for the client visits cancelled if making a house call during office hours. Doctors may also bill for procedures such as giving an injection or suturing a wound and for visiting a client in hospital. Amounts billed also vary depending on whether the doctor is the MRP (most responsible physician) or is just providing a consultation. (In the hospital, the MRP is the physician with the primary responsibility for caring for the client; this may be the client's family doctor but is usually a specialist.) Many doctors prefer to hang on to FFS, at least in part. Some of the primary health care reform models blend capitation-based funding (described below) with FFS.

Capitation- or Population-Based Funding

Capitation-based funding (also called *population-based funding*) pays the doctor for each rostered client in his or her practice. This funding format is often used by doctors in private practice who also operate under the umbrella of an alternative health care delivery format, such as a primary health care reform group. Physicians must receive approval from their provincial or territorial government to form such a group. Once physicians begin working in their selected primary care model, they are usually paid monthly.

With capitation-based funding, doctors receive for each client a set amount that is determined by the client's age, health care needs, or both. A doctor, therefore, would be paid more per year for an 89-year-old client with multiple health problems than for a 22-year-old healthy client. Whether the client visits the doctor once or 30 times in that year, the doctor receives the same amount of money. Additionally, doctors are paid extra for achieving certain milestones, such as immunizing a given portion of eligible clients and doing routine Pap smears and Pap smears for women in high-risk groups. (Physicians must track women in their practice and put procedures in place to do Pap smears in accordance with the criteria of the jurisdiction.) Setting such goals encourages doctors to be actively involved in disease prevention and health promotion.

Clients sign a form to say that they will seek medical nonemergent care only from their family doctor or members of the primary health care network group. This means these clients are rostered with that doctor or group of doctors. (For more details, see Chapter 7).

The fundamental components of capitation-based funding are summarized as follows:

- Physician payment is based on a given group of clients who are rostered, thus forming the foundation of the doctor's practice.

- The physician receives a guaranteed income based on the defined population base of his or her practice.

- The physician may enter into other compensation schemes; for example, a portion of his or her practice may still be FFS.

Capitation-based funding

A funding formula to pay physicians who participate in some type of primary health care reform group (see Chapter 7). The doctor receives a set amount (determined by the age and health status of each client) for each rostered client per year.

- Incentives provided to the physician incorporate a strong element of disease prevention and health promotion to result in better health outcomes for clients of the practice.

Blended Funding

Most physicians in Canada who engage in a form of funding other than FFS also partake in another method of payment. For example, a physician in a primary health care network group can have a certain portion of his or her practice non-rostered on an FFS funding scheme and another portion calculated on capitation-based funding.

Indirect Capitation

Indirect capitation is a funding model through which an organization (e.g., a regional health authority) receives a set amount of money to manage health care (including staff, services, administrative costs, and capital expenditures) for a population base. Employees within the organization may be compensated in various ways.

Global Budget

Doctors practising in underserviced areas are paid a certain fee for maintaining these practices. The global budget plan also usually includes ample vacation time and educational leave.

Salary

Doctors on salary receive a negotiated amount of money per time frame (usually a month). Larger hospitals, medical centres, clinics, and some nonprofit clinics often employ this model.

Specialists' Compensation

At teaching hospitals, specialists may have teaching responsibilities and receive a salary. Most specialists, even if on salary, maintain a private practice as well. In their private practice, they see a client upon referral from a family doctor until the problem for which the client was referred is resolved.

Specialists not employed by a hospital or other organization rely on fee-for-service and, therefore, bill the province or territory for services rendered. Specialists belonging to a primary health care reform group may receive other forms of compensation reflective of the payment formula for that particular group.

In most jurisdictions, after a certain period of time (often one year), if a client's health problem recurs, the client may call the specialist's office directly and return for another evaluation (called a *repeat consultation*). If a new problem occurs, or if the same problem returns *after* the designated time period, the client will need another referral (called a *consultation request*) from his or her family doctor. In most jurisdictions, a person cannot call a specialist's office and simply make an appointment. Channelling specialist visits through a primary care provider results in specialists' seeing only those clients who have legitimate problems and, thereby, creates cost savings.

Long-Term Care Accommodation

In 2007, over $16 billion was spent on long-term care, the fifth largest health care spending category (CIHI, 2008c). In Canada, approximately 250,000 older adults live in **nursing homes** (also called long-term care facilities), which provide total care for residents 24 hours a day, 7 days a week. Provincial and territorial governments oversee long-term care for all Canadians, with the exception of those individuals eligible for federal care through Veterans Affairs Canada, Workers' Compensation Boards, federal government acts, and medical health insurance.

Licensed by the provincial and territorial ministries of health, long-term care facilities (often privately owned) must meet standards regarding staffing levels, training, food preparation, pricing, and medical care, including the administration of medications. Unsubsidized and unlicensed residences also exist, but they offer limited or no nursing. These are usually regulated by municipal bylaws, which do not control the care provided.

Long-term care is provided for older adults at various levels—from those requiring minimal support but are unable to live on their own to those requiring total care and supervision for physical or mental reasons. Levels of care are classified as independent, semi-independent, and dependent (Case Example 6.4).

Nursing home
A facility or part of a facility that provides accommodation to persons usually over the age of 16 requiring intensive personal care under the supervision of a registered nurse.

Case Example 6.4

Seventy-two-year-old Olivia has had a stroke. She is fully cognizant and can manage some activities of daily living but needs assistance with dressing, eating, and moving about. Because she was unable to manage at home despite home care support, she is now in a nursing home, semi-dependent, and receiving a moderate level of nursing supervision and supportive care.

However, if Olivia had severe Alzheimer's disease (i.e., had no memory, wandered, and could not feed herself) and fell and broke her hip, she would be placed in a secure unit with maximum nursing supervision and be almost completely dependent.

The provincial or territorial government controls the number of long-term beds in the province or territory, so all beds must be approved by the government. Most governments subsidize nursing home care. However, Nova Scotia, until January 2009, required residents who could afford to cover the entire cost of their accommodation to do so; since then, the province has subsidized the payment.

Provincial and territorial governments subsidize public nursing home beds; however, in most provinces and territories, a flat rate is also charged to the client for basic accommodation, a fee called a co-payment. This co-payment covers the cost of room and board and possibly some operational costs, such as laundry services, administrative services, equipment costs, and mortgage expenses. The portion of costs a resident must pay may be dependent on his or her financial circumstances (Case Example 6.5). All jurisdictions have alternative funding options for those unable to pay, and no one can be denied accommodation or care.

Case Example 6.5

After falling and breaking her hip, 80-year-old Gertrude can no longer live independently at home. Arrangements have been made for her to move to Happy Meadows, a nursing home close by. Gertrude has concerns about being able to afford nursing home care, and is even more worried about what will happen to her life's savings and her house. "They will take all of my money," she laments. "What will happen to my house? I heard they take everything to pay for staying there!" What might happen to Gertrude?

The answer depends on what province or territory Gertrude lives in and what type of nursing home Happy Meadows is. In most jurisdictions, Gertrude's monthly income must be used toward payment of her accommodation. She need not worry about her house and savings, however. These assets are protected (although the amount of protection varies across jurisdictions) and will not be accounted for in the assessment of her ability to pay. If Gertrude's monthly income from her pensions is $2000 and the co-payment is $3000 per month, Gertrude will be unable to make the full co-payment. She will have to surrender the bulk of her income for the co-payment for her accommodation. The government will cover the balance, leaving her with enough money for personal expenses. Gertrude is eligible only for basic accommodation. Depending on the minimum accommodations available at Happy Meadows,

Continued on next page

Gertrude may be in a ward with several beds (up to six) or in a semi-private room with only one other person.

If Gertrude's monthly income were $3000 and the cost of her standard accommodation were $2500 monthly, Gertrude would be required to pay the full amount, leaving her with $500 left over to spend as she pleases.

In Newfoundland and Labrador, the approximate cost of a basic long-term care bed in the public system is $2800 per month, which the resident is asked to pay. If the resident cannot afford this fee, the regional health authority will perform a financial assessment to determine how much the client can afford. In Quebec, the co-payment for a basic room (one with three or more beds) is approximately $990 per month; in British Columbia, the 2009 minimum (basic) co-payment was approximately $940; and in Alberta, it was approximately $1354.

Government subsidies covering the cost of a nursing home bed apply only to basic (or ward) *accommodation*. As in hospitals, ward accommodation can mean a four- or even six-bed room. Many newer or renovated facilities, however, offer only semi-private and private accommodation. In these facilities, a semi-private room would qualify as basic accommodation. Some facilities include "preferred" semi-private rooms, which are divided by a partial wall, affording a greater level of privacy and dignity to each resident.

When a person must enter a nursing home and his or her spouse stays in the community, the province or territory adjusts the payment arrangements so that the spouse can retain enough money to remain in the community setting.

Across Canada, the aging population poses a challenge to governments and private nursing home facilities to ensure that an adequate number of long-term beds are available. The quality of long-term care is an ongoing concern, as well. Unfortunately, the media have reported many upsetting stories about neglect and cruelty in some nursing homes.

TECHNOLOGY

CT Scanners and MRIs

In 2007, 419 computed axial tomography (CT) scanners and 222 magnetic resonance imaging (MRI) machines were operational in Canada, up from 325 CT scanners and 149 MRI machines in 2003. However, during the same period, the increase in the number of tests performed far exceeded the increase in the number of scanners. A 27% growth in the number of CT scanners led to a 47%

growth in the number of exams, and a 12% growth in the number of MRI machines led to a 32% growth in the number of exams (CIHI, 2008d).

CT scanners and MRI machines are not evenly distributed across Canada, but their numbers are generally in line with provincial or territorial populations—and increasing. By the end of 2006, CT scanners per million population ranged from 10.2 in Ontario to 21.6 in Newfoundland and Labrador. MRI machines per million population ranged from 4.0 in Saskatchewan to 8.7 in Quebec (CIHI, 2008d).

Imaging services cost the health care system billions of dollars every year. In 2005–6, the operation of diagnostic imaging equipment cost an estimated $2.2 billion, up from $2.0 billion in 2004–5. Although the exact cost of Canada's imaging equipment is unknown, it is estimated that $90 million was spent on CT scanners and $78 million on MRI machines in 2006 alone (CIHI, 2008d).

Outsourcing

In many jurisdictions, health care services (e.g., diagnostic services, home care services) are contracted out to independent facilities. In Ontario, for example, some independent health care facilities have been licensed to perform MRI and CT scans for medically necessary procedures. To prevent queue jumping, clients must be referred to the facility for these procedures. The provincial government claims that contracting out these services costs 36% less than operating the same services within the hospital setting (Government of Ontario, 2003). These independent facilities may offer uninsured MRI and CT scans (e.g., to athletes or corporate executives whose firms cover such costs) only if they have signed a contract with the government to offer a designated number of insured scans per month, as well. Not until the insured scans have been completed can the company offer remaining spaces to the private sector.

Electronic Health Records

The maintenance of health information has increased dramatically over the past few years, but the ability to process, analyze, and use this information has not kept pace. The implementation of an **electronic health record (EHR)** network carries a high price tag but is essential to a modern health care system that is accessible, productive, and high quality. All levels of government in Canada are involved in creating an EHR network. The Canada Health Infoway, a federally funded, independent nonprofit organization, is responsible for its implementation.

The benefits of the EHR are significant. It offers improved safety, coordination, and care for clients and substantial cost savings and a high return on investment for the health care system. The implementation of a fully developed EHR will cost about $1 billion a year for 10 years, but cost savings achieved through

Electronic health record (EHR)
A secure accumulation of essential information about a client that is accessed electronically at different points of service (e.g., doctor's office, dentist's office, chiropractor's office, pharmacy) for purposes of client care.

the EHR are estimated at $6 billion annually (Health Council of Canada, 2007). Chapters 8 and 10 offer more information about EHRs.

CONCLUSION

Have you found the answers to the questions you were asked at the beginning of the chapter? How close were your estimates? To summarize, an intermediate assessment by a doctor will cost an uninsured client about $35. A knee replacement could cost as much as $7652; a hip replacement, $11,454; and having an appendix removed, $7200.

Now, consider your health card—just identification you must show when you seek health care services, right? Not really. Your health card is similar to a credit card but for health care services. Use it wisely.

What does the future of health care in Canada hold? It is near impossible to know, although change is a certainty. Resources are limited, and services may need to be rationed—an alien concept to Canadians. Excluding people from the treatment they need (or want) based on factors such as age, health status, or type of disease seems unthinkable, but it may become a reality. We must use health care resources wisely and continue to promote healthy lifestyles and disease prevention.

SUMMARY

❖ Presently, the federal government uses five models to make transfer payments to the provincial and territorial governments for health care services, in compliance with the principles of the *Canada Health Act*. The Act is the backbone of the health care system, although whether its principles keep pace with modern society and its health care needs is open to debate.

❖ Hospitals, drugs, human health resources, accommodation in long-term care and other such facilities, and technology account for the highest costs on the health care system. Governments, searching for the most cost-effective way to deliver high-quality health care, continually change funding mechanisms. For example, capitation-based funding as a payment model for primary care physicians has not yet been fully accepted as better than the fee-for-service model. The best solution at this point appears to be a blend of these models.

❖ Many health care services are not covered by the *Canada Health Act*, with the result that insurance companies and uninsured Canadians spend billions of dollars for them annually. The largest portion of private spending goes to dental care, medications, and care for older adults in long-term care facilities.

REVIEW QUESTIONS

1. Why do some Canadians regard health care as "free"? Do you feel that way? Why or why not?

2. Explain the concept of equalization payments, including why they are given and how they are calculated.

3. What types of services are covered by provincial and territorial insurance both in and out of hospitals?

4. What are the three largest expenditures for provincial and territorial health plans?

5. List five strategies for reducing the length of hospital stays and, thus, hospital expenses.

6. What are the key differences between prescription drugs and over-the-counter drugs?

7. How has advanced technology contributed to rising health care costs?

DISCUSSION QUESTIONS

1. Ask a grandparent or an older friend or relative whether health care has always been free. You will likely be told no. Before universal health care was introduced, Canadians were expected to pay for services. Ask your source how this affected his or her family. The philosophy of health was different then, too. Ask your source what his or her philosophy of health was then and what it is today.

2. Watch television, read the newspaper, or listen to the radio for a week to identify drugs advertised on commercials. Interview 10 people to find out (a) whether they have heard or seen the advertisements and (b) how likely they would be to ask their doctor to prescribe any of these medications if they thought the drug could benefit them. Then try to find out the price of each drug.

3. Research the types of long-term accommodation available in your community. How many kinds of long-term care facilities exist there? How does one access these services? How much does private, semi-private, and standard accommodation cost? How much does the client pay?

WEB RESOURCES

Canada Health Infoway Annual Report, 2007–2008

http://www2.infoway-inforoute.ca/Documents/Infoway_Annual_Report_2007-2008_Eng.pdf

A nonprofit organization created in 2001, the Canada Health Infoway collaborates with the provinces and territories, health care providers, and technology solution providers to accelerate the use of electronic health records (EHRs) in Canada. This link will take you to the organization's 2007–8 annual report.

Canadian Institute for Health Information

http://www.cihi.ca

An independent, nonprofit organization, the Canadian Institute for Health Information (CIHI) provides essential data and analyses on Canada's health system and the health of Canadians, with a focus on services, spending, and human resources in health care and on population health.

Spending on Health Care to Reach $5170 per Canadian in 2008

http://secure.cihi.ca/cihiweb/dispPage.jsp?cw_page=media_13nov2008_e

Focusing on how health care money is spent, this Canadian Institute for Health Information article provides the figures and projected figures for 2008 and analyzes spending trends. It also compares data on Canadian health care spending with international data.

WEB RESOURCES

Regulated Nurses: Trends, 2003 to 2007

http://secure.cihi.ca/cihiweb/dispPage.jsp?cw_page=AR_2529_E

This report draws on data from the Canadian Institute for Health Information's regulated nursing database, which covers the three regulated nursing professions in Canada.

Supply, Distribution and Migration of Canadian Physicians, 2007

http://secure.cihi.ca/cihiweb/products/SupDistandMigCanPhysic_2007_e.pdf

Produced by the health human resources team at CIHI to support health human resource planning and research efforts, this report provides demographic and descriptive statistics for physicians in 2007, including international entries and exits, as well as migration within Canada.

Public vs. Private Health Care

http://www.cbc.ca/news/background/healthcare/public_vs_private.html

This Web page discusses the differences among public, private, and two-tier health care and explains the forms of private health care and their presence in Canada today.

Organisation for Economic Co-operation and Development

http://www.oecd.org

The Organisation for Economic Co-operation and Development monitors events in its 30 member countries as well as those outside the OECD, and includes regular projections of short- and medium-term economic developments. It collects and analyzes data, which it then uses to help governments foster prosperity and fight poverty through economic growth and financial stability.

REFERENCES

Allan, G.M., & Innes, G.D. (2004). Do family physicians know the costs of medical care? *Canadian Family Physician, 50,* 263–270.

Canadian Broadcasting Corporation. (2006, December 1). Public vs. private health care. *CBC News.* Retrieved May 29, 2009, from http://www.cbc.ca/news/background/healthcare/public_vs_private.html

Canadian Broadcasting Corporation. (2008, December 1). Canadians fall through cracks without pharmacare: Report. *CBC News.* Retrieved May 29, 2009, from http://www.cbc.ca/health/story/2008/12/01/drug-plan.html

Canadian Health Services Research Foundation. (2002). Myth: Bigger is always better when it comes to hospital mergers. *Myth Busters.* Retrieved May 29, 2009, from http://www.chsrf.ca/mythbusters/html/myth7_e.php

Canadian Health Services Research Foundation. (2007). Myth: Generic drugs are lower-quality and less safe than brand-name drugs. *Myth Busters.* Retrieved May 29, 2009, from http://www.chsrf.ca/mythbusters/html/myth26_e.php

Canadian Institute for Health Information. (2005). *Hospital trends in Canada: Results of a project to create a historical series of statistical and financial data for Canadian hospitals over twenty-seven years.* Retrieved May 29, 2009, from http://secure.cihi.ca/cihiweb/products/Hospital_Trends_in_Canada_e.pdf

Canadian Institute for Health Information. (2007a). *Health care in Canada, 2007.* Retrieved May 29, 2009, from http://secure.cihi.ca/cihiweb/products/hcic2007_e.pdf

Canadian Institute for Health Information. (2007b). *Regulated nurses trends, 2003–2007.* Retrieved May 29, 2009, from http://secure.cihi.ca/cihiweb/dispPage.jsp?cw_page=PG_1710_E&cw_topic=1710&cw_rel=AR_2529_E%20style=

REFERENCES

Canadian Institute for Health Information. (2007c). *Supply, distribution and migration of Canadian physicians, 2007*. Retrieved May 29, 2009, from http://secure.cihi.ca/cihiweb/products/SupDistandMigCanPhysic_2007_e.pdf

Canadian Institute for Health Information. (2008a). *The cost of hospital stays: Why costs vary*. Retrieved May 29, 2009, from http://secure.cihi.ca/cihiweb/products/2008hospcosts_report_e.pdf

Canadian Institute for Health Information. (2008b). *Drug expenditure in Canada, 1985 to 2007*. Ottawa: Author.

Canadian Institute for Health Information. (2008c). *Health care in Canada, 2008*. Ottawa: Author.

Canadian Institute for Health Information. (2008d). *Medical imaging in Canada, 2007*. Retrieved May 29, 2009, from http://secure.cihi.ca/cihiweb/products/MIT_2007_e.pdf

Canadian Institute for Health Information. (2008e). *National health expenditure trends, 1975–2008*. Retrieved May 29, 2009, from http://secure.cihi.ca/cihiweb/products/nhex_2008_en.pdf

Canadian Institute for Health Information. (2009). *Drug spending estimated at $30 billion in 2008*. Retrieved September 1, 2009, from http://secure.cihi.ca/cihiweb/dispPage.jsp?cw_page=media_20090416_e

Department of Finance Canada. (2008). *Federal transfers in support of the 2000/2003/2004 First Ministers' Accords*. Retrieved May 29, 2009, from http://www.fin.gc.ca/fedprov/fmAcc-eng.asp

Department of Finance Canada. (2009a). *Canada social transfer*. Retrieved May 29, 2009, from http://www.fin.gc.ca/fedprov/cst-eng.asp

Department of Finance Canada. (2009b). *Equalization program*. Retrieved May 29, 2009, from http://www.fin.gc.ca/fedprov/eqp-eng.asp

Government of Ontario. (2003). *Ministry of Community and Social Services*. Retrieved May 29, 2009, from http://ogov.newswire.ca/ontario/!GPOE/2003/02/21/c2902.html?lmatch=%3C=_e.html

Health Canada. (2004). *Federal support for health care: The facts*. Retrieved May 29, 2009, from http://www.hc-sc.gc.ca/hcs-sss/delivery-prestation/fptcollab/2004-fmm-rpm/fs-if_16-eng.php

Health Canada. (2006). *Pharmaceuticals management and catastrophic drug coverage*. Retrieved May 29, 2009, from http://www.hc-sc.gc.ca/hcs-sss/delivery-prestation/fptcollab/2003accord/pharma-eng.php

Health Council of Canada. (2007). *Health care renewal in Canada: Measuring up? Annual Report to Canadians, 2006*. Toronto: Author.

National Center for Policy Analysis. (2007). *Therapeutic drug substitution*. Retrieved May 29, 2009, from http://www.ncpa.org/pub/st/st293/st293c.html

Organisation for Economic Co-operation and Development. (2008). *OECD Health data 2009: How does Canada compare*. Retrieved May 29, 2009, from http://www.oecd.org/dataoecd/46/33/38979719.pdf

Statistics Canada. (1997). Downsizing Canada's hospitals, 1986/87 to 1994/95. *Health Reports, 8*(4). Retrieved May 29, 2009, from http://www.statcan.gc.ca/studies-etudes/82-003/archive/1997/3023-eng.pdf

Statistics Canada. (2006, February 7). Health reports: Seniors' health care use. *The Daily* (No. 11-001-XIE). Retrieved May 29, 2009, from http://www.statcan.gc.ca/daily-quotidien/060207/dq060207a-eng.htm

CHAPTER SEVEN

Practitioners
and Practice
Settings

Learning Outcomes

1. Differentiate among conventional, allied, and alternative health care practitioners.

2. Discuss the regulation of health care professionals in Canada.

3. Explain what is meant by a *controlled act*.

4. Discuss the benefits of professional organizations.

5. Summarize the concept of primary health care reform.

6. Describe how various models of primary health care reform groups may differ.

7. Outline the principles behind the use of multidisciplinary teams in primary health care reform.

8. Discuss the benefits that a primary health care reform group offers to both clients and health care professionals.

KEY TERMS

Affiliating body, p. 252

Atherosclerosis, p. 228

Clinic, p. 250

Community-based care, p. 254

Congenital, p. 241

Controlled act, p. 232

Delegated act, p. 233

Deregulated, p. 227

Evidence-based, p. 225

Geriatrics, p. 240

Gestation, p. 242

Hydrocephalus, p. 242

Informed consent, p. 234

Intubate, p. 250

Modalities, p. 223

Placebo effect, p. 226

Profession, p. 223

Professional, p. 223

Professionalism, p. 223

Refraction, p. 242

Rostering, p. 257

Scope of practice, p. 227

Specialist, p. 238

Subdural hematomas, p. 244

Telehealth, p. 259

Title protection, p. 229

Urodynamic, p. 254

A variety of health care professionals and "informal workers" contribute to the provision of health care in Canada. Health care professionals typically include those who graduate from a university or college health care program; they diagnose or treat health problems (or do both) and provide related supportive services. Informal workers are those who provide "unofficial" assistance and care and include volunteers of community organizations and people caring for ill loved ones at home. Informal workers are an invaluable component of the health care workforce, particularly with the current move toward community-based care.

This chapter will look at some health care workers—who they are and what they do. It will briefly examine some of the professional organizations that support these people and the mechanisms in place to ensure that care is given by qualified individuals. It will also outline some of the practice settings, specifically those related to primary care, which are undergoing significant reform, affecting almost all health care professionals in one way or another.

The country is suffering from a critical shortage of almost all types of health care workers, including doctors and nurses. Over the past several years, both the federal and the provincial and territorial governments have taken steps to address these shortages, in particular by seeking ways to deliver primary care more efficiently so that all Canadians have equal and timely access to a primary care provider.

Primary health care reform aims to deliver continuous care in a timely fashion. Teamwork among all health care professionals helps to close the gaps in health care services so that client information, client care, and treatment are coordinated and complete.

Currently under scrutiny are how and where care is delivered and how efficiencies and cost-effectiveness can be created. Over the past decade, care of clients has moved from the hospital into the community. Because of new procedures and more community support for individuals recovering at home, hospital stays have been shortened (see Chapter 6). Primary care is continually evolving, with family doctors now delivering health care within a variety of models.

Health care professionals from diverse backgrounds use various **modalities** to treat clients. It is important to understand who these professionals are, what they do, how and where they work, and whom they work with. In recent years, health care professionals with different philosophical backgrounds and training have begun to work together in a concerted effort to ensure high-quality care for their clients. The chapter begins by defining *profession* and looking at some of the main categories of health care professionals.

Modalities
Prescribed methods or techniques.

WHAT IS A PROFESSION?

This chapter will use the terms **profession**, **professional**, and **professionalism**. Be sure to understand the words' different meanings.

Often, a professional association will oversee a profession, including any certification or licensing required to practise it. A large number of health care professionals belong to professional organizations at the provincial or territorial level. Benefits of membership include certification, awareness of educational and job opportunities, networking opportunities, and awareness of current professional developments.

Profession
An occupation that involves some branch of advanced learning.

Professional
A person practising an occupation that involves some branch of advanced learning.

Professionalism
A standard of skill and behaviour appropriate for a specific profession.

CONVENTIONAL MEDICINE

Conventional health care professionals (also called *traditional*, *mainstream*, or *orthodox* health care professionals) typically include doctors, nurses, nurse practitioners, midwives, dentists, pharmacists, podiatrists, dietitians, and others. They diagnose health problems, treat prediagnosed health problems, or do both, with scientifically proven therapies, medication, and surgery.

The allied health care field consists of a variety of health care professionals who work closely with primary care providers and are an invaluable part of the health care team. Allied health care practitioners are sometimes referred to as *paramedical practitioners*. Table 7.1 outlines the categorization of health care

Table 7.1	Health Care Professionals in Canada	
Health Care Professionals	**Allied Health Care Professionals**	**Alternative Health Care Professionals**
Dentists	Audiologists	Acupuncture practitioners
Doctors	Dental assistants/hygienists	Aromatherapists
Midwives	Diagnostic imaging technicians	Chiropractors
Nurse practitioners	Laboratory technologists	Homeopathic doctors
Pharmacists	Medical administrative assistants	Massage therapists
	Nurses (RNs/LPNs/RPNs/BScNs)	Naturopathic doctors
	Nutritionists/dietitians	Reflexologists
	Occupational therapists	Reiki practitioners
	Occupational therapy technicians	Therapeutic touch practitioners
	Optometrists/opticians	Traditional Chinese medicine (TCM) practitioners
	Osteopaths	Yoga practitioners
	Personal support workers	
	Physical therapists (physiotherapists)	
	Physiotherapy assistants	
	Podiatrists (chiropodists)	
	Psychologists	
	Radiographers	
	Respiratory technologists	
	Social workers	
	Speech therapists	

professionals, although this list is neither exclusive nor definitive. Titles, roles, and categorization may vary. For example, chiropractors may also be considered allied health care professionals.

ALTERNATIVE AND COMPLEMENTARY MEDICINE

Alternative medicine, sometimes referred to as *complementary medicine*, includes all health care practitioners not considered mainstream. Note, however, that although the terms are sometimes used interchangeably, a difference exists between alternative and complementary medicine. As its name suggests, complementary medicine supports, or complements, conventional medicine, while alternative medicine provides an option (i.e., an alternative), often to the exclusion of conventional medicine.

Although private insurance plans may cover some complementary or alternative therapies, complementary care and alternative care most frequently are not covered by provincial or territorial insurance plans and are not, as a rule, used in hospitals. Many of these therapies originate from spiritual, cultural, or religious beliefs and remain unproven by scientific standards. The complementary or alternative area of medicine includes acupuncture, traditional Chinese medicine, massage, homeopathy, meditation, aromatherapy, therapeutic touch, and spiritual healing (often used in Aboriginal communities).

Some critics of alternative medicine believe that treatment should be **evidence-based**—that is, proven to work—before it is used. If an alternative modality is scientifically proven to work, then it becomes accepted medical practice (Box 7.1).

Evidence-based
Proven, through high-quality scientific studies, to be effective.

Box 7.1	**When Mainstream Medicine Accepts Alternative Remedies**

"... since many alternative remedies have recently found their way into the medical mainstream [there] cannot be two kinds of medicine—conventional and alternative. There is only medicine that has been adequately tested and medicine that has not, medicine that works and medicine that may or may not work. Once a treatment has been tested rigorously, it no longer matters whether it was considered alternative at the outset. If it is found to be reasonably safe and effective, it will be accepted."

Source: Angell, M., & Kassirer, J.P. (1998). Alternative medicine—The risks of untested and unregulated remedies. *New England Journal of Medicine, 339,* 839–841.

As long as an alternative therapy is safe and results in some benefits for the client, many medical practitioners will accept it as a complementary option. Therapeutic touch, for example, claims to use balance and energy coupled with the healing force of the practitioner's hands to facilitate a client's recovery; however, no scientific evidence exists to prove it works. That is not to say that therapeutic touch does not benefit the client in terms of reducing stress and promoting relaxation. It will not, however, alter the course of a disease (Case Example 7.1).

Opposition to alternative medicine usually arises when people use it in place of scientifically proven treatments. Occasionally, a person will seek alternative

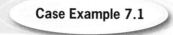

Case Example 7.1

Brigit, a 54-year-old woman, is diagnosed with breast cancer. If Brigit were to refuse medical and surgical treatment in favour of therapeutic touch, short of a miracle, the cancer would spread and Brigit would die.

However, if Brigit had surgery and was undergoing radiation or chemotherapy treatments and felt that therapeutic touch sessions helped her relax and cope with her diagnosis and conventional treatment, therapeutic touch could be considered complementary, and her medical doctors would be unlikely to pose any opposition.

Thinking It
Through

A client who was treated for breast cancer two years ago has just been diagnosed with metastases (the spread of cancerous cells from their original site). The doctor has recommended chemotherapy and radiation therapy, followed by surgery. Hopes for a cure are guarded. The client, based on her former unpleasant experience with the side effects of these treatment options, has decided to seek a homeopathic remedy. Considering these alternatives, what would you do if you were this client?

treatment when conventional medicine has nothing more to offer—for example, in the case of terminal cancer. Unfortunately, the alternative treatment may give false hope, impose significant costs, and waste precious time. On the other hand, if the treatment does no harm, it may provide optimism and even ease suffering.

Individuals may disregard conventional medicine for several reasons, including the following:

Placebo effect

An improvement in a person's condition without any actual treatment. Some evidence suggests that if people believe a specific treatment (e.g., a pill, which may be only a sugar pill) will cure them, a biochemical effect can minimize or alleviate symptoms.

- Mainstream medicine may at some point in an illness have nothing left to offer.

- The client may have suffered a bad experience with conventional practice.

- A client may hold a health belief system that contradicts mainstream medicine.

- A client may have at one time received an alternative treatment that appeared to have worked, convincing the client of the benefits of alternative medicine. In such situations, many physicians claim that the client would have recovered without any type of intervention because of the **placebo effect**.

Most conventional health care professionals support the complementary use of alternative therapies and conventional medicine; however, it is essential that the client, alternative practitioner, and medical practitioner work together to ensure no dangerous overlaps result. For example, herbal medicine can interfere with prescribed medications. St. John's Wort, a common herbal supplement taken to ward off depression, and prescription antidepressant drugs used together can result in an overdose. Many people use herbal medications (available over the counter at health stores and pharmacies) but fail to inform their doctor of such. They may believe that herbal medications are harmless, or they may be embarrassed or fearful to admit taking such medications, believing their physician will disapprove. Embracing both conventional and complementary medicine can medically and psychologically benefit a client, but that client must be open with and trusting of his or her health care professionals.

Chiropractic: Conventional, Complementary, or Alternative?

Chiropractors (doctors of chiropractic medicine) complete four to five years of postsecondary education to obtain a degree to practise this modality. Chiropractors diagnose and treat a wide range of conditions that deal primarily with disorders of the spine, pelvis, extremities, and joints and the resulting effects on the central nervous system. Taking a holistic approach to client care, chiropractors use various types of noninvasive therapies, such as recommending exercise routines to maintain and improve health. Chiropractors are not licensed to prescribe medicine or to do surgery. Chiropractic medicine is still considered by many to be on the cusp of alternative medicine (although others consider it mainstream)— in part because of the approach of many chiropractors to care and methods of treatment. For example, some chiropractors advise against immunization and will perform chiropractic adjustments on newborns and children.

Chiropractors and physicians typically share a mutual respect for each other's professions and work collaboratively as important components of the health care team. Chiropractors who encounter a medical problem they deem to be outside of their **scope of practice** will most often refer the client to a physician. A physician, in turn, may decide a client with a back problem could be treated more effectively by a chiropractor. Relationships between doctors and chiropractors are sometimes strained, perhaps because some chiropractors retain negative views of conventional medicine and of physicians' acceptance of chiropractic care, or vice versa. Immunizations have presented a contentious issue between the groups since many chiropractors (among others) do not recommend them. In general, the farther apart the philosophies of the practitioners, the less likely they are to understand and work with one another.

Until recently, several provincial and territorial plans covered a portion of chiropractic treatment, but it has since been **deregulated** by most. At this point,

Scope of practice
A range of skills, learned in school or through on-the-job training, that a practitioner can perform competently and safely. From a professional perspective, legal parameters usually (but not always) dictate what a practitioner may or may not do, based on the profession's education, training, and licensure.

Deregulated
No longer covered under the provincial or territorial health plan.

Treatment Versus Risk

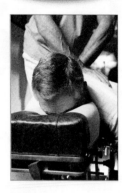

On September 1, 1996, Lana Dale Lewis, 45, of Toronto, suffered a stroke and was admitted to hospital, six days after chiropractic manipulation of her upper neck. She died from another stroke on September 12. Evidence at the coroner's inquest in 2002 was conflicting. Some experts testified that, in their opinion, Lewis's stroke was caused by natural disease—she had advanced **atherosclerosis**. Other experts blamed the neck manipulation for her stroke.

In January 2004, the jury ruled that Lewis's death was "accidental," in essence placing the blame on the chiropractic procedure. The jury made 17 recommendations to prevent similar deaths in the future, including the following: that further research study the relationship (if any) between neck manipulation and stroke; that clients provide "written and informed consent" to neck manipulations; that chiropractors keep written records of the exact procedure performed; and that an improved relationship be fostered between the chiropractic and medical communities.

A 2008 Canadian study has since concluded that no increased risk exists between chiropractic neck adjustments and stroke. While the researchers found an increased association between chiropractic care and stroke, they discovered the same association between a visit to the family doctor and stroke—an association likely explained by clients' seeking help from a chiropractor or medical doctor for neck pain (caused by an already damaged artery), rather than the care itself causing a stroke.

Atherosclerosis

A disease resulting from fatty deposits building up on the inner lining of arteries, eventually forming a mass called plaque. The artery may ultimately close completely, causing a heart attack or stroke.

Sources: Ontario Hospital Association. (n.d.). *Inquest into the death of Lana Day Lewis: Summary*. Retrieved May 29, 2009, from http://www.oha.com/Client/OHA/OHA_LP4W_LND_WebStation. nsf/resources/Lewis/$file/Lewis.pdf; Cassidy, J.D., Boyle, E., Côté, P., He, Y., Hogg-Johnson, S., Silver, F.L., et al. (2008). Risk of vertebrobasilar stroke and chiropractic care: Results of a population-based case-control and case-crossover study. *Spine, 33*(4 Suppl), S176–183; Alphonso, C. (2008, January 19). Chiropractors don't raise risk of stroke. *The Globe and Mail*. Retrieved May 29, 2009, from http://www.theglobeandmail.com

Photo credit: © iStockphoto.com/LattaPictures.

most private insurance plans will cover the cost of chiropractic treatments, in full or in part, up to a given number of treatments or dollar figure per year.

REGULATION OF HEALTH CARE PROFESSIONS

Some professions are regulated, meaning that legislation controls the conduct and practice of the profession and its members. In Canada, provincial and territorial legislation (e.g., British Columbia's *Health Professions Act*, Ontario's *Reg-*

ulated Health Professions Act) provides the legal framework for regulating most health care professions.

Regulated professions have self-governing bodies called colleges (e.g., College of Registered Nurses of Nova Scotia, the College of Massage Therapists of New-foundland and Labrador), which regulate the conduct and practice of their members. Each province and territory across Canada has 20 to 30 regulated professions, but professions regulated in some provinces and territories may not be regulated in all (Table 7.2). For example, psychiatric nurses in British Columbia are regulated by a college unique to their specialty—the College of Registered Psychiatric Nurses of British Columbia—while in Ontario, psychiatric nurses are under the umbrella of the College of Nurses of Ontario. Also, although Quebec is the only province to formally regulate counsellors, other jurisdictions have regulated health care professionals in various fields to provide the equivalent service. Note, however, that health care professionals in nonregulated fields may nevertheless practise.

Regulated professionals—those who belong to a professional body, are licensed to practice their profession, and are legally entitled to use a specific designation such as LPN (licensed practical nurse) or RT (respiratory therapist)—receive **title protection**, meaning only trained persons can legally use that title. For example, people who have cared for loved ones at home but have no formal training cannot call themselves licensed or registered practical nurses. Likewise, someone who dropped out of college halfway through a respiratory therapy program cannot call himself or herself a respiratory therapist. Nurses trained in other countries cannot call themselves registered nurses until they have met the standards (set by the college of nurses) of the province or territory they want to practise in. Along with title protection, regulated professions share other common elements (Box 7.2).

Title protection
Legal protection of a professional title and the legal right to use that title.

Box 7.2   Regulated Professions: Common Elements

- Educational standards
- Provincial and territorial examinations
- Practitioner's scope of practice, which outlines skills, acts, and services the practitioner is able to perform competently and safely
- Curbing of individual's practice if standards are not met
- Formal complaints process for the public
- Complaints investigation and follow-up
- Title protection
- Competence and quality assurance

Table 7.2   Regulated Professions in Each Province and Territory

Profession	Province/Territory												
	AB	BC	MB	NB	NL	NS	NT	NU	ON	PEI	QC	SK	YT
Chiropodists (podiatrists)	•	•							•		•	•	•
Chiropractors	•	•	•	•	•	•			•	•	•	•	•
Combined certified lab/X-ray technicians	•												
Counsellors (guidance counsellors, psycho-educators, and marital and family therapists)											•		
Dental assistants	•	•	•	•	•	•	•		•			•	
Dental hygienists	•	•	•	•	•	•	•		•	•	•	•	•
Dental technicians/ technologists	•	•		•					•		•	•	
Dental therapists							•	•				•	•
Dentists	•	•	•	•	•	•	•	•	•	•	•	•	•
Denturists	•	•	•	•	•	•	•	•	•	•	•	•	•
Dietitians/nutritionists	•	•	•	•	•	•			•	•	•		•
Hearing aid practitioners	•	•		•	•				•	•	•	•	•
Licensed practical nurses, registered practical nurses	•	•	•	•	•	•	•	•	•	•	•	•	•
Massage therapists	•	•			•				•				

Medical laboratory technologists

Medical radiation technicians

Midwives

Naturopathic physicians

Nurse practitioners (included under registered nursing in some provinces)

Occupational therapists

Opticians

Optometrists

Paramedics, ambulance attendants, emergency medical attendants

Pharmacists

Physicians

Physiotherapists

Psychiatric nurses

Registered nurses

Respiratory therapists

Speech language pathologists and audiologists

Traditional Chinese medicine and acupuncture practitioners

Source: Work Destinations. (2008). The forum of labour market ministers. Retrieved May 29, 2009, from http://www.workdestinations.org/occupation_list.jsp;jsessionid=A5362ED6600F22CD22A35E8204795FC6?lang=en.

Any health care profession can apply to the government to become regulated, but it must meet strict criteria. The minister of health and some type of advisory body within the province or territory usually oversee the lengthy and often arduous application process.

Regulation protects both the profession and the public by ensuring that those within a given profession are who they claim to be and do what they claim to do, in a competent and safe manner. Just as the possession of a legitimate driver's licence promises that a person knows how to drive and has passed a driving test, regulation proves a person has undergone training and gained some degree of skill or ability. Mind you, possession of a driver's licence does not guarantee driving excellence. That is to say, even in regulated professions, some health care professionals provide substandard services.

All regulated professionals must practise within a framework of skills and services defined by their governing body. Nurses have certain skills and acts they have been trained to do; doctors have a range of skills and services they have been trained to offer; and medical laboratory technologists likewise have a defined scope of practice. Even within a single profession, different levels of practice exist. For example, registered nurses with special training may perform acts that those without this training cannot, such as starting an intravenous line, working strictly with clients receiving chemotherapy, or managing wound care.

A medical doctor in family practice is not qualified to remove a gallbladder or do a hip replacement. A licensed practical nurse is not qualified to do a complete physical, but a nurse practitioner is. A massage therapist is not qualified to deliver a baby, but a midwife, nurse practitioner, or obstetrician is. In health care, many of these skilled procedures, some specific to certain professions, are called *controlled acts*.

CONTROLLED ACTS

As previously noted, each profession has a scope of practice statement that describes what the profession does and the methods it uses. Within some professions' scopes of practice are procedures or interventions called **controlled acts** (referred to as *reserved acts* in British Columbia), which only certain health care professionals may be allowed to perform. Considered potentially harmful if executed by an untrained individual, controlled acts vary slightly from one jurisdiction to another. Ontario's *Regulated Health Professions Act* (RHPA), for example, has identified 13 controlled acts (College of Physicians and Surgeons of Ontario, 2008). Specific acts may be within the scope of practice of any one (or more) profession, while other acts may not be within the scope of that same profession.

Examples of controlled acts include giving an injection, setting or casting a fracture, delivering a baby, and prescribing a medication.

Exceptions to Controlled Acts

Most provinces and territories allow controlled acts to be performed in certain situations by competent yet nonregulated individuals, including the following:

- Someone with appropriate training providing first aid or assistance in an emergency
- Students learning to perform an act under the supervision of a qualified person, as long as that act is within the scope of practice of graduates of the student's professional program
- A person, such as a caregiver, trained to perform an act (e.g., giving injections to a person with diabetes)
- An appropriate person designated to perform an act in accordance with a religion—for example, a rabbi may circumcise a male child

DELEGATED ACTS

As our health care system continues to evolve, so, too, do health care professionals' scopes of practice. Reforms in the health care system, in methods of delivery, and in which health care professionals are delivering the care have affected the traditional roles of health care professionals. The needs of clients also continue to evolve; more complex care is required more frequently. For client needs to be met, occasionally the acts, procedures, and treatments rendered by health care professionals must go beyond standard boundaries. To this end, health care professionals sometimes receive special training and share responsibilities. Under specific conditions, a health care professional who is not a physician may perform an act, treatment, or intervention that is typically outside of his or her scope of practice—that is, a **delegated act**.

Guidelines and protocol for delegation of medical acts vary across Canada. Generally, the delegated act must be clearly defined and supervised accordingly. Supervision can be direct (i.e., the delegating physician is physically present) or indirect (i.e., the delegating physician is available for consultation by phone). In health care organizations, the board of directors and the medical advisory committee (or their equivalents) must agree to the rules and procedures for delegated acts. A physician with expert knowledge has a commitment to his or her client to ensure that the person performing the act (i.e., the delegate) is properly trained and demonstrates competence in completing the act. In many cases, written rules dictate that the delegating physician must remain within proximity to the situation.

The delegating physician, the delegate, and the facility in which the act is performed share responsibility for the act. The physician who teaches or assesses the delegate's initial performance of the delegated act (and certifies the delegate as competent) is accountable for ensuring the act is, in fact, carried out competently. The person carrying out the act is liable if he or she performs the act ineffectually. Lastly, if the delegated act is carried out in a hospital or an equivalent facility, the board of directors is responsible for ensuring the availability of training for persons performing the act (Canadian Medical Association, 1988).

A physician may delegate an act to a nonregulated health care professional. For example, Sarah, a medical administrative assistant who graduated from a two-year college program, works in the office of Dr. Wong, a family physician. Dr. Wong decides to train Sarah to do allergy testing and give allergy injections. With proper training, then, Sarah can perform the delegated acts of giving clients their allergy shots and performing allergy tests as long as Dr. Wong is available onsite. Although Sarah has responsibility for her own actions, Dr. Wong is ultimately liable should anything go wrong.

Delegated acts, such as those performed by Sarah, can result in issues concerning physician payment. In most jurisdictions, certain criteria must be met for the physician to receive payment. These criteria apply whether a person is authorized to perform the act under the governing legislation (e.g., a registered nurse) or not (e.g., a nonregulated person the physician has trained to perform the act). For example, according to the College of Physicians and Surgeons of Ontario, the physician must personally carry out the procedure or delegate the procedure in accordance with the rules for delegated procedures. In the case of Sarah and Dr. Wong, the following guidelines would apply:

- The allergy injection must be administered by an employee of the physician.
- The physician must directly supervise the employee.
- The physician must be physically present in the office or clinic in which the delegate administers the act to ensure that he or she performs the procedure competently.
- The physician must be immediately available at all times to approve, modify, or otherwise intervene in the procedure as required in the best interest of the client.

Informed consent
Legally and ethically, clients must be given all relevant information about a treatment before agreeing to undergo the treatment. A client's consent without full disclosure of information is not considered informed consent.

Usually, the client must give **informed consent** to allow someone other than a physician to perform a procedure. In most cases, delegation will occur only with the client's consent and only after the physician has assessed the client, discussed the procedure, and answered any outstanding questions. The Web link for the Canadian Medical Association's *Guidelines for the Delegation of a Medical Act*, along with other resources pertaining to controlled acts, can be found in Web Resources at the end of this chapter.

Thinking It Through

A nurse or even an office manager in a health care office can be trained to carry out designated medical procedures. For example, a medical office manager may receive training to give allergy shots, or a nurse may be trained to do Pap smears. The physician, however, retains ultimate responsibility for the performance of these acts.

1. Do you think the delegation of acts should be allowed? Under what circumstances?

2. As a health care client, what type of assurance would you like that the person performing the procedure has received adequate training?

COMPLAINT PROCESS

Regulated professions have a system in place whereby the public can launch complaints against a health care professional. A designated committee investigates all complaints, protecting both the public, who can rest assured that legitimate complaints will be looked into and appropriate action taken, and health care professionals, who will have illegitimate or unfounded complaints against them dismissed. Health care professionals found to be at fault may face suspension, an order for additional training, the loss of their licence to practise, or even legal proceedings, such as a criminal investigation.

EDUCATIONAL STANDARDS

A regulator of a profession has the authority to set educational standards for the training of its professional members, including theoretical and practical components of their education as well as examinations for entry to practice. The educational process both prepares professional members and provides assurance to the public that the health care professional is competent to practise.

Professional bodies often use quality assurance programs to ensure the continued maintenance of standards. These programs provide health care professionals with a framework for this purpose and incentive to seek opportunities to maintain their professional competence. Often, proof that these standards have been met is a requirement for renewal of a professional's licence to practise. These programs aim to keep practitioners current and competent, protecting both the health care professional and the public.

LICENCE TO PRACTISE

In each province and territory, regulators of professions, in conjunction with educational facilities and in keeping with provincial and territorial requirements, oversee the licensing of their members. Regulated professions almost always require licence renewal annually.

Moving from one province or territory to another can cause issues for some professionals since not all regulated professions have agreements and standards in place for members to practise in other jurisdictions (Case Example 7.2).

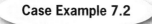

Case Example 7.2

Dr. Hiraki, a licensed general surgeon in Newfoundland and Labrador, wants to practise medicine in British Columbia. She must apply to the College of Physicians and Surgeons of British Columbia and follow its protocol before she is allowed to practise. Once licensed in British Columbia, Dr. Hiraki will be assigned a billing number, which she must use to bill the provincial plan for services rendered.

NONREGULATED PROFESSIONS AND OCCUPATIONS

Only about 20% of Canada's workforce labour in regulated professions (Human Resources and Skills Development Canada, 2007). All others work in the many professions and occupations that remain nonregulated across Canada, ranging from jobs that require university degrees and in-depth, specialized training (e.g., computer scientists, botanists) to those requiring very little education or training.

People who work within nonregulated occupations do not have federal or provincial legislation governing their occupations, although, in some provinces and territories, some professionals, such as electricians and plumbers, must complete strict examinations, both practical and written, to obtain a licence.

Like regulated professions, many nonregulated occupations have professional organizations or bodies that award certification when a person completes a set of written or practical examinations or both. Ontario and British Columbia have a professional organization for medical assistants and medical secretaries, although these remain nonregulated professions. Members of the Ontario Medical Secretaries Association (OMSA), for example, may write certification examinations and, if successful, may add the letters *CMS* (certified medical secretary) after their names to show that they have achieved a level of competence sanctioned by OMSA to practise within their field. Many jurisdictions offer a similar option for certification for dental technicians and dental administrative assistants.

To work as a medical secretary or administrator in a doctor's office or as a clinical secretary or coordinator in a hospital, a person requires a specialized knowledge base; however, an employer may hire someone with or without certification. A doctor, for example, could choose to hire a person with no experience as a medical secretary and provide on-the-job training, or he or she can hire someone who has graduated from a two-year diploma program in health administration. A hospital may require a clinical secretary to have a grade 12 diploma with some secretarial experience or, alternatively, a diploma from a two-year health administration program. The person or organization doing the hiring sets the requirements when a profession is nonregulated (Case Example 7.3).

Case Example 7.3

A doctor in Ontario decides that the person he hires as office manager must be a member of the Ontario Medical Secretaries Association. One applicant, Marika Smith, has written her certification examinations and can use the designation *CMS* (certified medical secretary). Because Marika has this designation, the doctor knows she has met minimal standards of competence to work as a medical secretary.

Many nonregulated disciplines have no specific standards to meet. For example, anyone can learn how to do ear candling or aromatherapy and put out a sign inviting the public to seek treatment.

HEALTH CARE PROFESSIONALS: WHO THEY ARE AND WHAT THEY DO

Health care traditionally has been dominated by physicians—from family doctors to specialists. However, a shift toward a team approach to health care is taking place, bringing to the fore the skills and expertise of many other health care professionals, particularly in the primary care setting.

Belonging to professions that are considered mainstream, or part of conventional medical practice, allied health care professionals support physicians in meeting clients' health-care-related needs. These professionals work independently as well as interdependently with other health care team members.

In addition, a host of other professionals do not typically render direct care but nevertheless provide valuable services for the implementation of health care—including administrative staff in health care facilities and health information management professionals.

Below are brief descriptions of select physician specialties and the functions of some other members of the health care team, including those with multiple titles, newer specialties, changing scopes of practice, or obscure job descriptions.

PHYSICIANS

Prior to attending medical school, would-be physicians must complete two to four years of undergraduate work, usually obtaining a bachelor's degree, and then write an entrance examination, called the Medical College Admission Test (MCAT), before applying for placement in one of Canada's 16 medical schools. MCATs examine applicants' writing, communication, and problem-solving skills, as well as their knowledge of science.

Medical school consists of three to four years of study, followed by a residency in the person's area of specialty (e.g., family medicine, internal medicine, general surgery). Prior to the 1970s, a doctor could go into general practice right after his or her internship year; however, family medicine is now considered a specialty.

Specialist
A physician trained in a specific field, usually concerning body systems or organs—for example, cardiology, internal medicine, orthopedic surgery—although some specialties (e.g., geriatrics) have a socioeconomic focus.

A doctor with specialized training in a specific area, called a **specialist**, usually sees clients only upon written request from a family doctor or another specialist. In fact, most provincial or territorial insurance plans will not cover the cost of a client visiting a specialist without the referral of another physician. A client will be referred to a specialist (also called a *consultant*) when a family doctor feels the client requires assessment and treatment outside the family doctor's scope of practice. The specialist will then treat the client until the condition has been resolved in one way or another, at which time the client returns to the care of his or her family doctor (see Chapter 6). In some cases, the specialist will continue to see a client who has ongoing problems requiring a specialist's care.

Box 7.3 lists the most common medical specialties in Canada.

Box 7.3   List of Common Medical Specialties in Canada

- Allergist
- Anaesthetist
- Cardiologist

- Dermatologist

- Emergentologist

- Endocrinologist

- Family doctor (general practitioner)

- Geriatrician

- Gynecologist (usually combined as an OB/GYN specialist)

- Laboratory and diagnostic medicine—a variety of specialist types (e.g., pathologist)

- Neurologist

- Obstetrician (usually combined as an OB/GYN specialist)

- Oncologist

- Ophthalmologist

- Otolaryngologist (ear, nose, and throat)

- Pediatrician

- Plastic surgeon

- Psychiatrist

- Surgeon (may specialize in a number of fields, such as general surgery, cardiac surgery, neurosurgery, orthopedic surgery)

- Urologist

Primary Care

Family Physicians/General Practitioners

Primary care physicians—doctors who specialize in primary care—are typically family doctors (also called general practitioners, or GPs). The family doctor has undergone training to take care of each person within the family, a commitment held until changed by death, relocation, termination of practice, or a parting of the ways because of client–physician incompatibility. With a wide knowledge base not limited to any specific disease or system or to any particular sex or age group, the family doctor provides ongoing care that includes counselling, health promotion and disease prevention, the delivery of babies (if the doctor so chooses), the care of chronic diseases, and care and support in the face of a terminal illness. His or her treatment of the client does not end when one particular health problem is cured.

Emergentologists

Some physicians, called emergentologists, have chosen careers practising full-time emergency medicine. This specialty has developed because many emergency departments (EDs, also often referred to as ERs, or emergency rooms) are hiring full-time physicians rather than staffing the ED with on-call physicians, as in the past. An emergentologist must hold a current certificate, have advanced CPR training, and, preferably, have taken courses in emergency and trauma medicine. The training qualifications of an emergentologist vary among hospitals. In small, rural settings, a family physician will often give up private practice to assume this role.

A stressful field, emergency medicine requires fast-paced, demanding triage and often split-second decision making regarding treatment. It is, in essence, primary care from an emergency perspective. The few Canadian universities currently offering emergency medicine programs include Dalhousie University in Halifax, Nova Scotia; the University of British Columbia in Vancouver, British Columbia; and the University of Western Ontario in London, Ontario.

Specialized Care

Geriatricians

Geriatrics
The branch of medicine dealing with the physiologic characteristics of aging and the diagnosis and treatment of diseases affecting the aged.

One of the newer medical specialties, **geriatrics**, focuses on the care of older people, typically those over 65. A geriatrician is usually an internist who has additional training in caring for older adults. In 2008, an estimated 216 geriatricians were practising in Canada—most not working in their specialty full-time—serving a population of 4.3 million seniors. That is 1 geriatrician for every 19,907 people (Steed, 2008).

Geriatricians care for and treat older adults who may suffer from such varied illnesses as Alzheimer's disease and other forms of dementia, heart problems, sensory loss (e.g., vision and hearing), and osteoporosis. Today, with high-quality medical management and new, effective medications to control and treat a number of conditions, people are living longer with multiple chronic conditions. Their doctors, however, are required to continually juggle medications and treatment options.

Geriatrics unfortunately does not attract a large number of physicians. The assessment and treatment of an individual with complex medical conditions is time-consuming, yet geriatricians are typically paid less than other specialists. Physicians entering into the specialty must enjoy dealing with older people and have a great deal of patience and empathy.

Both family doctors and geriatricians rely heavily on other members of the health care team to provide effective high-quality care to their older clients. Team members would include the following:

- Orthopedic surgeons (who repair damage related to the bones, for example, to the spine or extremities; hip fractures are particularly common in older people)

- Ophthalmologists (who treat diseases of the eye, for example, cataracts, which are common in older people)

- Pharmacists (who dispense prescription medications, act as a valuable resource to physicians, counsel clients, and help ensure they do not use medications that have negative interactions)

- Physiotherapists (who deal with mobility and joint issues)

- Respiratory technologists (who manage breathing problems related to such conditions as chronic obstructive lung disease)

- Chiropractors (who treat chronic musculoskeletal problems)

- Nurses (who provide ongoing care and support in the hospital and in the community)

Cardiologists

Cardiologists specialize in conditions and diseases of the heart, including abnormal heartbeats (i.e., arrhythmias), heart attacks, **congenital** heart defects, infections of the heart and heart muscle, and syndromes such as cardiovascular heart disease and congestive heart failure. The cardiologist treats from a medical perspective but does not do surgery. If surgery is required, the client is referred to a cardiac surgeon.

Gynecologists/Obstetricians

Specializing in women's health, gynecologists diagnose and treat disorders of the gynecological and reproductive systems. Obstetricians focus on the care of pregnant women and the delivery of their babies in both normal and high-risk situations. Closely related, these two specialties are usually undertaken together (resulting in the abbreviation OB/GYN in reference to these specialists).

In urban centres, babies delivered by obstetricians far outnumber those delivered by family physicians. In smaller towns and rural settings, family doctors have delivered their clients' babies for many years, a situation that is now changing for a variety of reasons:

- To cover the high cost of insurance to deliver babies, family doctors would have to deliver a relatively high number of babies, perhaps more than they would have an opportunity to over the course of a year.

- Delivering babies is time-consuming, disruptive to office hours, and disruptive to the doctor's private life.

Congenital

Present at birth but not attributed to hereditary factors; a condition that may have developed during pregnancy due to a variety of factors.

- Increasingly, midwives assume, in normal pregnancies and at the pregnant woman's request, care of her and delivery of her baby (CTV, 2004).

For the most part, a family doctor maintains the care of a pregnant woman until she reaches approximately 24 weeks of **gestation**, unless the pregnancy has complications, in which case she will be referred to an obstetrician earlier. Contrary to popular belief, the obstetrician does not provide care for the baby after its birth. A family doctor or pediatrician immediately assumes its care. For six weeks after the baby's birth, however, the obstetrician continues care for the mother.

Gestation
The period of time from a baby's conception until its delivery.

Neurologists

A neurologist treats conditions of the nervous system, including chronic and potentially fatal conditions such as Parkinson's disease and multiple sclerosis, sleep disorders, headaches, peripheral vascular disease, brain tumours, spinal cord injuries, and congenital abnormalities such as **hydrocephalus**. Neurologists do not perform surgery. When a client requires surgery, the neurologist refers him or her to a neurosurgeon. Often, a neurosurgeon and neurologist will manage a client's care together. For example, a client with hydrocephalus who needed surgical intervention would see a neurosurgeon for the surgery and a neurologist for ongoing medical management.

Hydrocephalus
Abnormal accumulation of cerebrospinal fluid (CSF) in the brain. The cause is usually genetic.

Ophthalmologists

Ophthalmologists, medical doctors who specialize in diseases of the eye, can carry out both medical and surgical procedures, such as cataract removal and ocular emergencies (e.g., glaucoma, eye trauma). Although ophthalmologists can perform **refractions** and prescribe glasses, these functions have largely been taken over by optometrists (who are not medical doctors).

Refraction
Testing of the eyes to evaluate their ability to see. An ophthalmologist or optometrist does a refraction to determine the type of lens a client needs in his or her glasses to maximize vision.

Oncologists

Oncology is the branch of medicine that deals with all forms and stages of cancerous tumours—development, diagnosis, treatment, and prevention. An oncologist specializes in the care and treatment of people with cancer. Because cancer treatment has become so highly specialized, oncologists may specialize in only certain areas, such as radiation therapy, chemotherapy, gynecological oncology, or surgery. For example, a radiation or chemotherapeutic oncologist may not be qualified to perform surgery, whereas a surgical oncologist would. Oncologists usually practise in large hospitals or medical centres specializing in cancer treatment.

Psychiatrists

Psychiatrists specialize in mental illness and emotional disorders, including depression, bipolar disease, schizophrenia, obsessive compulsive disorder (OCD), borderline personality disorder, bulimia, anorexia nervosa, and personal stress issues. As medical doctors, psychiatrists can order laboratory and diagnostic tests and prescribe medicine. They may work closely with other physicians (e.g., a family doctor or an internist) when physical problems become an issue or result from a mental or emotional disorder. Psychiatrists do not perform surgical procedures or even minor medical procedures, such as inserting a nasogastric (i.e., feeding) tube for an anorexic client.

Physiatrists

Physiatrists, medical doctors specializing in physical and rehabilitative medicine, work closely with other health care professionals, such as physiotherapists, occupational therapists, and geriatricians. Stroke and accident victims and postsurgical clients are among the types of clients that a physiatrist would see. Comprehensive care aims to restore the client to his or her maximum level of function. The family almost always plays a role in the restorative and rehabilitative process, as treatment is usually long and arduous. For this reason, social workers, psychologists, or psychiatrists may also participate on the health care team.

Surgeons

Surgeons complete their surgery residency in their field of choice usually over a period of four years or more after completing medical school. A general surgeon completes a number of rotations through various specialties (e.g., gastric, orthopedic, plastic, thoracic, vascular surgery) and then may select an area of interest, called an *elective*, much like the opportunity a student is given to choose a general education course in college. General surgeons are qualified to perform a wide range of procedures usually involving the gastrointestinal tract. Their scope of practice may be limited, however, by the presence of other surgeons with specific specialties at the same hospital or in the community (Case Example 7.4).

Case Example 7.4

Robert presents in the ER with a blockage in his bowel. Dr. Xiong, a general surgeon, is qualified to assess and operate on Robert, but if Dr. Silanka, a gastric surgeon, is available, the emergentologist may call on Dr. Silanka instead.

Cardiac or cardiovascular surgeons perform open heart surgery, which may involve, among other things, vascular procedures (i.e., those dealing with blood vessels) and procedures dealing with the valves of the heart. Whereas a cardiac surgeon performs procedures related to the heart, a cardiovascular surgeon specializes in surgery related to the heart and vascular system (e.g., coronary artery bypass). A cardiologist or cardiac surgeon can specialize even further in an area such as pediatric cardiology, which deals with conditions of the heart in children.

Neurosurgeons deal with conditions such as brain tumours, spinal cord injuries, herniated disks, and carotid artery disease, as well as trauma-related conditions like **subdural hematomas**.

Plastic surgeons are well known for performing cosmetic surgery (e.g., face-lifts, tummy tucks, breast augmentations), but a large component of their work includes reconstructive surgery—repairing damage to bones and soft tissues caused by accidents or cancer, or performing skin grafts and reconstructive surgery on burn victims. Most provincial and territorial health plans cover reconstructive surgery but not cosmetic surgery. For example, a woman who has had a mastectomy may have breast reconstruction surgery covered by her provincial or territorial plan, but a woman having a breast augmentation for cosmetic reasons would have to cover the cost of the procedure and recovery herself.

> **Subdural hematomas**
> A type of brain injury in which blood collects between the outer protective covering of the brain (i.e., the dura) and the middle layers of the brain covering (i.e., the meninges), most often caused by torn, bleeding veins on the inside of the dura as a result of a blow to the head.

NURSES

Many agree that the nurse, with multiple skills that transcend several disciplines, is the backbone of the health care system. For example, when a respiratory therapist is not available, the nurse does the inhalation treatments or sets up oxygen for a client. When the chaplain is not available, the nurse counsels and comforts the client and loved ones. When the clinical secretary is ill, the nurse assumes administrative responsibilities for the client care unit.

Nurse Practitioners

Nurse practitioners, registered nurses with extended training and skills, were introduced to the health care system in the late 1960s, with the intent that they would provide high-quality, low-cost health care, particularly in the north and in rural settings; however, nurse practitioners were not meant to replace the care of a medical or family doctor but only to supplement primary care for less-acute conditions. Nurse practitioners, called advanced practice nurses (APNs) in some jurisdictions, are regulated by the province's or territory's college of nurses (or its equivalent) or by their own governing body.

For a number of years, the concept of nurse practitioners was abandoned because of problems with funding mechanisms (e.g., controversy over whether governments or employers would pay for nurse practitioners), a perceived oversupply of medical doctors, doctors' opposition to nurse practitioners, and a lack of coordinated programs and legislation. During the 1980s, programs for nurse practitioners were, therefore, nonexistent. In the 1990s, a number of nurse practitioners who had graduated from programs several years before continued to practise in northern and rural regions and in community health centres. Over the past 10 years, nurse practitioner academic programs have been reintroduced in most jurisdictions across Canada, along with corresponding legislation to govern the profession.

Nurse practitioners practise independently but collaboratively with family physicians and other members of the health care team. In many provinces and territories, nurse practitioners diagnose and treat a specific range of health problems. Likewise, they can order specific lab and diagnostic tests and prescribe certain medications, which are outlined within their scope of practice. They work in primary care settings—family health groups, family health teams, family health networks, and clinics—and in hospitals under specialty designations (e.g., pediatrics, cardiology) and in emergency departments. In many jurisdictions, the precise role of the nurse practitioner is still being defined. Physicians remain in disagreement about how much and what kinds of responsibility the nurse practitioner can and should assume. Many physicians argue that since nurse practitioners are not doctors, they should work in collaboration with physicians—not independently of them. Some nurse practitioners agree; others feel they should be recognized as independent practitioners.

No agreements are currently in place among Canadian jurisdictions for nurse practitioners to have their credentials recognized in more than one jurisdiction. A newly crafted examination for nurse practitioners, however, is progress toward national acknowledgement of the field. Not all jurisdictions require nurse practitioners to write this exam as a requirement to practise. Nurse practitioners who move from one province or territory to another must contact the college of nurses in their new jurisdiction to determine licensing requirements there.

The doctor of nursing practice (DNP) designation, introduced in the United States in 2004, is expected to become a requirement for entry to practice for all advanced practice nurses by 2015. Canadian nursing leaders are currently examining the benefits and drawbacks of introducing a similar requirement in Canada.

Registered Nurses

Over the past few years, the diploma-prepared registered nurse (RN) has given way to a baccalaureate-prepared nurse, who must complete a four-year university program. Most jurisdictions have phased out their diploma RN programs. In the Northwest Territories, Aurora College graduates now hold a bachelor of science degree in nursing, obtained through linkage with the University of Victoria in British Columbia. Manitoba phased out its last diploma programs in 2009, and Alberta, in January 2010. The RN (prepared at either the diploma or baccalaureate level) usually assumes the most complex components of nursing care, as well as administrative and case management responsibilities. Many hospitals and other facilities employ RNs only in specific areas, such as intensive care units, where most of the nursing care demands skills only the RN is licensed to practise.

Diploma-prepared RNs may obtain a bachelor's degree in nursing by completing a two- or three-year program that, in many regions, can be taken on a part-time basis. Several universities offer the postdiploma degree program via teleconference, correspondence, and "satellite" classes held in various communities. Other postgraduate courses for registered nurses prepare them to assume a variety of roles and responsibilities. Advanced educational opportunities for RNs vary among provinces and territories.

Practical Nurses

To become a registered practical nurse, a person must complete high school (or the equivalent) and a two-year diploma program at a community or private college. The skill set and scope of practice of practical nurses have expanded dramatically over the past five years, with practical nurses now assuming many of the skills and responsibilities formerly limited to registered nurses. Their skill set includes doing dressings, dispensing medications, and, in some facilities, taking charge of units. The practical nurse collaborates with registered nurses and other members of the health care team to render client care.

Pharmacists

A licensed pharmacist dispenses medications in response to prescriptions. To practise pharmacy, a person must earn a bachelor's degree in pharmacy, complete an internship, and successfully pass a national board examination through the Pharmacy Examining Board of Canada.

Experts in their field, pharmacists provide other members of the health care team with valuable information about medications. The physician looks to the pharmacist for advice about current medications and interactions between medications. The client looks to the pharmacist for direction and advice about taking medications, their risks, and their side effects.

Currently, Alberta, Manitoba, and New Brunswick also allow pharmacists to write prescriptions under strict guidelines. Other jurisdictions are poised to soon follow suit. The Canadian Medical Association asserts that medical doctors and similarly educated health care professionals (e.g., nurse practitioners) should retain control of prescribing because they have the background, skill, and knowledge to take an adequate history, complete a physical examination, and correlate these findings with test results (Kondro, 2007). Pharmacists ask for only limited privileges—for example, to provide clients with a limited number of pills pending a doctor's visit to obtain a new prescription or to substitute a drug that a client has had an adverse reaction to.

MIDWIVES

Depending on the jurisdiction, women experiencing normal pregnancies may choose to see a midwife. Midwives provide prenatal care before the baby's birth, deliver the baby (either at the client's home or in the hospital), and provide post-partum care for up to six weeks after the birth.

Over the past 10 years, many jurisdictions have recognized midwifery through legislation and regulation and, in turn, have funded a midwife's care through the provincial or territorial health plan.

Strict guidelines dictate that the care of a pregnant woman must be turned over to a physician if her pregnancy becomes high-risk or shows signs of other problems (e.g., a multiple pregnancy, a previous history of complications, pregnancy-induced high blood pressure or diabetes). Toward the end of the preg-nancy, if the baby is in a breech position (i.e., feet first) or any other perceived or actual dangers exist (e.g., drop in the baby's heart rate, bleeding, umbilical cord hanging down into the birth canal), a specialist would be notified and the mother transferred to the hospital if she is not already there.

In jurisdictions that do not recognize or legislate midwifery, some women still seek out midwives for their care, delivery, or both. However, since these midwives are not regulated, their competence cannot be assured. In these ju-risdictions, the midwife cannot order prenatal tests or write prescriptions, and deliveries occur at the client's home, usually without medical intervention. It is advisable, therefore, in these conditions, that a woman choosing to use a mid-wife also remain under the care of her family doctor or obstetrician.

ALLIED HEALTH CARE PROFESSIONALS

OPTOMETRISTS AND OPTICIANS

Most optometrists first obtain an undergraduate degree, often in mathematics or science, before completing a four-year university program in optometry at one of Canada's two schools of optometry (in Waterloo, Ontario, and in Montreal, Quebec). The minimum requirement for entry to these programs is three years in a university science program attaining an average of at least 75%. Graduates of a school of optometry are awarded a doctor of optometry degree. To practise, optometrists must be licensed by their province or territory. Skilled in assessing eye function and conditions, they may use certain medications (e.g., eye drops to dilate the eyes for examination) in their practice and may prescribe glasses and contact lenses to clients who need them; however, clients with eye conditions requiring medical attention are referred to an ophthalmologist.

Ontario and British Columbia are in the process of proposing changes to expand the optometrist's scope of practice to include prescribing rights for topical eye medications and limited oral medications (e.g., antibiotics) for eyelid and corneal infections. Optometrists in Alberta have been prescribing certain medications for more than 10 years. Saskatchewan's, Manitoba's, and Nova Scotia's optometrists also can prescribe, although they face some limitations on steroids and glaucoma medications.

An optician completes a two- or three-year college program, sometimes followed by a practical component. Opticians can fill prescriptions for eyeglasses or contact lenses, fit glasses, help clients select frames, organize the grinding and polishing of lenses, and cut and edge lenses so they fit selected frames. They also do a considerable amount of health instruction related to contact lenses and glasses, including providing information about options such as lens coating and bifocal lenses. They may work independently or in a larger centre with other eye-care specialists.

OSTEOPATHS

Both a natural medicine and a treatment philosophy, osteopathy seeks to identify and treat restricted or constricted areas of the body. As a natural medicine, osteopathy applies the knowledge of the structure (i.e., anatomy) and function (i.e., physiology) of the body to all diseases, disorders, and dysfunctions. Osteopaths use a "hands-on" or "manual" approach to identify and correct problems. As a treatment philosophy, osteopathy demands that the body be addressed as an integrated unit and respect be given to all components of the client—body, mind, and spirit.

In Canada, osteopaths may be physicians with a full scope of medical practice rights as well as osteopathic manual training (these are regulated by the Royal College of Physicians and Surgeons of Canada), or they may be individuals without medical degrees but with extensive training in osteopathic manipulative treatment (these are currently nonregulated). Nonphysician osteopaths, sometimes known as *osteopathic practitioners* or *manual practice osteopaths*, compose the majority in Canada.

Although qualifications vary, in general, practitioners require an undergraduate degree and a licence. Many osteopaths complete a four-year degree in osteopathic medicine and a one-year residency. In Canada, several part-time programs teach the manual practice of osteopathy, and, in Quebec, the only province with a regulatory body specifically for osteopaths, a full-time program exists.

Osteopaths practise a holistic approach to client care. In Canada, they do not perform surgery or prescribe medicine and thus do not treat pathologic conditions requiring these types of interventions. Coverage for osteopathic treatment varies among jurisdictions. Many insurance companies, through extended coverage, cover the services of osteopaths who are licensed, registered, or certified by a government-recognized regulatory body.

Podiatrists (Chiropodists)

The only regulated professionals educated exclusively in conditions of the foot, podiatrists specialize in the recognition, assessment, and treatment of foot disorders. They treat sports injuries, foot deformities (related to the aging process as well as misalignments in children), infections, and general foot conditions, including calluses, corns, ingrown toenails, and warts. In North America, aspiring podiatrists must earn a bachelor's degree in science before embarking on a three- to four-year chiropody or podiatry program. Currently, only one chiropody school exists in Canada.

Personal Support Workers

In most jurisdictions, the personal support worker (PSW), formerly called a *nurse's aide*, requires formal training that may take three months to a full academic year to complete. PSWs work closely with their clients, providing personal care, psychological comfort, and assistance with daily activities. To meet the client's needs and render holistic care, the PSW collaborates with other members of the health care team. Their job is demanding, both physically and emotionally. PSWs, in many cases, spend more time with clients than do other team members, and clients come to depend on them for emotional and physical care.

Psychologists

Psychologists treat emotional and mental disorders, mainly through counselling. They administer noninvasive written and practical tests such as personality tests, IQ tests, assessment tests for attention deficit disorder (ADD), and diagnostic tests for the early stages of Alzheimer's disease or dementia. Since psychologists are not medical doctors, they do not have the authority to prescribe medications, perform medical procedures, or order lab or diagnostic tests. Often, a psychiatrist and a psychologist will work as a team for more effective and ongoing client treatment.

Physiotherapists and Physiotherapy Assistants

Physiotherapists graduate from a degree program. An essential part of the primary care team, physiotherapists work with clients to limit and improve physical impairments and disabilities and to prevent and manage pain. They work in a variety of settings such as hospitals, nursing homes, **clinics**, and private practices within the community. Some physiotherapists specialize in such areas as geriatrics, sports medicine, or pediatrics. Physiotherapists are regulated professionals, and their services are covered, with specific conditions, under most provincial and territorial plans, as well as most private insurance plans.

Clinic
A setting in which multiple health care professionals work collaboratively, usually in a similar field, to provide cost-effective, client-centred health care.

Physiotherapy assistants, members of the physiotherapy team, graduate from community or private colleges with either a certificate or diploma in the discipline. The physiotherapy assistant administers physical therapy treatments to clients under the direction of a physiotherapist.

Respiratory Technologists and Respiratory Technicians

To enter the field of respiratory technology, one must complete a postsecondary program in the field (usually three years), undergo a period of clinical training, and attain a licence from the College of Respiratory Therapists (or its equivalent) in his or her jurisdiction.

Intubate
To pass a tube into a person's trachea to facilitate breathing.

Respiratory technologists (RTs) and respiratory technicians work primarily in hospitals, within critical care areas such as the ER, intensive care and inpatient care units, and in clinics. Specialists in caring for people who have breathing difficulties, RTs respond to emergencies and are able to **intubate** clients and initiate the use of respirators. RTs are often required in the transfer of critically ill clients from one facility to another or from an accident scene to a hospital. They are also required in the delivery room when doctors suspect the baby has or may develop respiratory problems. RTs perform diagnostic testing, including arterial blood gases and pulmonary function tests. In the hospital setting, the RT is often responsible for setting up oxygen therapy or inhalation treatments when a physician orders these.

Respiratory technicians have a certificate or diploma in the field, which prepares them to work under the respiratory technologist and assume such responsibilities as testing clients, operating equipment to administer gases and drugs, monitoring clients, teaching clients how to use home equipment, and maintaining records.

Occupational Therapists and Occupational Therapy Technicians

Education requirements for occupational therapists (OTs) differ from one jurisdiction to another; however, all OTs must be registered with their provincial or territorial college. While some provinces and territories graduate OTs at a bach-elor's level, others require master's-level training. A national certification exam allows OTs to practise anywhere in Canada upon passing.

Occupational therapists (OTs) are health care professionals who help people learn or relearn to manage important everyday activities, including caring for themselves or others, maintaining their home, participating in paid and unpaid work, and engaging in leisure activities. Occupational therapists work with clients who have difficulties as the result of an accident, disability, disease, emo-tional or developmental problems, or aging. Clients can visit occupational thera-pists without a referral, or they may obtain a referral from their physicians.

Occupational therapists work in hospitals, private homes (usually through provincial or territorial home care programs), schools, long-term care facilities, mental health facilities, rehabilitation clinics, community agencies, public or pri-vate health care offices, and employment evaluation and training centres.

Occupational therapy assistants graduate from a community or private col-lege with a certificate or diploma in occupational therapy. They work closely with OTs to assist clients with their initiation and treatment plans (A. Jacobson, personal communication, April 7–9, 2009).

VOLUNTEER CAREGIVERS

It is only appropriate to note the tremendous support that friends and family provide to those who are ill. With current shortages in all categories of health care professionals, many clients depend on this group of people to fill in the gaps in their care that cannot otherwise be filled. The hours of care provided by these individuals are uncountable, the output unequalled, and the stress phenomenal. Many ill people could not manage without this supportive network. Volunteer caregivers work in partnership with professional caregivers.

ADMINISTRATIVE ROLES

HEALTH INFORMATION MANAGEMENT

Health information management (HIM) professionals manage health informa-tion in a variety of settings, including hospitals, long-term care and nursing homes, offices, clinics, and insurance and pharmaceutical companies. Educa-tional requirements for this role include a degree in health information and certification by the Canadian Health Information Management Association (CHIMA).

The responsibilities of these professionals are diverse and complex. Involved with almost every aspect of health information, from information retrieval to the destruction of information once it is no longer needed, HIM professionals are responsible for intricate communications systems, data collection and analysis, and information registries. The HIM professional is playing a pivotal role as Canada works toward the implementation of electronic health information systems.

ADMINISTRATIVE HEALTH CARE PROFESSIONALS

Every aspect of health care requires some level of administrative support. Being responsible for the day-to-day administrative management of a hospital unit, a clinic, or a physician's office requires skill, knowledge, patience, commitment, and a high level of professionalism. Increasing demands require people in this role to have a sound knowledge base in a variety of areas, including pharmacology, diagnostic and laboratory testing, medical terminology, anatomy and physiology, disease pathophysiology, and the principles of triage, among others. Administrative health care professionals must be flexible, friendly, empathetic, supportive, and comfortable around individuals experiencing health problems. They must have the ability to multitask and to work efficiently under pressure.

Administrative health care professionals may be prepared at either the diploma or degree level. Many colleges across Canada offer a two-year postsecondary diploma in health administration. Some private colleges offer one-year certificate programs that prepare graduates to assume basic responsibilities in the administrative field. Universities offering degrees in health administration prepare individuals to assume more complex roles or management positions. Some schools (e.g., Athabasca University in Alberta) offer postdiploma courses leading to a degree in health administration. British Columbia and Ontario are the only two provinces that have an **affiliating body** or association specifically for administrative health care professionals—the Medical Office Assistants' Association of British Columbia and the Ontario Medical Secretaries Association. The International Association of Administrative Professionals (IAAP) welcomes members from any administrative discipline and has chapters across Canada.

Affiliating body
An association that provides, among other things, direction, support, continuing education, and networking opportunities for its professional members (who may be regulated or nonregulated).

LABORATORY AND DIAGNOSTIC SERVICES

The field of medicine depends greatly on laboratory and diagnostic services. Many diagnoses cannot be confirmed without a lab or diagnostic test of some sort. Even to prescribe the appropriate antibiotic, doctors rely on laboratory tests. Highly qualified individuals, including physician specialists and laboratory technologists and technicians, populate this field. Many specialties exist within this area (e.g., pathology, hematology), as well, most of which are regulated in their individual province or territory.

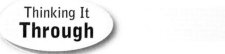

Thinking It **Through**

An older family member falls ill and requires constant supervision at home for a period of time. Home care options are limited.

Assuming that you work full-time and have a family of your own, what would you do to ensure your family member receives the care he or she needs?

PRACTICE SETTINGS

Most family doctors deliver care in an office, either in solo practice or in a group or clinic setting. Several types of clinic settings are described below. As a result of primary health care reform, family doctors often work in primary health care reform groups, which are discussed in more detail later in this chapter.

CLINICS

Urgent Case and Walk-in Clinics

Canadian residents can seek medical care from urgent care and walk-in clinics if they do not have a family doctor, are away from home, or cannot get an appointment with their primary care physician. These clinics reduce the burden on emergency departments by providing nonemergency care to clients who would otherwise clog the ER. Clinic visits also usually cost less to the health care system than do visits to the ER. Some urgent care clinics offer more immediate access to diagnostic testing, such as ultrasound, and minor procedures, such as suturing, whereas walk-in clinics often refer the client elsewhere for these procedures.

Ambulatory Care Clinics

In the most literal interpretation, ambulatory care clinics have traditionally encompassed any clinic that offers services and discharges the client immediately thereafter—that is, a clinic in which a client does not spend the night. Ambulatory care, therefore, may include day surgeries, visits to emergency rooms, cast changes, postsurgical assessment (perhaps after hip or knee surgery), or cancer treatment. And ambulatory care clinics may include several different types of facilities, including walk-in or urgent care clinics, privately owned clinics located in a medical building, and a doctor's private office.

Within the past five years, the term has referred more specifically to facilities that offer groups of services in one location—most frequently, a hospital.

Outpatient Clinics

Outpatient clinics offer services that vary from hospital to hospital and community to community in an effort to meet the unique needs of a particular area. An outpatient clinic can operate under the umbrella of an ambulatory care clinic—a clinic within a clinic. Services may include family doctor care, minor surgery, screening procedures (e.g., vascular screening), laboratory and diagnostic procedures, and foot care. Outpatient clinics in large hospitals offer a wider range of services.

Some hospitals divide clinics into areas of specialty and related services; others offer many disciplines within one clinic. For example, in Moncton, New Brunswick, the hospital has divided its ambulatory care clinics into five specialized areas: healthy living (includes services to assess and treat ongoing conditions, such as asthma, diabetes, chronic pulmonary disease), specialty procedures clinics (include **urodynamic** and eye clinics), treatments and orthopedics, diagnostic clinics (includes pulmonary assessment, electrocardiograms), and endoscopy and minor surgery.

Urodynamic
Referring to tests and assessments done to measure the function of the bladder and urinary tract.

Why Clinics Make Sense

Clinics have gained prominence for a number of reasons, including the following:

Community-based care
Care provided for the client in the home (e.g., incorporating visits from nurses or physiotherapists) or on an outpatient basis rather than in the hospital or another health care facility.

- Cost-effectiveness: The past few years have yielded a shift toward **community-based care**. New technologies have shortened surgeries and made them less invasive, allowing for earlier discharges and follow-up in clinics. It costs less to care for clients at home than to maintain them as inpatients. Many tests formerly done in a hospital are now done in a clinic on an outpatient basis. Having clients see a specialist or other health care professional in the clinic setting on a first-come, first-served basis usually costs less than having them make an appointment with a specialist or health care professional. Organizations can staff clinics more efficiently according to perceived need. As well, equipment booking, if handled centrally, can result in available equipment being maximized.

- Timely access, fewer client visits, convenience: With proper organization, clients can access more services faster, possibly in one clinic visit. The move toward multidisciplinary health teams has enabled clinics to readily provide the client with a variety of services (Case Example 7.5). With centralized resources, the client should have to make fewer visits, a result that is especially beneficial to those with multiple health problems and mobility or transportation issues.

Case Example 7.5

Diagnosed with diabetes six months ago, Jim is still learning how to live with the disease. He visits the ambulatory care clinic at 7:00 Monday morning. First, he goes to the lab and has blood work done. The nurse reviews with him his blood sugar levels for the past two weeks and how much insulin he is taking each day. He then sees the dietitian at 8:20 to discuss changes to his diet. At 9:30, he sees the doctor, who checks his blood pressure and general health and does an eye examination. The doctor reviews his insulin intake and diet, as well as his blood work—which is back from the lab and shows slightly elevated levels—and recommends some changes. Jim then returns to the nurse to discuss some of his personal concerns. He is finished at 12:00. At 12:20, he goes for a cardiac stress test, as he has been experiencing chest pains, which may or may not be related to his diabetes.

• Client focus: Specialized clinics are usually better prepared to work with clients and to consider their individual needs. The streamlined and client-friendly health education offered in these clinics involves the client. Clinic staff members typically have experience dealing with a specific condition and take the opportunity to learn from their clients, which increases their overall effectiveness in meeting clients' health care needs.

PRIMARY HEALTH CARE REFORM

Across Canada, thousands of Canadians have no family doctor and only limited access to other primary care providers. Even when a person does have a family doctor, getting an appointment can take days or even weeks, unless his or her condition is acute. In many jurisdictions, it is not uncommon for clients to wait up to six months for an annual physical examination.

In recent years, Canada has invested millions of dollars in health care and taken steps to strengthen the collaboration among the federal, provincial, and territorial governments to improve access to health care services and to enhance the services themselves (Box 7.4). Toward meeting their goals, the governments have changed how some practice settings are organized and how health care professionals are paid. The emphasis now and for the foreseeable future is on the development and implementation of primary health care reform initiatives (i.e., efforts to improve practice settings) and electronic health records (see Chapters 6 and 10).

> ## Box 7.4   Primary Health Care Transition Fund
>
> Canada's premiers met in September 2000 and agreed on the urgent need to make improvements to primary health care services through the use of multidisciplinary health care teams and other primary health care reform initiatives. The premiers allotted $800 million to the Primary Health Care Transition Fund, designed to assist health care professionals in moving into new models of health care delivery. This money supported primary care initiatives in the provinces and territories until 2006. Part of the money was also used to identify and address common barriers to health care across Canada. Ongoing funding, provided by various levels of government, is continually evaluated.
>
> The federal government aims to ensure that at least 50% of Canadians will have access to a multidisciplinary health care team by 2011—a goal that the Health Council of Canada believes should be accelerated.
>
> Source: Health Council of Canada. (2007). *Health care renewal in Canada: Measuring up? Annual report to Canadians 2006.* Toronto: Author.

PRIMARY HEALTH CARE REFORM GROUPS

Within primary health care reform groups, doctors are bound to an agreement to practise under specific guidelines to deliver primary care to a population base. These groups can vary in size, in composition of health care professionals, in services offered, and in name.

A number of family doctors can unite to create a primary health care reform group. They first need to choose what particular model to use (e.g., family health team, family health network). In most jurisdictions, the group then has to apply to the provincial or territorial government (or the appropriate body) for funding and permission to form the group. Each jurisdiction has a different name for its primary health care reform groups, and each jurisdiction's groups differ in such things as how many physicians are in the group, the inclusion of other health care professionals (e.g., nurse practitioners, dietitians, pharmacists), the responsibilities required by group members (e.g., on-call hours, clinic availability, Telehealth access), billing mechanisms such as blended funding (e.g., fee-for-service billing, capitation-based funding), and billing for certain services (e.g., smoking cessation, preventive care).

Once approved, the group will receive funding for the various services on offer—for example, a telephone helpline and an integrated computer system. The group must determine the types of team members to be hired (e.g., nurse practitioner, pharmacist, nutritionist). The province or territory may provide funding for the hiring of these team members, depending on the jurisdiction and the type and structure of care model the physicians adopt. Team members do not have to be physically located in the same building, although proximity to one another improves access for clients.

Once a team has been formed, the method of payment for the physicians changes from the typical fee-for-service system to another funding method, such as capitation-based funding, or to a combination of several methods. A more detailed discussion of payment for health care professionals' services can be found in Chapter 6.

Rostering

Most primary health care reform groups require that a certain percentage of clients formalize their relationships with the group by signing a form agreeing to become part of the doctor's practice. This is called **rostering**. If you have received and signed a form from your own family doctor, you have been registered or rostered into his or her practice. Signing the form is purely voluntary and not binding; a client may leave the practice at any time, or become unrostered. But being rostered entitles the client to all of the services and benefits offered by that particular primary health care reform group. Rostering may also affect how the doctor is paid (see Chapter 6).

If a rostered client visits another medical doctor for a routine health problem (i.e., not an emergency), the government will deduct from the family doctor's monthly stipend the fee for that visit (Case Example 7.6).

Rostering
The registering of a client in a primary health care reform group. Clients sign a form, which is nonbinding, stating that they will seek care only from a specific doctor.

Case Example 7.6

Although rostered with Dr. Gregory, George, who is experiencing extreme stress, goes to see Dr. Gresham, a family physician who also offers counselling services and psychotherapy. Dr. Gresham bills the provincial plan $100 for George's visit.

At the end of the month, Dr. Gregory gets a notice from his provincial ministry of health stating that $100 has been deducted from his monthly payment to compensate the ministry for the amount it was charged for George's visit to Dr. Gresham.

Being rostered is probably not appropriate for a person living in a temporary residence (e.g., a college student living away from home to attend school) because he or she may need to seek health care elsewhere.

SERVICES AND BENEFITS

For the Health Care Professional

Health care professionals enjoy the benefit of a supportive team environment within a primary health care reform group. These groups receive financial assistance from the government for training staff and for computer and information technology initiatives. In most groups, the physician can enjoy more time off, with the assurance that the clients in his or her practice will receive proper care while he or she is away. As well, other members of the health care team enjoy a better environment in terms of employment benefits, including paid vacation, sick time, and job security.

For the Client

Under the provincial or territorial health ministry's guidelines, primary health care reform groups must offer certain services to rostered clients, including access to a multidisciplinary team of health care specialists. For example, if a client needs to see a dietitian, one must be readily available.

Clients have access to a doctor at the clinic during extended evening and weekend hours. If the client's family doctor is away, the client can see another doctor within the group instead of having to visit a walk-in clinic or an emergency room. For after-hours assistance, the client has access to a telephone helpline connected to the family health group. The client's health records are in electronic form so that primary care providers have easy access to them if needed. (Communities across Canada are in various stages of implementing the electronic health record—see Chapter 6.)

Thinking It
Through

You move to a new town and set out to find a family doctor. You find one physician in solo practice who agrees to take you as a client because he cares for friends of yours. However, you also find a newly formed primary health care reform group with two physicians taking new clients.

Considering the benefits the primary health care reform group offers versus the close relationship you would be likely to develop with the physician in solo practice, which would you choose?

Telephone Helplines

Because telephone services are considered an important element in primary care, the government has invested significant funds into this initiative. Often called

Telehealth, or Teletriage, these helplines offer callers advice from health care professionals (usually registered nurses) 24 hours a day, 7 days a week.

Telephone helplines differ across the country in the type and scope of service they offer. Some offer only telephone advice, whereas others refer the client to another resource (e.g., a clinic, a nurse practitioner, a doctor, the ER). Some will forward the call to the physician on call for that group or ensure that the client's physician receives information about any care or advice the client received (Case Example 7.7).

Telehealth
A telephone help system, usually available 24/7 and funded by the provincial or territorial government, used to provide professional health care advice to Canadians who cannot readily access a doctor or other primary care provider.

Case Example 7.7

Helena lives in British Columbia and has a 3-year-old daughter, Gillian. Gillian wakes up at 2:00. She is warm, crying, and has diarrhea. Helena is not sure what to do. Should she take Gillian to the emergency department, or is it something that can wait until morning? Helena calls NurseLine, which offers British Columbians health information and advice from a registered nurse 24 hours a day, 7 days a week. The nurse tells Helena to sponge the baby, to try to give her some clear fluids, and to monitor her until the morning, at which time she can call her family doctor—which Helena does. In the meantime, NurseLine transmits an electronic report of the occurrence to the family doctor's office.

Although most helplines have follow-up procedures, these are not always foolproof. If a helpline attendant does not diligently obey such rules, using telephone helplines can be dangerous, as demonstrated in a rather extreme but not entirely unheard-of circumstance in Case Example 7.8.

Case Example 7.8

Theo called a telephone helpline at 2:00 Monday morning. He said he'd tried to kill himself by taking a bottle of aspirin and half a bottle of sleeping pills. The pills had only made him slightly drowsy. With a change of heart, he wondered what he should do. The nurse advised him to go to the nearest emergency department and offered to call an ambulance for him. He responded that he would go but that he had someone to drive him. The helpline did not follow up with Theo's family doctor about this call, which is not unusual in some

Continued on next page

circumstances. At 15:00 on Wednesday afternoon, a family friend found Theo semiconscious and dehydrated on the floor in his kitchen and called 911. Theo's kidneys had failed. Today he is alive but on dialysis. If Theo's doctor had been notified of the event Tuesday morning, he could have arranged for follow-up immediately and perhaps minimized the kidney damage.

Health Service Organizations

The concept behind health service organizations (HSOs) is similar to that of primary health care reform groups, except that the former's funding model more closely resembles the indirect capitation model, in which a third party receives and manages funding (see Chapter 6). In the case of HSOs, health care professionals operate within an organization and more or less ration care to their rostered clients, with the goal of rendering high-quality care while containing costs by ordering tests only when absolutely necessary. Because physicians get to know their clients, they can make informed decisions about necessary tests and investigations.

A successful HSO in Sault Ste. Marie, Ontario, called the Group Health Centre, is a nonprofit, alternatively funded ambulatory health organization constructed from a partnership between the Sault Ste. Marie and District Health Group and the Algoma District Medical Group (Group Health Centre, 2009). Approximately 60 physicians with varying specialties comprise the latter group. The corporation, governed by a board of directors from the community, owns its building, equipment, and furniture, and hires the staff (excluding physicians).

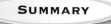

SUMMARY

❖ The delivery of high-quality, cost-effective health care remains a challenge across Canada. Problems we face include insufficient funding, a shortage of health care professionals, an aging population, aging diagnostic equipment, long waits to see specialists, clogged ERs, and high expectations of care.

❖ The professionals who deliver care in Canada—from administrative and support staff and allied health care professionals to the physicians—are the mainstay of our health care system. Strategies to increase the number of health care professionals, retain the ones we have, and maintain a high level of care are essential.

❖ In most provinces and territories, nurse practitioners and midwives have recently joined the ranks of regulated health care professionals delivering primary care—and various other modalities are following the same path. Regulation provides the public with a wider choice of health care professionals, with the assurances that the professional they choose meets legislated standards of practice.

❖ Some nonregulated professions are in the process of seeking regulation. As well, health care professionals—regulated and nonregulated alike—have support from a wide range of professional organizations, many of which offer education and certification to their members. A designation ensures a high standard of performance.

❖ The list of health care professionals is long and includes those practising conventional medicine as well as those practising modalities considered complementary or alternative. Increasingly, Canadians are appreciating the value of alternative and complementary health care professionals, often turning to them to supplement their medical care. All jurisdictions recognize the value of seeking the strengths of all professions and working collaboratively to enhance Canadians' health.

❖ A nationwide initiative, primary health care reform probably holds the answer to providing effective point-of-contact care to all Canadians. Models of primary health care reform include family health networks, family health groups, family health organizations, and family health teams.

❖ Working in health care today is frustrating, demanding, exciting, and rewarding. No matter what their discipline, all health care professionals are a dynamic and vital part of the health care team. Their involvement with the client, whether it be in a hospital or clinic setting, an office, or the community, is essential. Every day that you listen to the news or pick up the newspaper, you will likely hear or read about shortcomings and successes in health care. When embarking on a career in health care, be prepared for continued change in the system, in how and where you practise, in your scope of practice, and in your responsibilities.

REVIEW QUESTIONS

1. Outline the benefits that a regulated profession offers to the public.

2. Differentiate between a controlled act and a delegated act, giving an example of each.

3. What is meant by *title protection*?

4. What are the differences between an ophthalmologist, an optometrist, and an optician?

5. Explain the purpose of primary health care reform.

6. State the purpose of telephone helpline services. Explain how some differ in the services they offer.

DISCUSSION QUESTIONS

1. a. Choose three practitioners—one from each column—in Table 7.1 that you think have something in common. Summarize their scope of practice and the services they offer to the public. Discuss how these three professions might work collaboratively to benefit a client.

   b. Summarize how your own choice of profession can work collaboratively with the professions chosen in (a).

2. a. If your chosen profession is regulated, prepare a list of the responsibilities within the scope of practice. Using the controlled acts documented by your organization, list any that are pertinent to your profession. If no official scope of practice is outlined, discuss the job you are being prepared for and list the responsibilities that fall within your job description. Identify any delegated acts you might be asked to assume in your professional role.

   b. Investigate what professional organizations are available for you to join. Outline the procedure for joining and the benefits offered.

3. a. Locate a primary health care reform group in your community. Investigate what type of group (i.e., model) it is. Research the model based on these questions: Are clients rostered? What benefits does the group offer to the health care professionals and to the public? Does it offer a telephone helpline? Where are clients referred for emergency treatment?

   b. Save newspaper articles on primary care issues for one week. At the end of that time, summarize two of the articles and the initiatives within your community or province to deal with the issues.

4. Mario, 34, has been in hospital for a week recovering from a motor vehicle accident. He feels that a particular nurse did not treat the client in the next bed, Hu, properly. On three occasions, the nurse was very rough ambulating Hu, a stroke victim who could not speak clearly, and once used offensive language. After Mario got home, he started to worry about Hu's treatment and made a decision to complain about the nurse. What steps do you think Mario should take? What regulatory body would be involved?

5. Using the NPCanada Web site (see Web Resources), compare and contrast the responsibilities of a nurse practitioner and a primary care physician in your jurisdiction.

WEB RESOURCES

Baby Center: How to Find a Midwife in Canada
http://www.babycenter.ca/pregnancy/
antenatalhealth/testsandcare/
bookingappointment/

This Web site provides information on why, when, and
how to find a midwife in Canada. It explains what a
midwife does, offers tips such as what to look for in a
midwife, and gives the five questions to ask a midwife.

NPCanada.com
http://www.npcanada.ca

This Web site offers information about the scope of
practice of nurse practitioners, continuing education
resources, a job board, news stories about the field, and
provincial regulations.

Canadian Association of Occupational Therapists
http://www.caot.ca/default.asp?pageid=2

The Canadian Association of Occupational Therapists
provides services, products, events, and networking
opportunities to help occupational therapists achieve
excellence in their professional practice. This Web
page outlines the mission, vision, values, and strategic
objectives of the association.

CMA Leadership Series: Primary Care Reform
http://www.cma.ca/index.cfm/ci_id/44700/la_
id/1.htm

Published by the Canadian Medical Association
(CMA), *Primary Care Reform* is a magazine that offers
an overview of primary care reform initiatives across
Canada. A national, voluntary association of physicians,
the CMA advocates for high-quality health care on behalf
of its members and the public.

Guidelines for the Delegation of a Medical Act
http://www.ncbi.nlm.nih.gov/pmc/articles/
pmc1267562/pdf/cmaj00159-0083.pdf

This document outlines the Canadian Medical
Association's guidelines for physicians delegating a
medical act to a person other than a physician.

College of Nurses of Ontario
http://www.cno.org/international_en/intro/
expectations.htm

The College of Nurses of Ontario is the governing body
for the registered nurses and registered practical nurses
in Ontario. It regulates nursing and sets requirements to
enter the profession, establishes and enforces standards
of nursing practice, and assures the quality of practice of
the profession and the continuing competence of nurses.

**College of Occupational Therapists of Nova
Scotia**
http://www.cotns.ca

Established by the government of Nova Scotia, the
College of Occupational Therapists of Nova Scotia
oversees the practice of occupational therapists in the
province. A self-governing body, it registers, regulates,
and supports the ongoing competency of occupational
therapists.

Guideline on the Controlled Acts and Delegation
http://www.coto.org/pdf/Controlled_Acts.pdf

This set of guidelines from the College of Occupational
Therapists of Ontario addresses the concepts related
to controlled acts and the opportunity for occupational
therapists to be delegated to perform controlled acts.

**Guidelines for Delegated Medical Functions and
Medical Directives**
http://www.cpsns.ns.ca/publications/
GuidelinesforDelegatedMedicalFunctions2005.pdf

This document by the College of Physicians and Surgeons
of Nova Scotia and the College of Registered Nurses of
Nova Scotia provides registered nurses, physicians, and
health care agencies with a common base of information
related to the delegation of medical acts.

Primary Health Care
http://www.hc-sc.gc.ca/hcs-sss/prim/
index-eng.php

This Health Canada Web page provides links to
information on primary health care in Canada—what it is,
its potential, and how it is funded.

WEB RESOURCES

Medical Office Assistants' Association of British Columbia

http://www.medicalofficeassistantsofbc.com/page/page/1821867.htm

A nonprofit organization, the Medical Office Assistants' Association of British Columbia has seven provincial chapters committed to providing educational, personal, and professional growth opportunities for their members.

The Regulation of Counsellors Across Canada

http://www.bc-counsellors.org/files/SummaryReport(BRIEF).txt

This document contains an overview and policy questions for the National Symposium on Counsellor Regulation, held in 2005 in Vancouver, British Columbia.

REFERENCES

Canadian Medical Association. (1988). A CMA position. Guidelines for the delegation of a medical act. *Canadian Medical Association Journal, 138*. Retrieved May 29, 2009, from http://www.ncbi.nlm.nih.gov/pmc/articles/pmc1267562/pdf/cmaj00159-0083.pdf

College of Physicians and Surgeons of Ontario. (2008). *Delegation of controlled acts*. Retrieved May 29, 2009, from http://www.cpso.on.ca/policies/policies/default.aspx?ID=1554

CTV. (2004, April 21). Canada's Caesarean section rate highest ever. *CTV News* Retrieved May 29, 2009, from http://www.ctv.ca/servlet/ArticleNews/story/CTVNews/1082553935798_40

Group Health Centre. (2009). *Algoma District Medical Group*. Retrieved May 29, 2009, from http://www.ghc.on.ca/admg/content.html?sID=15

Human Resources and Skills Development Canada. (2007). *Labour mobility*. Retrieved May 29, 2009, from http://www.workdestinations.org/paged_category_drilldown.jsp?categoryId=44&crumb=41&crumb=43&lang=en

Kondro, W. (2007). Canada's doctors assail pharmacist prescribing. *Canadian Medical Association Journal, 177*(6), Retrieved May 29, 2009, from http://www.cmaj.ca/cgi/content/full/177/6/558

Steed, J. (2008, November 15). 10 innovative fixes for what ails us. *The Toronto Star*. Retrieved May 29, 2009, from http://www.thestar.com/printArticle/537348

CHAPTER EIGHT

The Law and Health Care

Learning Outcomes

1. Explain the division of powers between the Canadian federal government and the provincial and territorial governments in terms of legal jurisdiction.

2. Identify two examples of federal legislation affecting health care.

3. Discuss the legislative role of the *Occupational Health and Safety Act* and of workers' compensation in providing Canadians with a healthy and safe work environment.

4. Discuss recent challenges to the *Canadian Charter of Rights and Freedoms* regarding the right to health care.

5. Outline the basic principles of consent to treatment and the special considerations that apply to minors.

6. Discuss privacy of health information with reference to federal and provincial legislation.

7. Explain the security and access concerns surrounding electronic health information and the safeguarding of files.

8. Describe the role of self-governing health care professions in legal matters.

KEY TERMS

Act, p. 268

Age of majority, p. 301

Canada Health Act, p. 286

Circle of care, p. 296

Civil law, p. 269

Code of ethics, p. 307

Common law, p. 269

Confidentiality, p. 303

Conflict of interest, p. 291

Constitutional law, p. 267

Contract law, p. 273

Controlled Drugs and Substances Act, p. 278

Criminal law, p. 273

Drug-seeking behaviour, p. 280

Duty of care, p. 273

Electronic health record (EHR), p. 305

Electronic medical record (EMR), p. 305

Fiduciary duty, p. 291

Good Samaritan law, p. 310

Implied consent, p. 296

Incident report, p. 275

Informed consent, p. 293

Inpatient, p. 309

Jurisdiction, p. 276

Legislation, p. 267

Malpractice, p. 272

Minor, p. 297

Negligence, p. 272

Oral consent, p. 296

Personal Information Protection and Electronic Documents Act (PIPEDA), p. 302

Power of attorney, p. 297

Privacy, p. 303

Professional misconduct, p. 272

Proxy consent, p. 298

Quarantine Act, p. 284

Regulation, p. 268

Regulatory law, p. 268

Royal assent, p. 285

Statutory law, p. 268

Tort, p. 271

Whistleblower, p. 310

WHMIS legislation, p. 278

This chapter provides a practical overview of the relationship between the law and health care in Canada. It concentrates on basic elements of health care and the application of related legal issues, rather than on specific laws and legislation. Because laws vary among the provinces and territories, it is more meaningful to research those within your own jurisdiction to access specific information.

Hospitals, physicians, regional health authorities, and regulated professions are all governed by legislation, regulations, and guidelines, which affect how they function. This chapter begins by examining the division of legislative powers between the federal government and the provincial and territorial governments where health care is concerned. It also discusses the legal responsibilities of the federal government with respect to safety legislation and sections within criminal law that affect health care.

The chapter also addresses the legal right of Canadians to health care and discusses court challenges that have been launched (some successfully, some not) regarding the right of Canadians to timely medical intervention under the *Canadian Charter of Rights and Freedoms*.

Provincial and territorial **legislation** regarding private enterprise in health care varies. The chapter looks at restrictions imposed on Canadians with regard to seeking health care from private clinics and the right of Canadians to purchase private insurance for medically necessary services that the provinces or territories cannot provide within reasonable time frames.

The chapter also examines the legal guidelines and responsibilities of health care professionals regarding consent to treatment. The effects of the law on health care professionals, as well as on professionals' moral and legal obligations to clients, are also highlighted. Finally, this chapter addresses health information management, confidentiality, and current privacy legislation—and the challenges presented by electronic health records.

> **Legislation**
> Laws made by a provincial or territorial legislature or by Parliament. To become law, a bill (i.e., proposed legislation) that has been introduced to Parliament requires the agreement of the House of Commons, the Senate, and the Crown (i.e., the Governor General, the representative of the British monarch in Canada).

LAWS USED IN HEALTH CARE LEGISLATION

Law in Canada includes both statutory law (i.e., derived from acts) and common law (i.e., made by judges in deciding cases). Various levels of government are authorized to create laws. Some types of law apply to the health care industry more than others, including constitutional, statutory, regulatory, and common or case law, each of which is described in the sections that follow.

CONSTITUTIONAL LAW

Constitutional law addresses the relationship between the people and their government, and establishes, allocates, and limits public power. In Canada, cases challenging a person's right to health care have been based on the *Canadian Charter of Rights and Freedoms*, part of the Canadian Constitution. Under the Constitution, everyone has the following fundamental freedoms (*Canadian Charter of Rights and Freedoms*, 1982):

> **Constitutional law**
> The area of law dealing with legislation derived from or related to Canada's Constitution.

- Freedom of conscience and religion
- Freedom of thought, belief, opinion, and expression, including freedom of the press and other media of communication
- Freedom of peaceful assembly
- Freedom of association

A Canadian citizen denied any of these rights can challenge the person, persons, or organization denying him or her such rights based on the related section of the Charter. Challenges regarding the right to health care often occur under sections 7 and 15 (see pages 287–288).

STATUTORY LAW

Act
A usually comprehensive body of laws passed by Parliament or a provincial or territorial legislature.

A statute is a law or an **act**. **Statutory laws** are the laws passed in Parliament (i.e., at the federal level) or in the provincial or territorial legislatures. Statutory laws under federal authority include those dealing with immigration, taxation, and divorce. Statutory laws under provincial or territorial jurisdiction include those related to education, family, and health care.

REGULATORY LAW

Regulatory law
Laws made not by Parliament or by a legislature but by authorized persons or organizations to govern a particular group; these laws are ultimately subject to the provincial, territorial, or federal act that governs the administrative body, organization, or tribunal.

Regulation
A form of law, made by persons or organizations (e.g., an administrative agency) awarded such authority within an act (whether federal, provincial, or territorial), that has the binding legal power of an act.

Regulatory law possesses the legally binding feature of an act; however, regulatory law is not made by Parliament (i.e., at the federal level) or by provincial or territorial legislatures but rather by delegated persons or organizations, such as an administrative agency or a tribunal (e.g., the Public Utilities Board of Yukon and the Northwest Territories, the National Energy Board). The authority to implement **regulations**, however, must be specifically outlined in a federal, provincial, or territorial act—for example, in Manitoba, the *Regional Health Authorities Act* gives regional health authorities the power to make, implement, and enforce regulations. Federally, the *Food and Drugs Act* enables Health Canada's *Food and Drug Regulations*.

In health care, regulatory law affects hospital boards, health care institutions, and bodies governing health care professionals. Under provincial and territorial health care professions acts (e.g., Ontario's *Regulated Health Professions Act*), the minister of health oversees the manner in which health care professions operate and govern themselves and also retains the power to request a council make, amend, or revoke a particular regulation.

COMMON (CASE) LAW AND CIVIL LAW IN CANADA

In Canada, law in all provinces and territories except Quebec is based on common law. Common law, the law practised in Britain, governs almost all countries and regions either settled by or ruled by England. Quebec, however, operates under **civil law**, based on the French *Code Napoléon* or *Civil Code*.

Rather than being established within the legislature or being formally written like statutory law, **common law**, also called case law, results from the decisions of judges. These decisions are based on precedents—rulings other judges made in previous similar cases. Although Quebec's civil law system relies heavily on written laws, judges in Quebec courts often seek guidance from precedents set in earlier cases, as is done in common law systems. As well, common law may govern litigation conducted before the Federal Court of Canada, which sits both in Montreal and Quebec City.

Common law may serve to define obligations and legal rights or to further explain an element of, for example, the Charter or the *Privacy Act*, or a regulation under the *Occupational Health and Safety Act*. (See Box 8.6, which details a Charter case.)

CLASSIFICATIONS OF LAW: PUBLIC AND PRIVATE LAW

Laws are classified as public or private. Public law pertains to matters between an individual and society as a whole and, therefore, includes criminal, tax, constitutional, administrative, and human rights laws. For example, when an individual breaks a criminal law, his or her breach is considered a wrong against society, not just a wrong against another person or a select group of people. Public law is the same across Canada.

Private law governs matters concerning relationships between people and includes contract and property law, matters relating to inheritance, family law, tort law (e.g., negligence), and corporate law. As mentioned above, two systems deal with private law issues: civil law in Quebec and common law throughout the rest of Canada.

To illustrate the difference between public law and private law, if a nurse believed a client was better off dead and actively helped that person to die (active euthanasia), the police, acting on behalf of the state, would arrest the nurse and charge him or her under the Criminal Code (part of public law). If found guilty, the nurse could be sentenced to jail or be ordered to pay a fine (i.e., to the state). The victim's family could also launch a civil suit (under private law) against the nurse. If the family were awarded damages, the nurse would have to pay these directly to the family.

Some provinces and territories have specialized agencies called Criminal Injury Compensation Boards (see Web Resources at the end of this chapter) to which a victim (or the family of a victim) can apply for damages, bypassing the necessity of launching a civil suit, once an individual has been convicted in a criminal court. The government assesses the damages, which are awarded from public funds.

Civil law
A legal system in which laws governing civil rights, relationships within society and between people and property, and family relationships are written rather than being determined by judges.

In British Columbia, a landmark civil case fundamentally changed access to health care for hearing impaired persons across Canada and had implications for others with disabilities (Box 8.1). Also in British Columbia, parents of autistic children instigated legal action against the government in an effort to obtain payment for specialized treatment for their children (Box 8.2). These cases demonstrate how various interpretations of the law involving different levels of litigation (i.e., court proceedings) can produce different results.

Box 8.1   Equality of Care for the Hearing Impaired

Linda and John Warren and John Eldridge were born deaf. For many years, a private, nonprofit organization provided sign interpreters to help them communicate with health care professionals during doctors' appointments, hospital visits, medical tests, and the like. Sign language was their preferred method of communication.

In 1990, because of funding shortfalls, the organization that had provided the interpreter discontinued this service. Several appeals for financing proved futile, and the trio was left with no support to hire an interpreter. They claimed that the absence of a sign interpreter interfered with their ability to effectively communicate with health care professionals, increasing the opportunity for errors in diagnosis and treatment and impeding their ability to understand treatment options and to make informed decisions. Requests to the provincial and federal governments for support were denied. Launching litigation in the form of an appeal to the British Columbia Supreme Court on the grounds of discrimination, they asked the court to find that a "failure to provide sign language interpreters as an insured benefit under the Medical Services Plan violates section 15(1) of the Charter of Rights and Freedoms" (*Eldridge v. British Columbia*, 1997).

In 1992, the court dismissed the case, claiming that an interpreter was a supplementary service that the government did not have to provide (i.e., not medically necessary). A second appeal was dismissed two years later.

Undaunted, the individuals appealed to the Supreme Court of Canada. The Court ruled that the *Hospital Services Act* and the *Medical and Health Care Services Act* contravened section 15(1) (equality rights) of the Charter by failing to address the need for services for individuals to communicate effectively with health care professionals.

The Supreme Court directed that both acts—as well as those of other provinces and territories—be changed to accommodate these rights. Each province and territory dealt with this issue differently. Many jurisdictions made changes that affected other government departments. The case highlighted the rights of minority and marginal groups.

Source: Eldridge v. British Columbia (Attorney General), 3 S.C.R. 624, (1997).

Box 8.2   **Equality of Care for Children With Autism**

In 2004, a group of parents of autistic children charged that British Columbia discriminated against autistic children through its refusal to pay for select treatment. Two lower courts supported the group, but the Supreme Court of Canada threw the case out, claiming that no discriminatory action existed because the treatment was:

- Not medically necessary
- To a large extent, experimental
- Not provided by physicians, so funding was neither automatic nor guaranteed

The Supreme Court did state, however, that provinces and territories could pay for such services at their discretion. As a result of this case, some provinces now fund components of autism treatment under specific conditions—for example, for children up to age 6, as in Ontario.

In 2005, the Ontario Superior Court of Justice ruled that ending funding when children reached the age of 6 violated these children's rights. The province's Court of Appeal overturned this ruling in 2006. An appeal by families to the Supreme Court failed to get a hearing.

Sources: Parliamentary Information and Research Service. (2006). Library of Parliament. *Childhood autism in Canada: Some issues relating to behavioural intervention.* Retrieved May 29, 2009, from http://www.parl.gc.ca/information/library/PRBpubs/prb0593-e.htm; Canadian Broadcasting Corporation. (2006, July 7). Court: Ontario can stop autism funding once children turn 6. *CBC News.* Retrieved May 29, 2009, from http://www.cbc.ca/canada/story/2006/07/07/autism-ontario.html; CTV. (2007, April 12). SCC won't hear appeal for autism treatment funding. *CTV News.* Retrieved May 29, 2009, from http://www.ctv.ca

---

A person can sue a business, a dentist, a doctor, a hospital, a primary health care organization, or any individual for damages under private law, including the torts of libel and slander, breaches in privacy and confidentiality, and negligence suits.

TORT LAW

Tort law covers wrongful acts—whether intentional or not—that result in harm or damage to another person or another person's property. Health care professionals may find themselves accused of a **tort** if a client experiences physical or emotional injury resulting from something the health care professional did, whether intentionally or unintentionally. Unintentional torts may result from acts of outright negligence, misjudgement, or human error (Box 8.3). In Canada, an injured party who cannot prove negligence would rarely receive compensation.

Tort
A civil wrong committed against a person or his or her property.

Box 8.3   Examples of Unintentional Tort

- A person gets a wound infection while in hospital because the health care professionals failed to maintain infection control standards.

- A doctor misdiagnoses a case based on what he at the time considers sound evidence, resulting in unnecessary surgery.

- A respiratory therapist gives an inhalation treatment to a child using the wrong drug, which causes a serious allergic reaction.

- A client getting dressed after a colonoscopy falls, hits her head, and loses consciousness. The practical nurse had left the bedside to allow the client (who seemed cognizant and able) to get dressed. When the client awakens a day later, her mental status is noticeably altered. She is unaware of her immediate surroundings and has no memory of why she is in hospital.

Negligence

The civil wrong (i.e., tort) of **negligence**, also referred to as **malpractice**, occurs when a health care professional fails, whether intentionally or unintentionally, to meet the standards of care required of his or her profession. Negligence can result from forgetting to perform an action, not caring or confirming whether a particular action is performed, intentionally or unintentionally providing improper or substandard care, providing a client with unclear instructions, or failing to successfully instruct a client in how to follow a treatment plan. It may also result from **professional misconduct** (Case Example 8.1).

Professional misconduct
Behaviour or some act or omission that falls short of what would be proper in the circumstances. Examples include deviating from a profession's standards of practice or violating the boundaries of a professional–client relationship.

Case Example 8.1

Andrea, a physiotherapy assistant, has been asked to get 85-year-old Edgar up for the first time after his surgery. Suffering from Alzheimer's disease, Edgar is somewhat disoriented. Andrea manages to get him up for a short walk and then helps him back into bed. After leaving the floor, Andrea remembers that she failed to put up Edgar's side rail. Running late, she thinks, "Someone will have done it by now," and leaves the hospital. Edgar falls out of bed, breaking both legs. His family sues the hospital and Andrea, the assistant.

Duty plays a significant role in both medical ethics and medical law. Held more accountable in terms of their duty to their clients than people in many other professions, health care professionals often face litigation if it is proven that they failed to fulfill their duty to the client. Duty becomes part of the client–health care professional relationship as soon as the professional relationship begins. For example, Jeremy has made an appointment with a new nurse practitioner. Their professional relationship begins once the nurse practitioner has seen Jeremy, assessed him, and recommended a treatment plan. Before the appointment, Jeremy could not claim that the nurse practitioner was negligent in a health-related matter and bring legal action against him or her.

Results from a negligent incident may not be immediately apparent to anyone involved. For example, a subdural hematoma can occur several days after head trauma. Cases of adverse effects due to saline breast implants often come to light several years after being implanted.

Litigation and the Duty of Care

Almost all health care professionals are bound by a **duty of care** that is in keeping with their profession's standards of care. Litigation in such cases considers the standard of competency that a "reasonable person" (i.e., a person with similar training in a similar situation) is expected to meet. This standard generally remains constant within a profession but varies among professions (e.g., a registered nurse would be held to a higher standard of care than a personal support worker, depending, of course, on the situation).

CONTRACT LAW

Contract law concerns legally binding contracts—voluntary agreements between two or more parties. Contracts can exist between, for example, an employer and employee or a health care professional and a client. They also may be either expressed (i.e., openly spoken or written) or implied (i.e., unspoken but considered understood).

A breach of contract occurs when one of the parties fails to meet the terms of the agreement. A plastic surgeon, for example, can agree to perform a facelift on a client for a given price. If, for some reason, the physician fails to complete the procedure or if the client refuses to pay the agreed-upon price, one can sue the other for breach of contract. Another example: A private health care organization hires a dentist on a one-year contract. After two months, the dentist finds a higher-paying position and leaves. The health care organization can sue the dentist for breach of contract.

CRIMINAL LAW

The field of **criminal law** deals with crimes against the state or crimes deemed intolerable within society, such as murder, racism, and theft. In the health

Duty of care
The obligation to act in a competent manner according to the standards of practice.

Criminal law
The field of law dealing with crimes against the state or against society. Criminal law defines offences and controls the regulations concerning the apprehension, charging, and trying of those believed to have committed a criminal offence.

care field, examples of crimes punishable under criminal law include someone using another's health card fraudulently, a surgeon practising without a licence, a person trafficking narcotics, and someone performing euthanasia.

A person charged with a criminal offence may be found not guilty in a criminal court but later be found guilty in a civil court (Case Example 8.2).

Box 8.4 suggests ways to avoid legal problems in the health care environment.

Case Example 8.2

Jessica, a respiratory therapist, was charged with criminal negligence after she administered the wrong inhalation treatment to Hanna, a client. Hanna suffered a cardiac arrest because of an allergy to the medication administered. Jessica was found not guilty of criminal negligence, but when Hanna brought a civil charge against Jessica, the civil court upheld the charge and awarded Hanna $200,000 in damages.

In the **News**

Nondisclosure: A Criminal Offence?

In April 2009, Johnson Aziga, a Hamilton, Ontario, man, was found guilty in a criminal court of two counts of first-degree murder after causing the human immunodeficiency virus (HIV)-related deaths of two women by having unprotected sex with them and not divulging that he was HIV positive. This case is unprecedented in Canada, according to Crown Attorney Karen Shea.

Source: Canadian Press. (2009, April 5). Man spreading HIV convicted of murders. *CNews*. Retrieved May 29, 2009, from http://cnews.canoe.ca/CNEWS/Canada/2009/04/04/9006741-cp.html

Photo credit: THE CANADIAN PRESS/Hamilton Spectator—Gary Yokoyama.

Box 8.4   Strategies for Avoiding Legal Problems

- Most health care facilities require criminal checks both for potential employees and for students who apply to complete a work or co-op placement. Complete any such checks as requested and, if criminal activity exists in your background, tell your potential employer. Trying to hide something and having it surface later causes more harm. In most areas, criminal checks can be attained for a fee by contacting the nearest police station. The check may take several days or several weeks.

- Work only within your scope of practice. If asked to do something outside of your scope of practice or something you are not licensed to do, say no. If you feel unsure about how to perform a specific task within your scope of practice, ask for help. It is not a crime to seek assistance; it could be a crime if you do not.

- Complete, concise, and accurate documentation protects everyone—you, the organization you work for, and your client. Keep required charting current and accurate. Record all events, even those that seem trivial. In the event of litigation, the medical record may be the most important document in determining the outcome of a case.

- Most facilities maintain a formal process for the reporting of adverse events. These procedures usually involve completing a form called an **incident report**. Information on this form must be concise and accurate. In most cases, if the incident involves a client in the hospital setting, the information recorded on the incident report appears on the client's medical chart only if it relates directly to the client's health. The incident report itself is sent to the risk manager, who uses it to assess the occurrence and to implement measures to prevent similar future occurrences.

Incident report
A legal document outlining all relevant information concerning any negative occurrence in the workplace.

- Adhere to privacy and confidentiality laws. Think before you speak about work or information relating to work. Never access anyone's files (electronic or written) unless you have a legal right to do so. Being a friend or relative does not give you legal access to another's private health information. Remember, good news related to health information also must remain confidential.

- Always do your best. Never provide substandard care or treatment. Take the extra time to complete a task properly. An ounce of prevention goes a long way.

- Be an advocate for your clients. If you suspect that something is wrong, use the appropriate chain of command and talk to someone, rather than ignoring the incident. Your client may be afraid to address the situation personally or may feel that he or she will simply be ignored.

- Do not ignore unethical or illegal activities.

- Ensure that you have some type of liability insurance through your place of employment or your professional college or organization that will cover you for mishaps or wrongdoing.

FEDERAL AND PROVINCIAL JURISDICTIONAL FRAMEWORK

The law has played a role in health care since the *British North America Act* (now the *Constitution Act*) was passed in 1867, granting jurisdiction over some areas of health care to the federal government and jurisdiction over other areas to the provincial and territorial governments. A government's having **jurisdiction** means that it has authority over specific designated geographic and legislative areas and also possesses the right to draft, pass, and enact laws within its region.

Initially, the provinces assumed responsibility for "the establishment, maintenance, and management of hospitals, asylums, charities in and for the province, other than for marine hospitals" (Department of Justice, 1982). The federal government retained authority over health care for certain population groups, including members of the Royal Canadian Mounted Police (RCMP), inmates of federal penitentiaries, and Aboriginal peoples.

In addition to its fiscal influence over health care (see Chapter 4), the federal government controls certain components of health care activity covered by the Criminal Code of Canada. For example, the vague phrase "peace, order, and good government" (Department of Justice, 1982) allows the federal government to pass legislation on matters that would normally fall under provincial or territorial jurisdiction—in particular, the enactment of emergency powers, such as quarantine.

The next section examines federal authority in key areas of health care as it applies to the safety and protection of physicians, other health care professionals, and the general public.

WORKPLACE SAFETY

Several Canadian organizations—including the Canadian Centre for Occupational Health and Safety (CCOHS), the Workers' Compensation Board (WCB), and the Workplace Hazardous Materials Information System (WHMIS)—strive to maintain the health of working Canadians by ensuring that they have a safe and healthy workplace.

As a health care professional, you may interact with CCOHS and WCB in some manner, possibly by helping a client regain health in order to return to his or her workplace or to attain a level of health and mobility to transfer to a different career.

OCCUPATIONAL HEALTH AND SAFETY: JURISDICTIONS

In Canada, occupational health and safety legislation is divided among 14 jurisdictions: 10 provincial, three territorial, and one federal. The federal government manages labour affairs for certain sectors, including employees of the federal government and of federal corporations. The federal government also has jurisdiction over individuals working in occupations that cross provincial and territorial lines (e.g., transportation and communication) and in the federal public service sector.

Each province and territory hosts an occupational health and safety agency, which enacts its own legislation, generally called the *Occupational Health and Safety Act* or something similar. See Table 8.1 for a list of legislation covering occupational health and safety in each province and territory.

Table 8.1	Provincial and Territorial Health and Safety Legislation
British Columbia	*Workers' Compensation Act* Occupational Health and Safety Regulation, Part 5
Alberta	Occupational Health and Safety Code, Part 29 Workplace Hazardous Materials Information System, Sections 395 to 414
Saskatchewan	*Occupational Health and Safety Act* Occupational Health and Safety Regulations, Part XXII
Manitoba	*Workplace Safety and Health Act* Workplace Hazardous Materials Information System Regulations
Ontario	*Occupational Health and Safety Act* Workplace Hazardous Materials Information System Regulations
Quebec	*Act Respecting Occupational Health and Safety* Regulation Respecting Information on Controlled Products
New Brunswick	*Occupational Health and Safety Act* Workplace Hazardous Materials Information System Regulations
Nova Scotia	*Occupational Health and Safety Act* Workplace Hazardous Materials Information System Regulations
Prince Edward Island	*Occupational Health and Safety Act* Workplace Hazardous Materials Information System Regulations
Newfoundland and Labrador	*Occupational Health and Safety Act* Workplace Hazardous Materials Information System Regulations
Yukon	*Occupational Health and Safety Act* Workplace Hazardous Materials Information System Regulations
Northwest Territories and Nunavut	*Safety Act* Work Site Hazardous Materials Information System Regulations

Source: Canadian Centre for Occupational Health and Safety. (2005). Retrieved May 29, 2009, from http://www.ccohs.ca/

OCCUPATIONAL HEALTH AND SAFETY LEGISLATION: OBJECTIVES

Aiming to ensure a safe workplace for all Canadians and to support the rights of workers to such an environment, occupational health and safety legislation sets guidelines, provides for legal enforcement of these guidelines, and outlines the rights of employees, including the following:

- The right of the employee to be aware of potential safety and health hazards
- The right of the employee to take part in activities (e.g., by serving on committees or acting as a health and safety representative) aimed at preventing occupational accidents and diseases
- The right of the employee to refuse to engage in dangerous work without jeopardizing his or her job

Workers' Compensation Boards work hand-in-hand with the CCOHS but concentrate specifically on assisting injured employees by providing wages, rehabilitation, and training. Legislation related to these boards or commissions, drafted and administered by each province and territory, is typically named the *Workers' Compensation Act*. The Northwest Territories and Nunavut share a Workers' Compensation Board.

Workplace Hazardous Materials Information System

The CCOHS oversees the Workplace Hazardous Materials Information System (WHMIS), which became law through complementary federal, provincial, and territorial legislation in October 1988.

The national standards for **WHMIS legislation** were established by the federal *Hazardous Products Act* and the Controlled Products Regulations. Enforced by the federal, provincial, and territorial governments, this legislation applies to all Canadian workplaces in which identified hazardous materials are used. The national office for WHMIS operates as a division within Health Canada.

You may think that WHMIS legislation would apply only to industrial settings, but hazardous materials are present in many areas of the health care industry. Hospitals, for example, house hazardous substances used in diagnostic testing (radioactive products), chemotherapeutic agents, combustible agents (e.g., oxygen), infectious material, and medical waste.

Controlled Drugs and Substances Act
Federal legislation addressing Canada's drug laws, including a classification system for drugs.

DRUGS AND THE LAW

Canada's drug laws are covered primarily by federal legislation called the ***Controlled Drugs and Substances Act***. This Act replaced the *Narcotic Control Act* and the *Food and Drugs Act*, Parts III and IV, in May 1997. The new Act established different categories of drugs, called *schedules*. The classification system addresses the properties of drugs and their potential for harm. Schedule I, for example, includes cocaine, heroin, opium, oxycodone, morphine, and codeine; Schedule II addresses cannabis.

CONTROLLED DRUGS AND PRESCRIPTIONS

The *Controlled Drugs and Substances Act* outlines for hospitals and for health care professionals who can prescribe controlled drugs (e.g., doctors, dentists) and the conditions and terms of use for prescription narcotics. The prescribing of controlled substances occurs under combined federal, provincial, and territorial legislation.

Dispensing Controlled Drugs in Facilities

Most hospitals and other health care facilities maintain a closely monitored supply of restricted drugs such as phenobarbital, codeine, morphine, and meperidine (Demerol). These drugs must be prescribed by a physician and carefully issued to client care units by the pharmacy. Most jurisdictions require that health care facilities that stock such drugs keep them under double lock at all times.

Along with each bottle, vial, or ampoule of medication, client care units receive a form noting the precise number of pills or volume of solution. At the beginning and end of each shift, nursing units must count and record all controlled drugs. Every time a dosage is given to a client, the health care professional must record this information, either electronically or manually, in the narcotics control book. In an electronic environment, computer-controlled drug dispensers, for which each authorized health care professional possesses a unique password, track who acquired what drug, to whom it was dispensed, and when. In a manual environment, information, including the client's first and last name, the time the drug was given, and the dose, is recorded by hand. Each time a health care professional dispenses a partial dose, the "wasted" portion of the drug must be disposed of according to facility protocol, and the process witnessed and co-signed by a second nurse. If at the end of a shift, a single pill or ampoule is missing, it must be tracked and accounted for, which requires checking every medication administration record and every entry in the narcotics control book. The nurses may also have to review who had access to the locked-up drugs and when. In acute care settings, typically, only a registered nurse is allowed to handle or dispense controlled drugs. In nursing homes, however, licensed practical nurses (registered practical nurses, in Ontario) may, in some jurisdictions, dispense and sign for narcotics and complete a shift-end drug count with another nurse. Also, in most facilities, controlled drugs have an automatic stop date—a point at which the prescribing physician has to reassess the client and renew or discontinue the drug as required.

Prescribing Controlled Drugs

Under federal legislation, it is illegal for any medical practitioner to administer, prescribe, or provide a person with narcotics except for legal, therapeutic purposes. The legislation states that physicians must remain alert for behaviours that suggest clients are seeking drugs for unlawful purposes.

The two prescription drug classes most closely associated with illegal use are benzodiazepines (e.g., diazepam, lorazepam) and opioids (e.g., oxycodone, codeine, morphine) (Canadian Centre for Substance Abuse, 2007). These powerful drugs have addictive properties and are targets for illegal use and trafficking. Despite strict monitoring of the acquisition, storing, prescribing, and use of these drugs, misuse does occur. Individuals looking for controlled medication will often offer a variety of explanations as to why they want prescriptions renewed. Some explanations may be entirely legitimate; however, repeat requests from the same person may indicate **drug-seeking behaviour** and should be regarded with a degree of concern. Health care professionals may also find themselves approached by unfamiliar clients with atypical stories that cannot be verified. Case Examples 8.3 and 8.4 illustrate examples of common suspicious explanations.

> **Drug-seeking behaviour**
> A behaviour or activity focused on obtaining access to addictive controlled substances.

Case Example 8.3

Cecilia presents at a clinic, saying she lives in another province and needs pain medication. When asked for her health card (which, under the reciprocal billing arrangement, can be used to pay for her assessment—except in Quebec), she claims not to have it but states she will pay in cash.

Case Example 8.4

Manny comes to the office to try to have his prescription for diazepam (Valium) renewed before his current prescription runs out. He says, "I dropped my bottle in the sink, and the pills went down the drain."

Practitioners eligible to prescribe drugs are legally and morally bound to prescribe properly (i.e., to meet the client's health care needs while also adhering to the law) and to identify any circumstances raising suspicions about drug abuse. A prescriber suspecting drug abuse should take action—for example, by treating the client with another drug if the client overuses a prescribed narcotic or by reporting suspected criminal action (e.g., selling of drugs) to the police.

Thinking It Through

You work as an office manager for a family doctor. A client drops in claiming that she needs more sleeping pills because she was out of town for a week and forgot her medication in her hotel room. You know that the doctor has some samples in his locked cupboard. What would you do?

Regardless of the care prescribers take to avoid such situations, some clients will inevitably obtain prescription drugs for their own use or to sell. A province's or territory's college of physicians and surgeons can prevent physicians who prescribe too liberally from prescribing narcotics at all while still allowing them to practise medicine and prescribe other medications. Some physicians have knowingly prescribed drugs for illegal purposes, and some are addicted to drugs themselves.

Under federal legislation, prescribing practitioners must keep detailed records of all controlled substances prescribed and provide authorized inspectors access to these records upon request. In order to dispense controlled drugs, pharmacies must have an original signed prescription.

Health Canada routinely inspects pharmacies selling prescription drugs over the Internet or by mail order to ensure they comply with the *Food and Drugs Act* and *Food and Drug Regulations*. Such pharmacies must maintain an established licence to act as a wholesaler, and, under federal legislation, only certain categories of drugs may be sold in this manner.

PERMISSION TO USE ILLEGAL DRUGS

Some highly restricted drugs, such as marihuana, can be prescribed to control pain and nausea in individuals with AIDS or other serious illnesses. Several acts and regulations govern this particular drug, including the Marihuana Medical Access Regulations, the Regulations Amending the Marihuana Medicinal Access Regulations, and the *Food and Drugs Act* and *Food and Drug Regulations*.

Health Canada, under exceptional conditions (usually after other medications have proven ineffective), may grant a person permission to use marihuana. To apply for authorization to use this illegal drug, the client and his or her physician must fill out access forms and submit them to Health Canada. Clients have three methods to obtain their supply of the drug (Health Canada, 2008b):

1. Grow their own supply at home

2. Purchase it from a designated supplier

3. Purchase it from the government

People using marihuana for medicinal purposes vary in age and demographic profile. Rather than smoking marihuana, clients may ingest it in capsule form or inhale it using herbal vaporizers, the latter of which some health care plans (e.g., those in Ontario and British Columbia) now cover as medical devices. Vaporizers eliminate the particles in the smoke and allow for rapid-onset delivery. Health Canada emphasizes that marihuana, issued only under strict guidelines, is not proven as a therapeutic substance. Currently, more than 2778 persons hold an "Authorization to Possess" marihuana under the Marihuana Medical Access Regulations, and 1975 persons are allowed to cultivate marihuana for medical purposes (Health Canada, 2008a).

The use of other controlled substances available by prescription—including amphetamines, methamphetamines, and testosterone—is legislated under the *Food and Drugs Act*.

Thinking It **Through**

A large number of people claim that marihuana use provides pain relief and symptom control for a variety of complaints.

1. Should the government control the distributors of medicinal marihuana so tightly?

2. Should the process for seeking permission to use medicinal marihuana be relaxed?

At times, the provinces and territories challenge federal legislation, illustrating that, in many cases, the margins of law are not as clearly defined as they appear, as demonstrated by the case in Box 8.5.

Box 8.5   Supervised Use of Controlled Drugs: A Pilot Project

If someone told you a place existed in Canada where you could use heroin and other prohibited drugs legally, what would you think? Not only that such a place existed but also that someone would provide you with sterile needles and a clean, supervised place to rest and "shoot up." Would you believe that person?

Since 2003, a project called *Insite* has been operating in Vancouver with government support and funding, making it the first legalized injection site in North America. Insite, an initiative of Vancouver Coastal Health Authorities, provides impartial access to health care for individuals with addictions, mental illness, and related diseases. Controversially, it also gives people who use injection drugs clean needles and other supplies needed for their habit. Nurses supervise the injection process and offer support, counselling, and, when possible, referrals for medical help. The project aims to provide drug users with support and direction while also reducing the incidence of diseases such as hepatitis and HIV.

During the project's evaluation period, the facility was granted a temporary exemption for the use of drugs under the *Controlled Drugs and Substances Act*. As the exemption date for Insite drew nearer, Stephen Harper's Conservative government declared that funding for the project would be withdrawn and the project terminated because, it claimed, health care dollars could be better used.

In May 2008, the Supreme Court of British Columbia ruled that closing the site would mean ignoring the rights of addicts under Section 7 of the Charter—the right to life, liberty, and security—denying them the right to treatment and disregarding addiction as an illness. Insite was granted an immediate extension to stay open beyond the original federal exemption, which ended in June 2008. The ruling has forced the federal government to update its laws to ensure that the provinces and territories can provide appropriate treatment for addicts. The ruling also served to preserve the autonomy of the provinces and territories to render health care without interference from the federal government and to shift the view of drug abuse from being not only a criminal offence but also a health problem.

Source: PHS Community Services Society v. Attorney General of Canada, BCSC 661 (2008). Retrieved May 29, 2009, from http://www.courts.gov.bc.ca/

Thinking It Through

In its decision to keep the Insite project open, the Supreme Court of British Columbia asserted that addiction is an illness.

1. Do you agree that people who suffer alcoholism and drug addiction should be treated the same as people battling any other illness?

2. Do you think that a project like Insite can succeed in directing addicts to treatment facilities as well as in reducing the spread of HIV and AIDS?

Advertising Prescription Drugs

In Canada, advertising prescription drugs directly to the consumer (referred to as direct-to-consumer advertising, or DTCA) is illegal. In fact, the only countries whose laws currently allow this practice are New Zealand and the United States

(Mintzes, 2006). Canada's *Food and Drugs Act* contains the legislation against such advertising; however, both pharmaceutical companies and communications firms are lobbying the government to have it changed.

Some drugs can be advertised in Canada under the following two conditions:

1. "Reminder advertisements": Manufacturers can advertise drugs, using their brand names but not directly mentioning their uses. You have probably seen television ads for "Celebrex" or "Viagra," which merely hint at the drug's intended use and end by suggesting you "ask your doctor."

2. "Disease-oriented ads": Rather than mentioning a brand name, these commercials discuss a condition, suggesting that the consumer consult his or her physician for available medication (Mintzes, 2006).

Of course, Canadians watch a lot of American television. American drug ads name the drug, state its uses, list all of the side effects or associated risks, and then suggest that viewers consult their physicians.

Thinking It Through

Canada strictly regulates the content of drug advertising, whereas the United States allows pharmaceutical firms to include the name of the drug, its uses, and its side effects. Drug ads in both countries end by advising consumers to "consult their doctors."

1. Do you think that, because Canadians can view American drug ads, which include information restricted in Canada, Canadian restrictions are pointless?

2. Should Canada allow more content in Canadian drug ads both to better inform Canadians and to give the Canadian pharmaceutical industry a level playing field with American firms?

HEALTH CANADA EMERGENCY POWERS

Quarantine Act
Updated in 2005, this legislation gives the federal government powers to assess individuals and possibly detain those who may pose a health risk to Canadians.

The Constitution states that the federal government has an interest in "peace, order, and good government." As a result, the federal government retains the power to enact laws to manage health-related emergencies of national concern, such as the 2003 SARS epidemic, West Nile virus, and avian influenza. The speed at which these infectious diseases spread has taken many countries by surprise, including Canada, prompting the federal government to renew the severely outdated **Quarantine Act**. Even 10 years ago, immigration, air travel, and the import and export of food and other products did not pose the same level of threat as they do today in terms of furthering the spread of disease. As a result of today's global village, many people believe it is only a matter of time before a world-wide pandemic of some description occurs. The 2009 outbreak of the H1N1 virus fuelled fears of a full-blown pandemic. The World Health Organization (WHO) put the world on alert, adjusting the phase of pandemic alert accordingly (see Chapter 4).

THE QUARANTINE ACT

A new *Quarantine Act* (Bill C-12) received **royal assent** and became law in May 2005. Previous legislation had remained unchanged since 1872! Administered by the federal minister of health, the *Quarantine Act* complements International Health Regulations (discussed next) by allowing Canadian authorities to respond more rapidly to health threats at Canadian borders and better preparing authorities to deal with threats and risks to global public health. The Act is also designed to complement existing provincial and territorial public health legislation.

Provisions under the Act address concerns and threats in society today. The federal government now can:

- Divert aircraft or cruise ships to alternative landing sites
- Designate quarantine facilities anywhere in Canada
- Restrict or even prohibit travellers who represent a serious public health risk from entering Canada (Public Health Agency of Canada, 2004)

The Act also created two new occupational categories: environmental health officers and screening officers. These officers have the authority to assess, screen, and detain individuals who pose a health risk; to investigate and detain ships; and to examine goods and cargo crossing into or out of Canadian borders. Importantly, however, this Act does not restrict the movement of Canadians from one province or territory to another.

INTERNATIONAL HEALTH REGULATIONS

International Health Regulations outline strategies to prevent the global spread of infectious diseases and to minimize any resulting disruption to the world economy.

In 1951, the first International Sanitary Conference was held in Paris, France, to develop protective guidelines against the spread of disease. That same year, the member states of the World Health Organization adopted these guidelines;

in 1969, they were revised and renamed the International Health Regulations. The regulations have since undergone numerous modifications, the last in 2005, to address evolving concerns, including the reappearance of infectious diseases thought to have been eliminated.

The regulations initially monitored six serious infectious diseases: cholera, plague, yellow fever, smallpox, relapsing fever, and typhus. By 1969, only three diseases remained reportable: cholera, plague, and yellow fever. But by the 1990s, others had resurfaced—cholera outbreaks occurred in South America, plague in India—and new diseases, such as Ebola and hemorrhagic fever, were added to the watch list. All of these diseases are considered global threats because of the ease of transmission in today's world.

International regulations offer many benefits in monitoring and containing risks. Under the World Health Organization's constitution, all member states are bound by law to adhere to International Health Regulations, which provide ways to identify a global public health emergency and outline measures for quickly gathering and distributing information and global warnings, including travel warnings. Some countries, however, remain resistant to the idea of reporting outbreaks for fear of any negative effects on their economy.

HEALTH CARE AS A RIGHT

Because Canada has a publicly funded health care system and legislation at various levels of government to manage health care, Canadians believe that access to public health care is their right. Certainly, under the **Canada Health Act**, access to health care is a *legal* right. This right, however, remains limited by the principles and conditions of the Act. Notably, the *Canada Health Act* does not *guarantee* health care as such. It states that qualified Canadians are eligible for prepaid health care for medically necessary services—that is not a guarantee. The Act is federal legislation, and the provinces and territories are not bound by law to adhere to its principles, although the federal government can impose financial penalties on uncooperative jurisdictions. Application of the Act, therefore, varies among jurisdictions, depending on interpretation, resources, finances, and so on. The cases discussed previously concerning hearing impaired people and autistic children illustrate how Canadians push to have the right to equal access to health care clarified and broadened.

Medically Necessary: What Does It Mean?

The term *medically necessary* appears throughout the *Canada Health Act* because the principles of the Act developed from the legal right of Canadians to "medically necessary" procedures. At first glance, the term seems straightforward: when one is sick, the services needed to make one well; when one is well, the services needed to maintain that health. However, *medically necessary* is a subjective term at best, in large part because services vary not only among provinces and territories but also *within* provinces and territories. A resident of northern Saskatchewan, for example, does not have access to the same type of health care services as a resident of Saskatoon.

In recent years, decreasing financial and human resources have increased limitations regarding who should receive what medical care (medically necessary or not) and when. As a result, services previously deemed medically necessary have been removed from public insurance plans (i.e., deregulated), resulting in such services being offered privately, a matter discussed later in this chapter.

More recently, with strained resources resulting in long waits for just about every aspect of health care, people have turned to the Charter for legal means to gain improved access to health care services. Canadians want the right to buy insurance for services covered under the public plan and the right to seek services outside of Canada using public insurance. Interestingly, Canada remains one of the few industrial nations that does not offer its citizens a choice between public and private health care. In Canada, it is still illegal to purchase insurance to cover medically necessary procedures.

THE CANADIAN CHARTER OF RIGHTS AND FREEDOMS

The *Canadian Charter of Rights and Freedoms*, embedded in the Canadian Constitution, was passed into law in 1982 and amended by the Constitutional Amendment in 1983. The Charter guarantees Canadians certain rights and freedoms but is tempered by the phrase "subject only to such reasonable limits prescribed by law as can be demonstrably justified in a free and democratic society" (*Canadian Charter of Rights and Freedoms*, 1982). The Charter does not specifically identify health care, nor does it guarantee in specific terms that Canadians have a right to health care. The Charter does, however, demand that health care be provided to all persons *equally* and *fairly*.

The following sections within the Charter have met more legal challenges than others relating to the right of Canadians to health care:

- Section 7—life, liberty, and security of person. To determine whether a person's rights have been violated, the court must consider three things: (1) the medical resources available at the time of the person's illness, (2) the demands made on those resources, and (3) the urgency of the individual's medical needs. Under the law, everyone has the right to fair assessment, but this right does not guarantee access to specific services.

- Section 15—equality. Section 15(1) states, "Every individual is equal before and under the law and has the right to equal protection and equal benefit of the law without discrimination and, in particular, without discrimination based on race, national or ethnic origin, colour, religion, sex, age or mental or physical disability." A defendant must prove discrimination (i.e., that he or she has been treated unequally) on the basis of one or more of the criteria outlined in this section.

Several notable challenges regarding people's right to health care have been prompted by long waits for access to surgical services. Probably the most significant is the case of *Chaoulli v. Quebec* (Box 8.6).

Box 8.6   Court Challenge: *Chaoulli v. Quebec*

In *Chaoulli v. Quebec (Attorney General)* (2005), the Supreme Court of Canada ruled that Quebec's ban on private insurance in the face of long wait times violated the Quebec *Charter of Human Rights and Freedoms*. Although binding only in Quebec, the landmark decision has potentially opened the door to changes within the health care system across the nation. Certainly, it has resulted in changes within the province of Quebec.

Physician Jacques Chaoulli and his client, businessman George Zeliotis, challenged the courts, demanding that two sections of the province's *Healthcare and Hospital Insurance Act* be struck down.

Dr. Chaoulli had opted out of Quebec's medical care system. The Quebec *Health Care Act* effectively prevents anyone opting out of the provincial plan from providing private medical care within a public hospital. Dr. Chaoulli challenged the courts for the right, therefore, to provide medical care out of his van, which he had equipped as a mobile emergency room.

As well, the Quebec *Health Insurance Act* prohibits Quebec residents from buying private insurance to cover medically necessary procedures covered by the provincial health insurance plan. George Zeliotis required a hip replacement and was put on a lengthy waiting list. While on the list, he suffered increasing immobility and pain, which, he claimed, interfered with his sleep and compromised almost every aspect of his quality of life. He stated that he should have the right to govern his life, including the right to make decisions that would enhance his quality of life. In his case, that meant he should have access to timely health care. Mr. Zeliotis asked the Quebec government for permission to purchase private insurance to enable him to access surgery more quickly.

In 2005, the Supreme Court of Canada ruled in favour of Dr. Chaoulli and George Zeliotis. The Court held that long waits for medically necessary health care violated an individual's rights and that individuals should be allowed to purchase private insurance, enabling them to access private health care services outside the public system. The Supreme Court essentially removed restrictions prohibiting individuals from using private insurance to pay for services offered by the public system. The Court held that removing this restriction would guarantee freedom of choice for individuals and improve accessibility of care. The Court ruling was achieved in a 4 to 3 decision by a panel of 7 justices.

Source: Chaoulli v. Quebec (Attorney General), 1 S.C.R. 791, 2005 SCC 35 (2005). Retrieved May 29, 2009, from http://scc.lexum.umontreal.ca/en/2005/2005scc35/2005scc35.html

Many Canadians believe the door to more privatization of health care across the country has been opened, although only marginally. Others believe a challenge against the Charter to make health care accessible through private insurance is forthcoming. At this point, private health care exists in various forms across Canada and has for some time, particularly in Quebec, Alberta, and British Columbia. As well, the Quebec ruling in the *Chaoulli* case has opened the door for other such cases challenging provincial and territorial governments for the right to private insurance coverage for medically necessary procedures.

Thinking It **Through**

Canadians from coast to coast to coast must endure long waits for access to medical care and treatment.

1. Should the provincial and territorial governments have to pay for treatment elsewhere (even out-of-country) if it cannot be provided within a designated time frame?

2. What criteria should be used to define a "reasonable wait," given that every case differs?

THE LEGALITY OF PRIVATE SERVICES IN CANADA

As mentioned, Canada remains one of only a very few countries prohibiting private insurance for medically necessary procedures. However, the Supreme Court's ruling on *Chaoulli v. Quebec* (see Box 8.6) may have opened the door for consumers to purchase insurance for core publicly funded health care services.

Those in favour of a purely public health care system worry about the impact private insurance would have on the publicly funded system, fearing that it would result in a two-tier health care system in which those with less money would receive inferior care and have to endure longer wait times than would people who can afford to purchase private insurance.

Consequently, controversy continues over whether a place for expanded private health care exists beyond complementary and supplementary services in Canada, although it already exists in various forms across the nation. For example, Workers' Compensation Boards, the RCMP, Indian and Northern Affairs Canada, and the Correctional Service of Canada pay for medical services in private surgical clinics for their population groups. Considered justifiable in the case of Workers' Compensation Boards, private health care is deemed essential to ensure workers are treated and returned to their occupations as soon as possible to keep compensation payments down.

All provincial and territorial governments fund certain types of medical care in private clinics under specified conditions—for example, cataract surgery, hernia repairs, and knee surgery. Governments also pay for other services, such as diagnostics, in private clinics with which they hold contracts. And Canadians everywhere can purchase private insurance for non–medically necessary health care.

PHYSICIANS OPTING OUT OF THE PUBLIC PLAN

It is common belief among Canadians that doctors *legally* must take part in socialized medicine, adhering to the practice of charging the provincial or territorial plan for their services. However, doctors may work in either a public or a private system or in both. Operating entirely outside the public system, though, is not a practical option. Opting out means de-registering themselves from the public plan and billing clients directly for services. In Manitoba, Ontario, and Nova Scotia, opted-out doctors cannot charge the client more than the public plan would pay for services rendered, which effectively removes any incentive for opting out. Alberta, British Columbia, New Brunswick, Quebec, and Saskatchewan will not reimburse people who use the services of an opted-out physician, making it even more unattractive for a doctor to opt out. Opted-out New Brunswick doctors can ask clients to sign waivers stating that they will pay doctors' fees that are above what the provincial plan pays. Prince Edward Island will not provide funding for physicians (opted-in or -out) who charge more than what the Prince Edward Island health insurance plan pays for a specific service (Flood & Archibald, 2001).

Thinking It **Through**

You receive a brochure advertising a comprehensive medical workup, including a physical exam, dietary counselling, routine blood work, and some diagnostic tests, within a week of making an appointment. The cost is $1000. You could have these assessments done by your family doctor, and the services would be covered by your provincial or territorial health plan—but you would have to wait several months for an appointment. What would you do?

INDEPENDENT HEALTH CARE FACILITIES

Hundreds of independent health care facilities across Canada (e.g., diagnostic centres, laboratories, physiotherapy clinics, surgical clinics) offer diagnostic and therapeutic medical services.

These private facilities depend on referrals from doctors and, theoretically, can compensate doctors for referring clients to them, which causes legal concern. Doctors may also own such a private facility and refer his or her own clients to the clinic. The question raised is both legal and ethical in nature: Would self-interests distort a physician's clinical judgement? See Case Example 8.5.

Case Example 8.5

If Dr. Harper owns a clinic that operates magnetic resonance imaging (MRI) and other diagnostic equipment, would he refer clients to that clinic more liberally than he would if he did not possess a financial interest in it? Would unnecessary procedures be done at a public expense? Similarly, if Ribera Medical owned a string of physiotherapy clinics and offered Dr. Harper $25 for each client he referred, would Dr. Harper suddenly find a large number of clients needing physiotherapy? When such a personal interest exists, a doctor may be influenced by the fact that by referring more clients to the facility, he or she makes more money, creating a conflict of interest.

In Canada, common law governs **conflict of interest** concerns. The law binds physicians to behave with honesty and integrity (i.e., to act according to a **fiduciary duty**) with regard to their medical practice. That is not to say that Dr. Harper cannot refer clients to his own clinic, but by law, he must disclose

Conflict of interest
The possible clash of two or more concerns. For example, a personal financial interest in a business may influence one's professional decisions.

Fiduciary duty
A duty binding professionals to act with honesty and integrity, and in the best interests of their clients, with regard to their professional practice.

to clients his interest in the clinic; however, tracking violations of this law is difficult. Medical organizations, such as the Canadian Medical Association or the provincial and territorial physicians' regulatory bodies, probably carry more weight than other officials in terms of creating and enforcing regulations and guidelines that address these issues.

As is the case with most aspects of health care, provincial or territorial legislation directs the operation of private health care facilities in Canada. In Ontario, for example, the Independent Health Facilities Program (implemented under the *Independent Health Facilities Act*) licenses, in some cases funds, and coordinates quality-assurance assessments for private facilities. As well, these facilities are subject to routine inspection, often by the provincial or territorial college of physicians and surgeons.

In Alberta, the *Health Care Protection Act* oversees surgical services provided outside of hospitals. Private surgical facilities must have the approval of both Alberta Health and Wellness and the College of Physicians and Surgeons of Alberta; must secure a contract with a regional health authority to provide insured services; must comply with the principles of the *Canada Health Act*; must be a required service within their geographic location; and must not negatively affect the public health system.

Private clinics, such as the False Creek Surgical Centre in Vancouver, British Columbia, provide services ranging from diagnostic ultrasound to general surgery. A state-of-the-art surgery facility with three operating rooms, six recovery beds, and five overnight-stay rooms, this centre legally provides services for Workers' Compensation Boards and other designated groups as well as for private citizens (False Creek Surgical Centre, 2009).

Organizations such as Timely Medical Alternatives assist Canadians in accessing any type of health care services—some of which can be obtained within Canada, while others are outsourced to the United States. In most cases, clients pay for these services themselves.

Ottawa-based La Vie Health Centre, Calgary-based Foothills Health Consultants, and Toronto-based Medcan Health Management are just a few of the clinics across Canada that offer services aimed at the prevention of and early detection of health problems. For a price, a person can enroll for a one-day comprehensive assessment that includes a three- to four-hour block of time dedicated to testing, screening, and receiving advice, health education, and planning (e.g., working out a diet or exercise plan) from health care professionals. Because this service does not involve medically necessary procedures, it does not contravene the *Canada Health Act*. All of the services offered by these organizations are available at publicly funded doctors' offices through the provincial and territorial health plans but will entail waits and multiple visits to health care professionals.

INFORMED CONSENT TO TREATMENT

Throughout Canada, before a health care professional may treat a client, he or she requires the **informed consent** of the client. In order to provide informed consent, a client must understand, consent to, and accept the treatment and its foreseeable risks. When doubt exists about a person's capacity to understand the information provided, in most cases, the health care professional must determine whether the person is capable of giving consent to treatment. Importantly, an individual's capacity to give consent can change. Persons quite capable on one day may be incapable on another day, depending on their mental and physical state. If a previously capable client becomes unable to understand the nature of an intervention, the issue of consent must be readdressed.

Consent must be both informed and voluntary:

- Informed: Clients must understand the treatment or procedure—the nature and purpose of the proposed treatment, the risks, side effects, benefits, and expected outcomes. Clients must also understand the implications of refusing the recommended treatment and be made aware of alternatives, if any, to the proposed treatment so that they have choices. The health care professional has an obligation to use language that is at an appropriate level and to discuss the information when the client is not stressed or unhappy (this may require a second explanation of the intervention when the client is in a calm frame of mind).

- Voluntary: Clients must not feel compelled to make a decision for fear of criticism, nor must they feel pressured toward any particular decision by the information provider or anyone else. Sometimes in health care, only a fine line exists between coercing (i.e., bullying) and making a recommendation, especially when the health care professional feels strongly that the client should consent to a treatment, and the client is leaning toward refusing it (Case Example 8.6).

Case Example 8.6

Jennifer has terminal cancer. She asks the doctor, "What is really best for me? You have more knowledge and experience than I do, so let's go with what you think is best." In this case, Jennifer is clearly looking for the physician's expertise to help her make a decision.

Continued on next page

Alternatively, Jennifer might say, "Dr. Mather, I am not sure I want the chemotherapy. You sound almost angry with my decision. I know you think I should have it. . . . I'm confused." Is Dr. Mather pushing Jennifer to accept chemotherapy? Jennifer's decision to refuse the treatment could be based on wanting to enjoy a higher quality of life during the time she has left rather than living longer and enduring the side effects of chemotherapy. In such cases, Jennifer may want to seek a second opinion or ask her doctor to list the reasons he thinks she should embark on a treatment regime.

The Supreme Court of Canada supports the basic right of every capable person to decide which medical interventions he or she will accept or refuse (*Ciarlariello v. Schacter*, 1993). Involving clients in their health care should be a fundamental policy of all health care professionals. Not only does it show respect for the client and his or her right to autonomy; it also improves client compliance with treatment regimes.

Each province and territory has enacted its own legislation addressing informed consent. Policies, therefore, vary somewhat among the jurisdictions. Relevant legislation may include the *Adult Guardianship Act*, the *Mental Health Act*, and the *Health Care Consent Act*. Increasingly, physicians and other health care providers are advised to obtain written consent for even minor medical services such as immunizations.

All health care professionals in a position to provide care to a client (e.g., physiotherapists, respiratory therapists, laboratory technicians, nurses, doctors) have both legal and ethical obligations regarding that client's consent to proposed care. The ethical components of consent are discussed in Chapter 9.

Thinking It
Through

A woman with four small children is asked to sign a consent form each time one of her children receives an immunization.

1. Is the physician correct in having her sign a consent form for every immunization?

2. Since the woman and her family form part of the physician's practice and receive routine care (and immunizations amount to routine care), should her consent be implied?

TYPES OF CONSENT

Written Consent

All major medical interventions require signed, written consent as confirmation that the appropriate process for obtaining consent was followed and that the client has agreed to the proposed intervention. Ideally, the person signing the consent form understands what the intervention is, including its risks and benefits. In reality, however, how much the client has been told is hard to prove, and how much he or she understands is hard to determine. Although written consent provides health care professionals with evidence of consent, a signed consent form may be weighed against any conflicting evidence and, therefore, may not provide a solid defence.

Most consent forms have to be signed by the client, dated, and witnessed. People qualifying as a witness to consent vary among jurisdictions and health care organizations. For medical procedures, including minor or major surgery, a physician or registered nurse will usually witness the consent. The witness must ensure the client understands what he or she is signing. If any doubt remains, the appropriate person (e.g., usually the physician, nurse, or technologist doing the procedure) should speak to the client and provide clarification (Case Example 8.7).

Case Example 8.7

Prepared to sign a consent form for a hysterectomy, Mary reads through the form the nurse has brought her. The type of surgery named on the form is a *pan-hysterectomy*. Mary looks at the word and comments, "I'm not sure what that means, but I'm sure it's all right. The doctor said he was going to take out my uterus."

Importantly, some facilities have a policy that physicians must witness the signing of consent forms for procedures they are performing on a client. In other facilities, a registered nurse may obtain and witness a consent unless a client has concerns or questions beyond those the nurse can address.

Unfortunately, if Mary signs the consent form as it stands, she will lose more than her uterus. A pan-hysterectomy is the surgical removal of a woman's ovaries, fallopian tubes, and uterus. If possible, the nurse should explain the term and have the surgeon discuss the upcoming surgery with Mary to ensure that Mary understands what she is consenting to.

Note that a multicultural environment may present challenges surrounding consent because of religious, cultural, gender, or social concerns, as well as language barriers. Most hospitals maintain a list of volunteer interpreters should the need arise; however, interpreters capable of delivering health-related information clearly and accurately are not always available. Often, medical staff must rely on a family member to translate for the client. As a result, what is presumed to be "informed consent" may not be.

Oral Consent

Equally binding as written consent, **oral consent** is given by spoken word over the phone or in person. At times, someone other than the client offers consent to surgery; however, two people (usually health care professionals) must validate that consent has been given. For example, if a husband gives telephone consent for a procedure for his wife, assuming she is unable to give consent, two health care professionals must be on the telephone to validate the husband's consent— that consent was given, that he has had all of his questions answered, and that he fully understands the circumstances under and for which consent is being provided. Protocol may vary among facilities and jurisdictions.

When a health care professional receives oral consent, he or she should carefully document it in the client's chart, describing the intervention discussed, stating that the client has acknowledged understanding of the intervention, and noting that the client has agreed to it orally. Written consent remains the preferred alternative, however, for complex treatments.

Implied Consent

Implied consent

Consent assumed by the client's actions, such as his or her seeking out the care of a health care professional or his or her failure to resist or protest.

Circle of care

The individuals and health care professionals legitimately involved in rendering a client's care.

Implied consent occurs by virtue of the fact that an individual seeks the care of a physician or other health care professionals (i.e., a client's **circle of care**). If you have ever received an immunization or other treatment from your family doctor without having signed a consent form, the immunization or treatment has been provided under the umbrella of implied consent. As previously mentioned, however, more and more health care professionals are requesting written consent, even for immunizations.

By allowing themselves to be admitted to hospital, clients imply their consent to certain interventions (e.g., allowing the nurse to give them a bath or to take their vital signs). However, when possible, oral consent should be obtained (e.g., "Roger, I am going to begin your exercises now. Is that okay?"; "Emiko, I would like to change your dressing in about an hour. Are you okay with that?"). Clients may provide or deny consent through their actions, such as by nodding ("yes") or shaking their head ("no"). A client's refusal to treatment should be documented in detail on his or her medical record, along with any reasons provided.

Who Can Give Consent

A capable person receiving the intervention most often gives consent for the treatment. If the individual proves incapable of providing consent (e.g., is not mentally competent or is unconscious), the person's legal representative or next of kin (subject to provincial and territorial law) assumes the responsibility. In most jurisdictions, the person who legally has **power of attorney** for personal care or who is named as proxy for health care decisions for the client or a person related to the client usually takes on this duty.

In the absence of a legally assigned person, most provinces and territories will allow a spouse (whether legal or common law) or another family member to legally provide consent. Some jurisdictions outline a designated order, depending on the availability of particular relatives—for example, a spouse will have such control before a father or mother, who would have control before a sibling, who would have control before an aunt or uncle, and so on.

In Alberta, when a person is deemed unable to give consent (unless mentally incompetent), the only person who can legally provide it is a guardian under the *Dependent Adults Act* or someone named under the *Personal Directives Act*. Under Alberta's *Mental Health Act*, however, a family member can make a decision on behalf of a mentally incompetent individual. In urgent situations, when no legal alternative exists, nor is there time to appoint one, two consenting physicians can sign certificates indicating the need for treatment—ideally, after consultation with the next of kin or other appropriate persons.

Contrary to popular belief, in most jurisdictions, no specific age defines a **minor** when it comes to providing independent consent to treatment or to requesting treatment without a parent's knowledge. As long as the minor fully understands the treatment and its risks and benefits, he or she can make an informed decision about accepting or rejecting the treatment, and health care professionals must respect his or her wishes. When a minor's consent is accepted, the minor is referred to as a *mature minor*. Frequently, a minor's consent to treatment is made in conjunction with the parents. *Emancipated minors*—those married, living on their own, or showing independence from their parents in some way—may also validly consent to medical care.

When required, either parent who has legal custody of the minor (or a legally appointed guardian) can provide consent for treatment. If children are travelling, the legal guardian or parent can provide written permission to another adult travelling with the minor to consent to medical treatment in case of an emergency.

In extraordinary circumstances, a province or territory can seek temporary guardianship and order that treatment be implemented (In the News: When

Power of attorney
A legal document naming a specific person or persons to act on behalf of another in matters concerning personal care, personal estate, or both.

Minor
A person under the age of majority in a particular province or territory.

the Law Overrides Religious Rights). Although the Charter holds that Canadians have the right to freedom of religion, when children are, in the view of the courts, too young to hold and express beliefs or to understand the consequences of receiving treatment or not receiving treatment, courts usually uphold requests made to intervene on the children's behalf.

In the **News**   **When the Law Overrides Religious Rights**

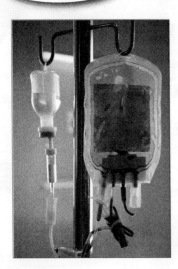

In early 2007, a Jehovah's Witness woman gave birth to sextuplets in British Columbia. Two infants died soon after birth, and physicians at the hospital determined that more would die unless they received blood transfusions. The parents adamantly refused the procedure. The British Columbia hospital successfully applied to the provincial government, gaining temporary guardianship of the three sickest babies. Two of the babies received blood transfusions against the express wishes of the parents. The babies were later returned to their parents.

Source: Canadian Broadcasting Corporation. (2007, January 31). B.C. intervened to save 3 sextuplets after 2 died. *CBC News*. Retrieved May 29, 2009, from http://www.cbc.ca/canada/british-columbia/story/2007/01/31/bc-sextuplets.html

Photo credit: © **Drliwa**/Dreamstime.com.

Even in emergency situations, if at all possible, health care professionals should obtain consent from a client before providing treatment. Under some circumstances (e.g., the individual cannot communicate because of a language barrier or because he or she is unconscious), a health care professional can administer emergency treatment without the client's permission if, in the professional's opinion, delay in treating the person will result in serious harm or injury. In such circumstances, however, the health care professional must provide clear, detailed, and concise written documentation explaining the decision to give treatment in the client's medical record.

Proxy consent
Consent given by a person authorized by a health care client to give consent on his or her behalf.

Finally, a power of attorney, an important legal document, provides a person the legal power to act on behalf of another in matters of estate, personal care, or both. A power of attorney for personal care or a **proxy consent** specifically grants a person (usually a loved one) the right to make health care decisions for another if the second is deemed incapable. Such a document can be, and often is, separate from a power of attorney for matters of finance or estate. See Web

Resources at the end of this chapter for samples of various legal forms, including power of attorney packages.

THE HEALTH RECORD

Any person who has received health care in Canada at any time possesses a health record, an accumulation of information relating to his or her interactions with health care services. If you work in the health care industry and deal directly with clients, you will likely be in a position to access and record health information relating to services provided for the client. Most information today is electronically recorded and stored.

Depending on the nature of the facility and those involved in the client's circle of care, a health record may consist of information gathered from many sources. A health record in the hospital setting will have more components than one in a dentist's office, a chiropractic clinic, or a physiotherapy clinic. In the hospital setting, the record will contain such items as:

- An admission sheet
- A client history
- Laboratory reports
- Medication records
- A client intervention screen (which shows all treatments a client is receiving)
- Consultation reports (i.e., reports written by a specialist) and an operation record if applicable
- Progress notes
- Interdisciplinary notes (e.g., notes about day-to-day care for the client, most often recorded by nurses)

Clinics or offices may also maintain a variety of reports: laboratory reports, consultation reports, history sheets (sometimes called a *cumulative profile*), and a record of what happened at each encounter (e.g., details of visits to the family doctor, including the reason for the visit and the treatment received).

THE IMPORTANCE OF ACCURATE RECORDING

In most disciplines, health care professionals must, by law, record information clearly, concisely, and thoroughly. Possibly one of the most important tasks of those in the field of health care, careful recording provides valuable information that can ensure continuity of client care. As a legal document, health records also may prove pivotal in a legal situation (Case Example 8.8).

Case Example 8.8

A woman with abdominal pain was diagnosed as having uterine fibroids and, as a result, underwent a total abdominal hysterectomy. It turned out that she actually had endometriosis. Although the hysterectomy was still the best course of action, the woman sued the physician because the procedure rendered her infertile. In his consultation report (written at the request of the referring doctor), the doctor had written that the client had clearly stated she wished to have a hysterectomy and was not planning to have children. The doctor, however, did not include this information in his progress notes (i.e., notes taken during client visits). The woman claimed that she had made no such statement.

The court ruled that the doctor should not have proceeded with the procedure because of doubts regarding the woman's wish to preserve her fertility. The outcome of the case would likely have been different if the physician had clearly documented on the hospital progress notes that the woman wanted the hysterectomy.

OWNERSHIP OF HEALTH INFORMATION

The health care facility or doctor's office that collects the information and creates the health record owns the client's physical chart. Physicians, dentists, other health care professionals, and health care facilities that maintain such records act as custodians of that information.

The health information itself, however, belongs to the client. Clients retain the right to request a copy of their information, including consultation reports and copies of reports generated by other physicians at the request of third parties, such as insurance companies. However, clients may not physically remove the record from the facility or alter its data. Office staff should supervise clients viewing their charts to avoid any unauthorized making of changes that may pose legal problems for the health care professional or the facility. Changes, including additions, may be made, but only if the health care professional agrees. Such revisions to data in the chart must be dated and initialled.

When a third party requests a client's health information, the client must provide written consent for its release, or a court of law may order the release of such information.

Clients moving or changing physicians often request a copy of their chart, which may be given to the client or sent directly to the new physician by registered mail or courier, usually for a fee based on the amount of photocopying required (accounting for both time and paper). Clients should be advised in advance of the cost to receive a copy of their chart. Because of security and privacy issues, clients' health information should never be sent via e-mail.

Under some circumstances, usually to avoid serious negative effects on the client's mental, emotional, or physical health, a physician may deny a person access to his or her medical information or may selectively remove information from a client's chart before providing the client with a copy of it. Although existing provincial or territorial legislation aimed at safeguarding health information usually supports denying a client access, the physician must be able to justify any such decision. A client can usually appeal a denial.

STORAGE AND DISPOSAL OF HEALTH INFORMATION

If a physician moves, ceases to practise for some reason, or retires, the medical information he or she accumulated must be retained and stored in such a manner that clients and other health care professionals providing care for that client can access them (with the client's permission) as needed. If another health care professional assumes responsibility for the practice at the same location, the clients' charts often remain at that location. Clients must receive notification of the change of provider.

When physicians or other health care professionals form a group, they should immediately clarify ownership of the charts—for example, does each own the charts of the clients he or she regularly sees, or do all of the records belong to the organization?

When a health care professional leaves a practice and no one assumes direct responsibility for the records (e.g., no one takes over the practice), a custodian—a person or business legally allowed to store or otherwise keep medical records—may take over the charts. Medical file storage companies can charge clients several hundreds of dollars for photocopies of their files. Provincial and territorial governments and regulatory bodies specify guidelines for the storage of records, including how long they must be maintained.

The Canadian Medical Protective Association advises that physicians retain medical records for at least 10 years from the date of the last entry or, in the case of minors, for at least 10 years from when the **age of majority** is reached. Physicians are encouraged to retain records for a longer period, if at all possible (Canadian Medical Protective Association, 2008).

The ultimate destruction of medical records must be accomplished in a manner that will ensure the information can never again be accessed. For example, a health care professional cannot just delete medical information from his or

Age of majority
The age at which a person is considered an adult; depending on the province or territory, age 18 or 19.

her computer; rather, the hard drive on which the information is stored must be professionally wiped clean.

FEDERAL LEGISLATION AND PRIVACY LAWS

Each of Canada's provinces and territories implements its own privacy legislation. Some provinces, including Alberta, Manitoba, Saskatchewan, and Ontario, have privacy legislation specific to health care service providers. (See Web Resources at the end of this chapter for a link to privacy legislation for each of the provinces and territories.)

Two related federal acts—the *Privacy Act* (1983) and the *Personal Information Protection and Electronic Documents Act* (2004), known as **PIPEDA**—contribute to this protection.

Privacy Act

Enacted in July 1983, the *Privacy Act* requires federal government departments and agencies to limit the private information they collect from individuals. As well, the Act restricts the use and sharing of any collected information. The *Privacy Act* also allows individuals to access any information federal government organizations have about them.

Personal Information Protection and Electronic Documents Act

PIPEDA protects personal information preserved in the private sector. The Act supports and promotes both online and traditional commercial activities by protecting personal information that is collected, used, or disclosed under certain circumstances. It defines *personal information* as "information about an identifiable individual" and includes any factual or subjective information, recorded or not, in any form. For example, the following would be considered personal information:

- Name, address, telephone number, gender
- Identification numbers, income, or blood type
- Credit records, loan records, existence of a dispute between a consumer and a merchant, and intentions to acquire goods or services

Known as consent-based legislation, *PIPEDA* requires any organization collecting and using personal information to present clients with consent forms that fully disclose how their personal information will be collected and managed, and to have these forms signed. For example, a dentist's office collecting information for research purposes for commercial gain must reveal to the client all personal information gathered and seek permission before using it.

Personal Information Protection and Electronic Documents Act (PIPEDA)

A federal act ensuring the protection of personal information in the private sector.

Since January 2004, all Canadian businesses have had to comply with the privacy principles set out by *PIPEDA*, except those businesses in provinces with privacy legislation similar to *PIPEDA* (e.g., British Columbia, Alberta, Quebec). *PIPEDA* protects information throughout Nunavut, the Northwest Territories, and Yukon because most organizations, other than hospitals and schools, remain under federal jurisdiction there.

PIPEDA does not usually affect hospitals and other health care facilities since most are not overtly involved with commercial activities. The legality of exempting some publicly funded organizations from *PIPEDA* legislation has been questioned, however, because some functions within health care facilities (e.g., a privately owned diagnostic clinic operating within the hospital) mimic those of a private organization.

In most jurisdictions, personal information collected by health care facilities remains under the protection of province- or territory-generated, public-sector legislation (e.g., in Ontario, the *Personal Health Information Protection Act* [*PHIPA*]; in British Columbia, both the *Freedom of Information and Protection of Privacy Act* [*FIPPA*] and *Personal Information Protection Act* [*PIPA*]). Some jurisdictions, such as New Brunswick, Newfoundland and Labrador, Nova Scotia, and Prince Edward Island lack specific privacy legislation for private-sector organizations and use *PIPEDA* instead.

CONFIDENTIALITY

All health care professionals must legally and ethically keep all health information confidential. First developed 2500 years ago (Box 8.7), the concept of **confidentiality** refers to the health care professional's moral obligation to keep a client's health information private. Conversely, the concept of **privacy** refers to

Privacy
The client's right to control access to their body and personal information.

Box 8.7   Confidentiality: An Age-Old Concept

The concept of confidentiality was outlined in the Hippocratic Oath 2500 years ago as follows:

"Whatever, in connection with my professional practice, or not in connection with it, I see or hear, in the life of men, which ought not to be spoken of abroad, I will not divulge, as reckoning that all such should be kept secret. While I continue to keep this Oath unviolated, may it be granted to me to enjoy life and the practice of the art, respected by all men, in all times. But should I trespass and violate this Oath, may the reverse be my lot."

Source: The Internet Classics Archive. (n.d.) *The Oath, by Hippocrates*. Retrieved May 29, 2009, from http://classics.mit.edu/Hippocrates/hippooath.html

the client's right for his or her health information to remain confidential and to be released only with his or her consent.

Any health care professional involved directly in a client's case—the circle of care—legally has access to that client's information. In the hospital setting, the circle of care may include the doctors, the nurses, social workers, physiotherapists, and other members of the health care team who are instrumental in the client's care and rehabilitation. Administrative personnel also have access to a person's health information and likewise must keep it confidential. Almost all places of employment—particularly in the health care sector—require employees to sign a confidentiality waiver (see Web Resources at the end of this chapter for a link to a sample waiver) and to adhere to the principles and policies within the document.

Many hospitals now use codes to protect clients' health information. In this system, any individuals with whom a client will willingly share his or her health information receives a code, which they must supply when calling the client care unit to ask for updates on the client's health.

In today's busy environment, breaches of confidentiality occur more easily and more frequently than one might think. Professionals involved in a case may discuss clients while sitting in the health care facility's cafeteria or riding in the elevator. While the content of these discussions may be legitimate (i.e., need to be discussed), such conversations should not occur in public places where they can easily be overheard—possibly by a relative, friend, or acquaintance of the client being discussed or simply by someone not entitled to that person's health information.

Often occurring by accident, breaches of confidentiality include revealing good news and news that will be readily available sooner or later. As a rule, health care professionals should never discuss health information with anyone other than members of the health care team responsible for the client's care. It is unacceptable to mention to a friend that Sally just had a baby boy or that Pang broke his leg and has a cast.

Health care professionals, both morally and legally, must keep a client's health information secure and restricted to only those who have the need to know and the right to access that information; however, under some circumstances, health care professionals may have a moral and legal responsibility to *release* confidential health information (e.g., when an individual has harmed or is in danger of harming him- or herself or others). Also, some health conditions, such as communicable diseases, must be reported to the local public health authority.

A client who discovers a breach of confidentiality can bring a lawsuit against the individual responsible for the breach, whether the breach was intentional or not (Case Example 8.9).

Case Example 8.9

While at a party, Alicia, a student nurse, was conversing with Ruby, who commented on how fast their mutual friend Heather delivered her baby boy last week. "Imagine," said the friend. "Heather's delivery lasted only three hours. That's really fast for her first baby." Alicia responded, "But that wasn't her first delivery, and second babies usually come much faster." The damage was done. Heather had had a baby 10 years prior, as a teenager. She'd given the baby up for adoption and told no one. Now the secret was out, causing hurtful and damaging information to circulate among Heather's friends. Think of the possible implications if Heather's husband did not know about her history!

Most health care organizations (public and private) require employees to sign a confidentiality form or waiver at the onset of employment. This form outlines the rules, regulations, and expectations the organization has of the employee from a legal and ethical perspective.

ELECTRONIC HEALTH INFORMATION REQUIREMENTS

Both electronic and hard copy records are subject to the principles of confidentiality and the protection of health information. However, the electronic environment poses unique challenges to maintaining confidentiality and privacy standards.

Electronic health records and electronic medical records are separate collections of the same material. Whereas **electronic medical records (EMRs)** are housed in one facility and pertain only to care received at that facility, **electronic health records (EHRs)** provide the "bigger picture." Compiled in a central database accessible to authorized persons for the purpose of providing care, electronic health records contain information from several different sources.

Since an electronic health record contains information from various sources, several people will have accessed the information. The more people involved, the more likely it is that a breach of confidentiality can result. As with all electronic information, the potential exists for information theft by hackers or by individuals who gain unauthorized access to information because of carelessness with passwords. The physical components of computers present the opportunity for files containing health information about thousands of people to be carried off by one person—quite within the realm of possibility compared with someone trying to walk off with thousands of files in hard copy format.

Electronic medical record
Health information obtained and stored at one facility, perhaps a dentist's, chiropractor's, or doctor's office.

Physical units storing health information may even go missing. Four computer tapes containing confidential information about residents of New Brunswick and British Columbia who had received treatment outside of their own province disappeared while en route from New Brunswick to Health Insurance B.C. The information, on magnetic tapes, was not encrypted. For three weeks, the fact that the tapes had not arrived in British Columbia went unnoticed. Not until two months after they had gone missing did the Ministry of Health notify the Office of the Information and Privacy Commissioner for British Columbia. The devices were being transferred to British Columbia as part of the reciprocal agreement whereby provinces reimburse one another for health services administered in other provinces (with the exception of Quebec) (Canadian Press, 2007).

The consent rules that apply to information stored in hard copy format apply, too, to information managed electronically, according to *PIPEDA* and territorial and provincial health privacy legislation. The information custodian must disclose to the client who will have access to the information and any auxiliary purposes for which the information may be used. The client also has a right to know what safeguards the facility has in place to protect the information. Some information custodians believe that once people give consent to have their information stored on an electronic health record, implied consent allows for other uses of that information. Not so. Any new, previously undisclosed initiative requires renewed consent from the client.

Many health care facilities use client information for research purposes. Strictly speaking, the health care facility should obtain the client's consent, as well as provide clear and accurate information about the research.

With the support of the Canadian Health Information Management Association, several organizations, including the Canada Health Infoway, are working toward introducing electronic health information systems at a national level. (These organizations are discussed in more detail in Chapter 10.) Jurisdictions across Canada have reached various stages of implementing electronic health information systems. As these systems evolve, so, too, will concerns about and solutions for dealing with privacy, confidentiality, and security.

HEALTH CARE PROFESSIONS AND THE LAW

REGULATED HEALTH CARE PROFESSIONALS

Most health care professionals in Canada belong to a regulating body that assumes a high level of responsibility for the ethical, moral, and legal conduct of its members. All regulated professions have a system in place for dealing with complaints against their members and for dealing with members charged with an offence. Likewise, they have an obligation to protect their members when claims prove unfounded, and they do so in a collaborative manner when violations involve the courts.

Clients who have complaints against health care professionals may launch a legal complaint as well as a complaint to the related regulatory organization. In the case of the latter, the organization's regulatory committee will assess the complaint and, if it finds the health care professional at fault, impose a penalty that may range from a reprimand or a suspension of the health care professional's licence to the permanent cancellation of his or her licence. The offending individual may also be subject to legal penalties.

Although litigation against health care professionals happens far less often in Canada than in the United States, it is becoming increasingly common here; therefore, all health care professionals should purchase some type of liability insurance. Many health care professionals obtain malpractice or liability insurance through their professional college or the organization they work for.

Every profession has a **code of ethics** (see Chapter 9) that provides moral and ethical guidelines for health care professionals to follow in their professional practice. However, codes are not legally binding documents. Rather, they advise the public what to expect from the health care professional. Adhering to the principles of one's professional code of ethics is a good way to avoid unethical or illegal practice.

Code of ethics
A set of values and responsibilities serving to guide the behaviour of the members of an organization or a profession.

Sorry, I Made a Mistake

In most cases, an admission of error in medical care leads to litigation. Apology laws, which first appeared in the United States in the 1990s, offer another option. The first Canadian apology legislation was passed in 2006 by British Columbia and Saskatchewan, followed in 2008 by Manitoba and Alberta. Ontario's apology legislation, Bill 108, passed its third reading on March 10, 2009. Apology laws allow health care professionals to apologize for errors without fear of legal retaliation.

Fashioned after a successful approach in Minnesota (now in 16 states) called *Sorry Works*, which gives physicians legal immunity for their apologies (Friedman, 2005), offering an apology reduces the tendency of clients to resort instantly to litigation and allows health care professionals to deal with their clients humanely—by recognizing the importance that an apology can play in settling disputes.

As part of the "Sorry Works" approach, if a client or health care professional suspects or knows an error has been made, both parties meet. The situation is reviewed and discussed, and an apology is made. The health care professional commits to take steps to minimize or remove the likelihood of the action being repeated. Clients receive an opportunity to provide feedback and recommendations. The most frequent result is a healthier client–health care professional relationship based on enhanced trust, a sense of respect for one another's position, and a feeling of safety.

Ending a Physician–Client Relationship

A physician becomes legally responsible for the care of a person when active treatment begins. If a physician or other health care professional refuses or ceases to care for a client without due process (e.g., notifying the client), he or she can be charged with abandonment. Unfortunately, a variety of situations will cause a client and a physician to part ways, such as significant disagreement between the client's expectations and the physician's ability to meet those expectations or aggressive or unacceptable behaviour on the part of the client.

In most jurisdictions, the physician must address the termination of a client–physician relationship in writing (often called a *Dear John letter*). The administrative assistant working for the doctor usually bears the responsibility of handling this correspondence, which is most often sent by registered mail or courier to gain proof that the letter was received. Physicians must continue to provide care for any such client until the client has found another doctor—a challenge, given the current shortage of doctors in Canada.

Conversely, clients can simply walk away from their doctor—with no formal separation process—never to return.

Physician Authority: Involuntary Confinement

In all jurisdictions, under a provincial or territorial *Mental Health Act*, doctors have the power to temporarily commit a client to a mental health facility under certain circumstances, whether acting either independently or in conjunction with the client's family.

Clients who pose a danger to themselves or others and who are noncompliant with requests to receive treatment may be subject to a physician enacting this authority. Most regions require the physician and a judge to sign a form, which designates a time frame (e.g., 72 hours) in which time the client will receive an evaluation. Afterward, the client can be discharged; discharged and, if need be, readmitted on a voluntary basis; or readmitted as an involuntary client. In the case of the last situation, to protect the rights of the client, a physician other than the one who signed the original form would have to provide an assessment. In most jurisdictions, the client and his or her family must also have access to a trained rights advisor or advocate, who may provide an avenue for appeal of the decision for involuntary commitment.

Nonregulated Health Care Professionals

The current landscape and structure of health care in Canada increasingly uses nonregulated health care professionals, primarily in community-based care. Nonregulated care providers include individuals who are not part of a professional body or under the umbrella of an act such as the *Regulated Health Professions Act*. Paid nonregulated care providers include personal support workers, health care aides, personal care assistants, and homemakers. Unpaid nonregulated care providers are usually family members or friends of the person requiring care.

Predominantly employed by heath care facilities, institutions, and community service agencies, paid nonregulated health care professionals often must have received some type of formal training, either through a community college, private college, or related organization. Registered or practical nurses usually supervise these professionals in their workplace. For the most part, hiring agencies provide liability insurance for nonregulated health care professionals. Personal attendant caregivers, usually hired by the family of an ill person, however, may or may not have liability insurance, sometimes creating a grey area in which the family and the caregiver have little legal protection (Case Example 8.10).

Case Example 8.10

Leroy, a self-employed personal attendant, provides assistance to Amar, a paraplegic. One day, when Leroy is helping Amar transfer from his wheelchair to his bed, Amar falls, fracturing his arm. Amar sues Leroy for negligence. Amar personally hired Leroy, who has no formal training, no insurance, and no money. If Leroy had been a personal support worker employed by a community agency, the agency would likely have had liability insurance to cover the incident.

Generally speaking, nonregulated health care professionals can provide only personal care. In the case of regulated professionals, scope of practice guidelines and controlled acts legislation clearly outline the responsibilities they can assume as well as the activities and procedures they can perform.

Other Legal Issues in Health Care

Client Self-Discharge From a Hospital

Unless confined under legislation, any **inpatient** can leave a hospital at any time without a physician's permission. Typically, a doctor will decide to discharge a client when he or she feels that hospital care is no longer required because the client can manage at home or in an alternative facility. The doctor writes a discharge order on the client's chart, and the client leaves.

When a client decides to leave a hospital without a doctor's permission, the facility should have the client sign a form releasing the hospital, the physician, and other members within the client's circle of care from responsibility for that client's well-being. Once the client leaves, he or she assumes all responsibility for any unforeseen effects of this action.

Good Samaritan Laws

Good Samaritan law
A law protecting individuals who attempt to offer help to a person in distress.

Good Samaritan laws legally protect anyone who offers to help someone in distress if something goes wrong—as it did in Case Example 8.11.

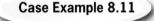

Case Example 8.11

Greg was having a heart attack. Ishim found him on the ground with no vital signs. Trained in first aid, Ishim began CPR. Greg survived but suffered a punctured lung as a result of a rib that was broken when Ishim initiated cardiac compressions. In provinces with a Good Samaritan law, Ishim would likely be protected if Greg tried to sue him for causing the broken rib and collapsed lung.

Currently, Ontario, British Columbia, Alberta, Quebec, and Nova Scotia have Good Samaritan legislation. In fact, under Quebec's Civil Code, every citizen must act as a *bon père de famille*, meaning that every person must act wisely and in a reasonable manner to help someone in distress if it does not pose a serious threat to the person. In other words, any person responding to an urgent situation is expected to do so within his or her scope of practice, knowledge, and level of expertise. A person with no medical training would be held less accountable than would a nurse or a doctor.

Whistleblowing

A **whistleblower** is a current or past employee or member of an organization who reports another's misconduct to people or entities with the power and presumed willingness to take corrective action. Unfortunately, whistleblowers often suffer a backlash, such as demotion, suspension, or termination for their efforts.

Provinces and territories remain at various stages of addressing the issue of whistleblowers; however, overall, whistleblowers currently receive little protection in Canada. The federal government provides legislation to protect public servants. Bill C-11, the *Public Servants Disclosure Protection Act* passed in 2005, covers the entire federal public sector and Crown corporations.

However, whistleblowers in both the public and private sectors must rely chiefly on the protection offered by common law. Under common law, an employee owes his or her employer the general duties of loyalty, good faith, and, in appropriate circumstances, confidentiality (Government of Canada, 2000). When an employee breaches these duties by revealing a confidence or some information, believing it is in the public interest, the employer usually takes disciplinary action, which may include dismissal. In the face of such punishment, employees may seek protection from the courts or, if they are governed by a collective agreement, through a grievance procedure.

SUMMARY

❖ Health care remains a legal responsibility primarily of the provincial and territorial governments.

❖ The federal government maintains legal authority over spending, issues related to criminal law, and issues related to laws that uphold "peace, order, and good government." For example, the control of narcotics and other drugs is regulated by the federal government. Under the Constitution, Health Canada can also exercise emergency powers through the *Quarantine Act* in the event of a national disaster or pandemic.

❖ As the Canadian health care landscape changes, so do the expectations for our health care system. Many Canadians regard health care as a fundamental right, even though it is not specifically identified in the *Canadian Charter of Rights and Freedoms*. Challenges relating to the right to health care, however, often arise under sections 7 and 15 of the Charter.

❖ Canada has always harboured some level of private health care, maintained restrictions on what types of health care can be delivered privately, and governed the services Canadians can purchase with private health insurance.

❖ Thousands of independent and private facilities across the country offer diagnostic and therapeutic medical services. Canadians can access them for services deemed not medically necessary and cover the costs of these services with private health policies. All private facilities are licensed by the province or territory in which they operate. Moreover, many are under contract with provincial and territorial governments for providing medical services to Canadians paid for with public funds.

❖ Confidentiality, consent to treatment, and the protection of health information are issues covered, in some cases, by both federal and provincial and territorial legislation. The *Personal Information Protection and Electronic Documents Act* (*PIPEDA*) federally regulates how organizations may collect, store, and use personal information, including medical records, for commercial purposes. Hospitals and other health care facilities are largely exempt from this legislation but subject in most jurisdictions to similar legislation that specifically concerns health information.

❖ Recent challenges to health care include the management of health information in an electronic environment and the provision of timely and high-quality health care.

REVIEW QUESTIONS

1. Explain the federal government's authority under the *Quarantine Act*.

2. What is the purpose of occupational health and safety legislation?

3. Identify some drug-seeking behaviours.

4. Why is the term *medically necessary* controversial?

5. What impact did the ruling in the *Chaoulli* case have on health care in Quebec?

6. Under what circumstances would a physician who owns a private health care facility be in conflict of interest?

7. What are three elements of informed consent?

8. Describe the purpose of a power of attorney for personal care.

9. How long must a health care professional or facility retain medical records?

DISCUSSION QUESTIONS

1. Explore privacy legislation in your own jurisdiction, comparing it with the regulations in *PIPEDA*. Summarize the responsibilities of the health information custodian with respect to the acquisition, use, and storage of health information.

2. Using the Internet to research confidentiality agreements and the guidelines of *PIPEDA*, create a confidentiality form that would be appropriate to use in an area of health care you might want to work in (e.g., physiotherapy clinic, doctor's office, hospital, dental office).

3. Hildy, a laboratory technician, was preparing two biopsies for examination by the pathologist. She put the samples down without labelling them. When she got around to attaching the clients' names, she felt certain she labelled them correctly. Ten days later, Mrs. Prince was informed she had cancer of the stomach. Fortunately, before surgery was booked, further investigation revealed that the diagnosis was incorrect. Mr. Ing, however, went undiagnosed for three additional months before it was determined that his biopsy had been wrongly labelled.

    a. Under what type of law should this incident be addressed?

    b. Who do you think should be held responsible: Hildy, the laboratory, or both? Why?

    c. What actions do you think Hildy should have taken?

    d. What do you believe to be the possible implications of this case in terms of physical or emotional harm to either client?

4. In March, Chidora learned that he needed cardiac bypass surgery, which was scheduled for the following August. Chidora's father had died from a heart attack, and Chidora was frightened that he might die before the surgery could be done. Despite his doctor's assurances that he was not in immediate danger, Chidora remained unconvinced. Assuming that Chidora lives in your province or territory, explore the available options for him, including:

    a. Visiting a private clinic

    b. Having the surgery performed out of the country without provincial or territorial coverage

    c. Using the Charter to appeal for prompt, paid-for access to the surgery

WEB RESOURCES

Occupational Health and Safety (Reports on Canadian Laws)

http://www.hrsdc.gc.ca/en/lp/spila/clli/ohslc/
01Occupational_Health_and_Safety.shtml

This Human Resources and Skills Development Canada Web page contains links to issues related to occupational health and safety acts—from changes to the legislation to the prevention of violence in the workplace.

Association of Workers' Compensation Boards of Canada

http://awcbc.org

Founded in 1919 as a nonprofit organization, the Association of Workers' Compensation Boards of Canada was established to facilitate the exchange of information between Workers' Compensation Boards and Commissions.

Canadalegal.com

http://www.canadalegal.com/forms/
wills-and-power-of-attorney.asp

This site provides examples of various legal documents, including powers of attorney.

Criminal Injury Compensation Boards

http://www.courtprep.ca/en/witnesstips/cic.asp

Courtprep.ca offers Canadians information about the country's legal system. This Web page provides information on topics including who is eligible for compensation and how to file a claim.

Canadian Privacy Legislation

http://www.privacysense.net/privacy-legislation/
canadian/

This Web site provides links to the privacy legislation of each of the provinces and territories.

Canadian Medical Association: Privacy Resources

http://www.cma.ca/index.cfm/ci_id/8402/la_id/1.
htm

This Web page gives a brief background to the *Personal Information Protection and Electronic Documents Act*. It also provides links to privacy-related Web sites.

Good Samaritan Act [RSBC 1996], Chapter 172

http://www.qp.gov.bc.ca/statreg/stat/G/96172_
01.htm

Good Samaritan laws legally protect anyone who offers to help a person in distress if something goes wrong. This Web page presents British Columbia's *Good Samaritan Act*.

Quarantine Act

http://www.phac-aspc.gc.ca/media/nr-rp/
2006/2006_10-eng.php

Designed to strengthen Canada's public health system, the new *Quarantine Act* became law in 2005.

Confidentiality Agreement for Physician Office Employees

http://www.oipc.bc.ca/pdfs/Physician_Privacy_
Toolkit/Confidentiality_Agreement_for_Physician_
Office_Employees.pdf

This confidentiality agreement is used by the British Columbia Medical Association, the Office of the Information and Privacy Commissioner for British Columbia, and the College of Physicians and Surgeons of British Columbia.

REFERENCES

Canadian Centre for Substance Abuse. (2007). *Prescription drug abuse FAQs*. Retrieved May 29, 2009, from http://www.ccsa.ca/2007%20CCSA%20Documents/ccsa-011519-2007.pdf

Canadian Charter of Rights and Freedoms (1982).

Canadian Medical Protective Association. (2008). *Retaining medical records*. Retrieved May 29, 2009, from https://www.cmpa-acpm.ca/cmpapd04/docs/resource_files/infoletters/2005/com_il0520_2-e.cfm

Canadian Press. (2007, December 11). Confidential medical records go missing. *CTV News.* Retrieved May 29, 2009, from http://www.ctv.ca/servlet/ArticleNews/story/CTVNews/20071211/medical_records_071211/20071211?hub=Health

Ciarlariello v. Schacter, 2 S.C.R. 119 (1993).

Department of Justice. (1982). *Constitution Acts 1867–1982*. Retrieved May 29, 2009, from http://laws.justice.gc.ca/en/const/c1867_e.html

Eldridge v. British Columbia (Attorney General), 3 S.C.R. 624 (1997).

False Creek Surgical Centre. (2009). *Our facility*. Retrieved May 29, 2009, from http://www.nationalsurgery.com/facility.html

Flood, C.M., & Archibald, T. (2001). The illegality of private health care in Canada. *Canadian Medical Association Journal, 164*(6). Retrieved May 29, 2009, from http://www.cmaj.ca/cgi/content/full/164/6/825#T135

Friedman, R.A. (2005, July 26). Learning words they rarely teach in medical schools: 'I'm sorry!' *The New York Times.* Retrieved May 29, 2009, from http://www.nytimes.com/2005/07/26/science/26essa.html?_r=1

Government of Canada. (2000). Bill S-13: *Public Service Whistleblowing Act*. Retrieved May 29, 2009, from http://dsp-psd.tpsgc.gc.ca/Collection-R/LoPBdP/LS/362/s13-e.htm

Health Canada. (2008a). *Marihuana for medical purposes: Statistics*. Retrieved May 29, 2009, from http://www.hc-sc.gc.ca/dhp-mps/marihuana/stat/_2008/june-juin-eng.php

Health Canada. (2008b). *Medical access to marihuana*. Fact sheet. Retrieved May 29, 2009, from http://www.hc-sc.gc.ca/dhp-mps/marihuana/law-loi/fact_sheet-infofiche-eng.php

Mintzes, B. (2006). *Direct-to-consumer advertising of prescription drugs in Canada*. Health Council of Canada. Retrieved May 29, 2009, from http://www.healthcouncilcanada.ca/docs/papers/2006/hcc_dtc-advertising_200601_e_v6.pdf

Public Health Agency of Canada. (2004). *New Quarantine Act reintroduced in Parliament* [News release]. Retrieved May 29, 2009, from http://www.phac-aspc.gc.ca/media/nr-rp/2004/2004_54-eng.php

Ethics and
Health Care

Learning Outcomes

1. Define *ethics*, *morals*, *values*, and *duties*.

2. Develop a reasonable understanding of your own moral and ethical beliefs.

3. Discuss four ethical theories that shape health care decisions.

4. Explain the ethical principles that are important to the health care professional.

5. Demonstrate an understanding of professionalism and of the ethical boundaries required of the health care professional.

6. Discuss ethical considerations relating to end-of-life issues.

7. Discuss ethical considerations relating to the allocation of resources in health care.

8. Briefly discuss the moral and ethical issues related to euthanasia, abortion, and genetic testing.

Health care professionals are held to a high level of accountability because the personal and sensitive nature of health care demands it. Entering a health care profession means entering into a moral and ethical contract with your clients, your peers, and other members of the health care team. It requires you to employ the highest standards of professionalism and ethical behaviour and to make a commitment to excellence in how you practise in your chosen field. You must respect the rights, thoughts, and actions of your clients. You must advocate for them, put aside any biases you have, and assist them in their quest to achieve wellness. Finally, you must work collaboratively with all health care team members, respecting their areas of expertise and scopes of practice.

People will often make ethical decisions that differ from ones you might make in the same situation. To help you understand why people can make different ethical decisions, this chapter briefly outlines four ethical theories that form the basis for most ethical decisions. Recognizing the perspective from which a person makes ethical decisions will help you to show tolerance when you disagree. You will learn that understanding and supporting the client does not require you to compromise your own beliefs and values.

Health care professionals have a duty to adhere to six ethical principles that have particular relevance to the health care profession. This chapter addresses these principles from the perspective of clinical and administrative practice, emphasizing the importance of ethical behaviour, professionalism, and client autonomy.

WHAT IS ETHICS?

Ethics is the study of standards of right and wrong in human behaviour—that is, how people ought to behave, considering rights and obligations, as well as virtues such as fairness, loyalty, and honesty. Various systems, approaches, and conceptual frameworks deal with how human actions are judged. Ethics examines the criteria we use to determine which actions are right or wrong (Alberta Health Services, n.d.; Online Ethics Center for Engineering, 2006; Sheldon Chumir Foundation for Ethics in Leadership, n.d.).

Ethics also involves values, duties, and moral issues. Ethics is neither religion nor determined by religion—if it were, nonreligious persons would be considered unethical. Ethics remains separate from the law although ethical and legal issues are at times closely connected. Ethical choices do not always fit with what is legal, and things that may be legal—or legal decisions—are not always ethical. Moreover, being ethical does not mean following social norms; behaviour considered ethical in one society may be deemed unethical in another (e.g., polygamy).

The term *ethics* also refers to a code of behaviour or conduct. Our behaviour reflects our belief system, which is shaped by many factors, including how we are parented, our home environment, and societal factors such as religion, friends, and school. Continually influenced by events and experiences, our ethical viewpoints change over time. Ethical standards are moulded by morals, values, and a sense of duty—all elements critical to ethical practice in health care.

MORALITY AND MORALS

Almost always linked to ethics, **morality** extends from a system of beliefs about what is right and wrong. It encompasses a person's values, beliefs, and sense of duty and responsibility. **Morals** are what a person believes to be right and wrong regarding how to treat others and how to behave in an organized society.

Morality
A code of conduct put forward by a society or some other group, such as a religion; also, a code of conduct accepted by an individual to guide his or her own behaviour, or one that, given specified conditions, would be put forward by all rational persons (Gert, 2008).

For example, a person may have a moral belief that one must always tell the truth, regardless of the consequences.

Whereas individual morals serve to define personal character, ethics can be described as an individual's collection of morals or, alternatively, a social system in which a collection of morals from a number of people are applied. Ethics, as a professional code of conduct, encompasses the profession's morality and moral beliefs. People bring their own moral code to their profession; it influences how they behave as professionals as well as the degree to which they honour their professions' codes of ethics.

The differences between morals and ethics are subtle and may be best illustrated in an example. Suppose a client and physician have agreed to apply a do-not-resuscitate (DNR) status to the client's infant because of that infant's clinical condition. Amy, a registered nurse working in the pediatric unit, does not morally agree with the decision, believing that all attempts to save the infant's life should be applied, including cardiopulmonary resuscitation (CPR). However, ethically (i.e., out of respect for the client's choice, or his or her autonomy), she must abide by the decision of the client and the doctor and refrain from initiating CPR should she be present when the infant has an arrest.

Health care professionals who understand their own values and moral standards come better prepared to deal with issues that may arise in their professional role. As well, they typically possess a better sense of their commitment to practise in an ethical manner.

Many grey areas exist in ethics and in beliefs regarding what is morally right. Often, no absolute right or wrong exists, and the health care professional's personal beliefs may affect how he or she deals with difficult situations or reacts to clients. Morally charged topics include the right to die, withholding treatment, DNR orders, withholding information from a client, and interfering with the client's right to **self-determination**. Understanding and feeling comfortable with your own beliefs in such areas can make accepting the decisions of others—even when they differ from what you would do—easier. Respecting the decisions of others does not mean compromising your own values.

Self-determination
The freedom to make one's own decisions.

You are more likely to be faced with less dramatic moral issues. Is it proper to accept a gift from a client, or will the act bind you to providing the client with preferential treatment? Is it morally acceptable to cover up a medication error that did not cause harm to a client? Is it acceptable to chart on care not given because you were so busy that you only had time to do the basics? Is it okay to take hospital supplies home for personal use as long as there are plenty left for the clients? How you decide what is acceptable and unacceptable behaviour will depend on your moral code as well as your values.

VALUES

Values, beliefs important to an individual, guide a person's conduct and the decisions he or she makes. People can have personal values, social values, and work values. A person who greatly values friendship may consider his or her relationship with a particular person more important than, for example, a material object. And although one may value friendship in general, one friend may be more valued than another. Context may also influence values and, therefore, behaviour (Case Example 9.1).

Case Example 9.1

Tony, an occupational therapy student, clearly values professional conduct at work more than he does personal conduct at school. At work, he maintains an excellent attendance record, is never late, and does his job well. However, at school, he talks in class, hands in assignments late, does not study for tests, and has poor attendance—especially on Friday afternoons. As well, he often misses a day of classes prior to an exam or test. He may place more importance on work for several reasons, including earning money for rent and other amenities. He may not (at least yet) value his education or see it as a means to an end—establishing a career and becoming financially secure.

In health care, particular value is placed on certain virtues—truthfulness, respect for others, competency, and the right to life. For example, one cannot effectively establish therapeutic relationships with clients or trusting relationships with colleagues without truthfulness (the foundation for trust) and respect for others.

At times, another person will make a decision that violates your moral beliefs and values. After all, health care professionals face situations that challenge deep-rooted values and interfere with the preservation of life, as illustrated in Case Example 9.2.

Case Example 9.2

Jennifer seeks an abortion to terminate a pregnancy resulting from rape. Her primary nurse, Sanga (a new graduate), cannot understand how Jennifer could make that decision. Sanga values life more than anything. Had it

Continued on next page

been her, abortion would have been out of the question, regardless of the circumstances. However, Sanga also values trust, respect for others, and integrity. For that reason, she can give Jennifer the care and support she needs and respect Jennifer's right to make the decision best for her.

SENSE OF DUTY

Duties

Obligations a person has in response to another's claims on them. A duty may result from a professional or personal obligation or may relate to one's own morals or values.

Duties often arise from others' claims. If a client depends on you (i.e., has a claim on you) for your professional services, you have a duty, or obligation, to deliver these services. As a member of the health care profession, you also have a duty to behave in an ethical, moral, and competent manner. Alternatively, duties may be self-imposed. For example, a person who values honesty will make it his or her duty to be truthful.

Health care professionals, by the very nature of the field they work in, have a moral and ethical duty to care for their clients in a competent manner as well as a legal obligation, called the "duty of care." As discussed in Chapter 8, the legal component of this duty requires health care professionals to provide clients with a reasonable standard of care in accordance with their professions' standards of practice. In terms of a moral obligation, health care professionals are expected to provide care even in situations that may threaten their own lives or health; however, they may not be legally bound to do so.

Thinking It **Through**

Suspected of carrying the SARS virus, Al has been placed in isolation. You have been asked to provide his treatment. Despite precautions, the risk that you will acquire the virus still exists. You recognize that the SARS virus has had deadly consequences for health care professionals (more so than the H1N1 virus to date).

1. Would you carry out your professional responsibilities because it is your duty to, or would you refuse to treat Al because of the risks involved?

2. Would your decision differ if Al was suspected of having the H1N1 virus?

ETHICAL THEORIES: THE BASICS

Health care professionals face making ethical decisions that affect them individually, that affect other members of the health care team, and that affect their clients. These professionals also face exposure to ethical situations in which decisions made by others may affect them, perhaps not directly but emotionally.

An **ethical theory** guides people toward making an ethical decision. The discussion of ethical theories that follows, although not in-depth, will help you see how individuals make difficult decisions.

Ethical theory
A framework of ideas that provides a template for making decisions to justify a set of actions.

TELEOLOGICAL THEORY

Teleological theory, also referred to as *consequence-based theory*, defines an action as right or wrong depending on the results it produces. Theoretically, the result must bring about the most benefit for the most people. Consider Case Example 9.3, a real-life situation.

Case Example 9.3

Postsurgery, it is discovered that a sponge was left inside a client. The client, a man with metastatic cancer, has a limited life expectancy. The staff members present, along with Nima, an operating room technician, decide it is in everyone's best interests to say nothing. The sponge will not hurt the man, but opening him up and removing it would hasten his death and cause him more pain. The family, already trying to cope with the man's impending death, would be distressed over the incident. It is a simple mistake—why get the surgeon and nurses into trouble?

In Case Example 9.3, to say nothing becomes the group's ethical decision. The individuals involved determine what they think would be the best result and make their decision accordingly. Of less importance to them is that, in taking this chosen action, they will conceal the truth (not to mention the legal implications of their decision—by law, in most jurisdictions a client must be told when a medical error has occurred).

Similarly, an expected result may inform a client's decision to accept or refuse treatment (Case Example 9.4).

Case Example 9.4

Bruno, a 75-year-old man with prostate cancer, discusses treatment options with his oncologist. If treatment offers a high chance of recovery with quality of life, he will likely accept it. If the expected result is uncertain or involves suffering, he is more likely to refuse treatment.

Deontological Theory

Deontological developed from the word *duty*. In the case of **deontological theory**, a moral and honest action is taken, regardless of the outcome. If, in Case Example 9.3, the team had used a deontological approach and did the "right" thing, they would have removed the sponge, or they would have told the family what had happened, explained the risks, and allowed them to make the decision. In Case Example 9.4, health care professionals might struggle with Bruno's decision to refuse a treatment that would prolong his life because they strive to preserve life.

Virtue Ethics

Virtue ethics looks at the ethical character of the person making the decision, rather than at his or her reasoning. This theory operates under the belief that a person of moral character will act wisely, fairly, and honestly and will uphold the principles of justice. Therefore, virtue ethics, unlike teleological and deontological theories, does not provide guidelines for decision making.

In Case Example 9.3, several people were present for the postsurgery discovery. Person A may have decided that it would be best not to divulge the incident about the sponge, while Person B may have decided the incident must be exposed. Each person would make an individual decision based on his or her own set of values and morals. A common decision often, however, must be reached. When people disagree about the course of action to take, sometimes the majority will rule; other times, one person may have the authority to make a call. However, each person should still feel comfortable with his or her own actions because each person might have to take responsibility for such actions. In the case example, the individuals involved may feel it is not their place to question the surgeon's decision, believing that showing loyalty to the physician fulfills their professional ethical obligations. Then again, the act is both illegal and contrary to hospital policy, so these individuals may take a personal risk by complying with the decision not to report the incident. Ultimately, each person must weigh the situation, determine to whom he or she owes the greater loyalty, and decide according to his or her own conscience.

Divine Command

The most rigid ethical theory, **divine command ethics** follows philosophies and rules set out by a higher power. For example, Christians must live by the Bible's Ten Commandments, a list of religion-based moral laws. Muslims follow the rules outlined in the Koran, such as maintaining a just society and engaging in "appropriate" human relationships. In Case Example 9.3, followers of divine command ethics would without question decide that the incident should be reported because honesty makes up a significant part of the divine command theory.

Thinking It Through

Dr. Swarovski decides to lie to Jake (an older client with no relatives or emotional support system) about the nature of his illness—amyotrophic lateral sclerosis (ALS), which causes progressive paralysis eventually leading to the inability to swallow or breathe. The physician believes that she is sparing Jake unnecessary grief, at least for the short term.

1. Is Dr. Swarovski justified in her decision to lie to Jake?

2. Would it make any difference if Jake had family or friends to support him?

ETHICAL PRINCIPLES AND THE HEALTH CARE PROFESSION

Common to all ethical theories, **ethical principles**—acceptable standards of human behaviour—provide guidance for decision making and, therefore, form the basis of ethical study. Ethical principles can be personal or professional in nature. In the best-case scenario, individuals practise similar principles in both their personal and professional lives. Personal principles predominantly guide a person's actions and form the foundation from which professional principles evolve. People who believe in showing kindness and helping those in need in their personal life will likely do the same in their professional life. Those with an uncaring, indifferent attitude toward others in their personal life are unlikely to show support, respect, or adequate care to a client.

> **Ethical principle**
> An acceptable, usually highly valued and moral, standard of human behaviour—for example, honesty, truthfulness, and fairness.

Outlined below are a number of ethical principles that lend themselves particularly well to health care. These important elements of ethical decision making almost always appear in the codes of ethics adopted by health care professions.

BENEFICENCE AND NONMALEFICENCE

The foundation of health care ethics, **beneficence** refers to showing kindness to or doing good for others. No matter what ethical theory is used, beneficence guides the process toward a morally right outcome. All health care professionals have a duty to do good, to prevent harm, and to not cause harm (sometimes called *nonmaleficence*). Often treated as a separate principle from beneficence,

nonmaleficence refers specifically to causing no harm, whereas beneficence encompasses the duties to prevent harm and to remove harm when possible.

Similar to beneficence, the principle of **double effect** requires a person to choose the option that achieves the most favourable outcome or that causes the least harm. When secondary, potentially negative outcomes or side effects can be predicted, these must not be the intended outcome of the action. For example, Augusta, who has terminal cancer, takes high doses of morphine sulphate controlled-release (MS Contin), which has proven to be the only means of controlling her pain. However, she now experiences respiratory distress—a known side effect of MS Contin—which could well lead to her death. Despite this, making Augusta comfortable is considered, ethically and morally, the action of choice.

RESPECT

Another key ethical principle is respect. All clients have the right to be treated with respect by those who care for them. Colleagues also have this right, as do you. Respecting others involves honouring their right to autonomy (see below), being truthful, not withholding information, and honouring their decisions, whether stemming from personal, religious, cultural, or societal influences.

AUTONOMY

Autonomy comes from the Greek *autos*, meaning self, and *nomos*, meaning governance. The ethical principle of **autonomy** underscores a person's right to self-determination. Autonomy recognizes the right of a mentally competent individual, given all of the relevant facts, to make independent decisions without coercion (i.e., pressure or force). Health care professionals may try to influence a client's decisions, often unintentionally, thinking they know what is best. However, clients have the right to choose their own course of treatment or to refuse treatment altogether.

TRUTHFULNESS

Truthfulness, a valued principle that clients should expect of a health care professional, contributes to building a bond of trust vital to any client–health care professional relationship. Without this bond, an effective relationship is impossible. Rarely justifiable, withholding the truth shows disrespect and works against a person's autonomy and rights.

Fiduciary relationship
A relationship based on trust.

A special relationship, called a **fiduciary relationship**, exists between health care professionals and their clients. To some degree, the health care professional retains a position of power over the client, considering the client's dependence on the health care professional for his or her care. In such a relationship, clients should expect the health care professional to care about them as well as for them, to be honest, and to be trustworthy.

Thinking It **Through**

Mekhi has a serious illness, but a treatment option that will potentially cure his illness is available. His doctor tells him about the treatment, but, fearing Mekhi may decide to refuse the treatment, he does not inform him of the serious side effects that he will likely experience.

1. Do you think the physician is showing respect for Mekhi?
2. What ethical principles has the physician breached?

FIDELITY

The principle of **fidelity**—faithfulness or loyalty—requires health care professionals to adhere to their professional codes of ethics and the principles that define their roles and scopes of practice, as well as to fulfill their responsibilities to clients by practising their skills competently. The term *fidelity* comes from a Latin root word meaning to be faithful. Fidelity, therefore, requires faithfulness and loyalty to clients, colleagues, and employers (Case Example 9.5). Health care professionals are also expected to uphold the rules and policies of the organization (or person) for which they work. In the workplace, **role fidelity** becomes an important ethical principle for health care professionals as they work to honour clients' wishes and to earn the trust essential to the professional–client relationship.

Role fidelity
In health care, meeting the reasonable expectations of members of the health care team, clients, their families, and employers by being loyal, truthful, and faithful, by showing respect, and by earning and maintaining trust.

Case Example 9.5

Cecelia, who owns a number of urgent care clinics, is on a bus and overhears a conversation between two young women in the seat in front of her. "That clinic is the worst," says one. "They expect me to do everything they ask, and they want it done, like, yesterday." "Yeah," responds the other, "I know what you mean. I bet you hate working there. It sounds like that manager is a real dragon. I'd never go to that clinic—unless I was dying and there was

Continued on next page

nowhere else to go!" Cecelia recognizes one of the women as an employee. Needless to say, the clinic staff will be subject to a discussion about loyalty the next day.

JUSTICE

The principle of justice applies, in one way or another, to most ethical situations. In health care, for example, it raises questions such as the following: Do all clients get the appropriate (i.e., just) treatment? Are health care resources fairly distributed? Are the client's rights honoured? The three main types of justice are distributive, compensatory, and procedural. Distributive justice deals with the proper and equitable (i.e., distributed according to priority and need, not necessarily equally) distribution of health care resources. Compensatory justice concerns compensation for wrongs done (e.g., if a client suffers as a result of a negligent act, compensatory justice holds that the client should be appropriately compensated for damages, whether emotional, financial, or physical). Procedural justice points to acting in a fair and impartial manner (e.g., seeing clients on a first come, first served basis; not giving preferential treatment to a friend).

The *Canada Health Act* entitles all Canadians equal access to **prepaid health care** and physician and hospital services. However, with resources stretched to their limits and long waiting lists for many services, equal access, as well as other principles of the Act, is compromised. Health care professionals, therefore, must do what they can to provide the best services to their clients.

Health care professionals must practise within the boundaries of the law and report any actions that break the law or compromise the health or safety of a client. Most organizations set up a process for reporting unethical or illegal behaviour. It is important to learn this process and to follow it, no matter who—an employer, a peer, or a superior—one finds acting unethically. By simply having knowledge of an illegal or immoral act and not reporting it, a person may be considered guilty in the matter. Consequences can range from a tarnished professional and personal reputation to legal action and client harm. In Case Example 9.3, therefore, Nima may disagree with the decision not to report the missing sponge, but, by not reporting it, she could share the guilt in any ensuing legal action.

Justice in health care also considers the allocation of health care resources, which raises questions about whether health care services are spread evenly across Canada. The allocation of resources is discussed in more detail later in this chapter.

CLIENTS' RIGHTS IN HEALTH CARE

Numerous moral controversies surround **rights in health care**, such as the right to die, the right to self-determination, the rights of a fetus, the rights of women to abortion, smokers' rights, and the rights of an individual to health care. Under the *Canada Health Act*, Canadians have certain rights to health care (see Chapters 3, 5, and 8). The *Canadian Charter of Rights and Freedoms*, in some situations, can also assist Canadians in ensuring they receive their health care rights (although the concept of health care rights in the Charter is vague). For example, the Charter can uphold rights related to discrimination but not rights related to specific medical treatments, although, as discussed in Chapter 8, some recent health-related challenges under the Charter have proven successful.

Technology has raised questions about an individual's right to certain health care services and procedures, including, for example, in vitro fertilization (IVF). Depending on the jurisdiction, the cut-off age in Canada for IVF ranges from 45 to 50 years old. But is it fair to place such limits on who may receive the procedure? Should older women be given a right to it? If a woman travels outside of the country for in vitro fertilization, should her provincial or territorial health plan cover her medical expenses? Should the number of embryos implanted be limited?

In vitro fertilization in older women and the implantation of multiple embryos into a woman's uterus, regardless of her age, both present significant risks to both mother and baby (or babies). Multiple births—particularly when three or more fetuses exist—are dangerous and often result in premature delivery, placing the babies at risk for a variety of problems, including cardio-respiratory difficulties, cerebral palsy, blindness, learning disabilities, and developmental delays. These complications, when they arise, cost the health care system millions of dollars over the life of the child. Ethical storms brewed when the following two cases were brought to light, prompting discussion about implementing clear guidelines for in vitro fertilization.

Rights in health care
Entitlements, things that can and should be expected of health care professionals and the health care system. Rights may be tangible (e.g., the right to receive a vaccination covered under the provincial or territorial plan) or intangible (the right to be treated with respect).

In the **News** **How Many Is Too Many?**

In January 2009, an American woman, Nadya Suleman, gave birth to six boys and two girls, conceived through in vitro fertilization, at 30 weeks gestation. All of the babies have survived. The single mother already had six children at home, ranging in age from 2 to 7 years. Debate immediately arose over the ethics of using in vitro technology in such a manner. The American College of Obstetricians and Gynecologists claimed that physicians should think twice before proceeding with what is termed "high order" multiple gestations

Continued on next page

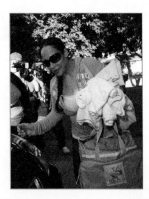

(i.e., more than three embryos implanted in one woman at one time). No laws exist in the United States or Canada to limit the number of embryos implanted; the physician involved may choose to set such limits him- or herself.

Sources: Ayres, C. (2009, January 28). American woman gives birth to live octuplets. *Times Online*. Retrieved May 29, 2009, from http://www.timesonline.co.uk/tol/life_and_style/health/article5600866.ece; Associated Press. (2009, January 30). Mom of octuplets already has 6 children. *CBC News*. Retrieved May 29, 2009, from http://www.cbc.ca/world/story/2009/01/30/octuplets-family.html

Photo credit: CP Photo/Aguilar/Stefan/INFphoto.com.

In the **News**   Should Age Be a Factor?

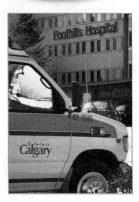

In February 2009, a 60-year-old Alberta woman, Ranjit Hayer, delivered twins by Caesarean section at Foothills Hospital in Calgary. She conceived through in vitro fertilization that was performed in India because clinics in her home province refused her the procedure. She is the oldest woman known to have borne children in Canada. Ethical questions arise regarding how old is too old for in vitro fertilization. Will this mother be around to care for her children? Will she be capable of caring for them as they grow? According to Hayer and her husband, who had been trying for decades to have children, in India, children are considered a blessing, and few married couples do not have them. The couple views the birth of their twin boys as having completed their family.

Sources: Canadian Broadcasting Corporation. (2009, February 5). 60-year-old Calgary mother welcomes twins. *CBC News*. Retrieved May 29, 2009, from http://www.cbc.ca/canada/calgary/story/2009/02/04/cgy-twins-60yearold-mother.html; Lang, M. (2009, February 6). Calgary woman, 60, gives birth to twins. *Calgary Herald*. Retrieved May 29, 2009, from http://www.calgaryherald.com/Calgary+Woman+Gives+Birth+Twins/1259096/story.html

Photo credit: CP PHOTO/Jeff McIntosh.

Clients' rights fall into three categories: the rights Canadians have *within* health care, the right *to* health care, and the right to *timely* health care (Flood & Epps, 2002).

1. Rights *within* health care, established in law in most provinces and territories, include clients' right to their own medical records, the right to

confidentiality concerning their health affairs, and the right to informed consent. Other rights are more vague, such as the right to be treated with respect, compassion, and dignity, the right to privacy, and the right to a reasonable quality of care, including **continuity of care**. Usually contained in the codes of ethics of health care professions, these latter rights tend to be described more as elements health care professionals must deliver, rather than as rights the client is entitled to.

> **Continuity of care**
> Health care based on the treating practitioners' having all required information to optimize the care the client receives; this requires their having access to the individual's health records and maintaining excellent communication among all parties involved in the client's care.

2. Although difficult to enforce and, at times, subjective, the principles of the *Canada Health Act* address Canadians' right *to* health care (with limitations). Services offered within each province and territory vary, with some jurisdictions offering services above and beyond the requirements of the *Canada Health Act*. Some newer procedures, however, remain uncovered by provincial or territorial plans, resulting in those who cannot afford them doing without, thus creating the basis for the argument that a person's right to adequate health care is violated.

3. A growing movement claims that Canadians should also have the right to *timely* health care—that is, reasonable wait times for both urgent and nonurgent medical services. Improving wait times for services would require further government financing, increased human health resources, and a redistribution of health care services; thus, it is an issue not easily addressed. Currently, no legislation guarantees a person's right to prompt medical care, and only limited legal avenues exist for a client to pursue this issue. Despite commitments from the federal, provincial, and territorial governments to shorten wait times, waiting lists are, in most regions, actually getting longer (see Chapter 10).

Many countries have developed a clients' bill of rights—a statement of the rights clients are entitled to when they receive medical care, including information, fair treatment, and autonomy over medical decisions. Legislation supports these bills of rights in countries such as Norway, New Zealand, the United States, England, Spain, Sweden, and Italy. In some other countries, clients' bills of rights exist only as guidelines.

In Canada, provincial and territorial governments have adopted a range of approaches:

- Quebec implemented legislation defining clients' rights in 1991.
- In Ontario, a private member's bill (Bill 27), called the *Tommy Douglas Act*, was introduced in 2002 to provide a clients' bill of rights that would standardize levels of care and ensure whistleblower protection for health care professionals who report inadequacies within the system. This bill, however, was defeated by the Conservative government later that year.

- In New Brunswick, the *Health Charter of Rights and Responsibilities Act*, the first such act in Canada, was introduced to the legislature in April 2003 (Legislative Assembly of New Brunswick, 2003).

- Other provinces have set health care goals, objectives, and expectations in planning and policy documents for clients' bills of rights, but these have not been formally legislated.

Most hospitals create their own clients' bills of rights. Many include a section outlining the responsibilities of the client, which include providing health care professionals with accurate health information, taking an active role in their health care, being courteous to health care professionals, other clients, and staff members, and respecting hospital property.

In the **News**   **Wait Lists: Do They Work?**

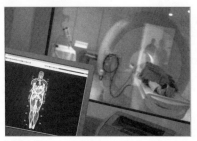

To deal with a client's right to timely care involving hospitalization, most provinces and territories now post wait times online. Individuals can log on to find out the length of wait for admission for certain procedures and can possibly seek the necessary service in an area with a shorter list. Controversy over the usefulness of these wait lists and whether wait times are becoming shorter persists. In many jurisdictions, wait times appear not to have improved. The following Web site provides links to the wait time sites of the various jurisdictions: http://www.hc-sc.gc.ca/hcs-sss/qual/acces/wait-attente/index-eng.php

Source: Health Canada. (2007). *Wait times in Canada.* Retrieved May 29, 2009, from http://www. hc-sc.gc.ca/hcs-sss/qual/acces/wait-attente/index-eng.php

Photo credit: © **Haak78**/Dreamstime.com.

DUTIES AND RIGHTS

If a client has a right *within* health care or *to* health care, for the most part, the health care professional has the responsibility, or duty, to grant that right. At the heart of clients' rights in health care is the principle of autonomy, which has prominence over most other things. Thus, duties, rights, and autonomy are necessarily joined.

To fulfill one's duty to honour clients' rights, the health care professional must either act to carry out a responsibility or refrain from acting or interfering in a situation. In other words, a client's right to something may require one to take steps to provide a service (e.g., educate the client to aid his or her decision making); alternatively, it may require one to do nothing (e.g., refrain from pointing a client toward a particular treatment option). Clients' rights include noninterference regarding some aspects of their health care.

Autonomy and the Client

The principle of autonomy serves as the basis for the principles involved in informed consent and self-determination regarding treatment choices. As discussed in Chapter 8, clients must be mentally capable and fully informed about their situation to be able to make autonomous and knowledgeable decisions about their health care. It falls upon the health care professional to ensure that clients have the appropriate information, to help clients understand the information, and to answer clients' questions regarding their situation. Clients also have the right to seek a second opinion.

Client autonomy is a controversial topic in health care. The original Hippocratic Oath placed physicians in the position of the informed authority whose "job," or ethical and professional responsibility, it was to do their best for the client, to preserve life at all costs, and to make decisions in the best interest of the client—essentially awarding physicians unquestioned trust and authority. Doctors of the past were regarded with such reverence that clients followed their advice with little or no discussion. While this approach did not recognize the client's right to autonomy, it was considered to be in the client's best interest. Attitudes toward client autonomy have changed over the years, ultimately resulting in a version of the Hippocratic Oath (Box 9.1) more aligned with modern concepts, philosophies, and practices.

Box 9.1   A Modern Version of the Hippocratic Oath

I swear to fulfill, to the best of my ability and judgment, this covenant:

I will respect the hard-won scientific gains of those physicians in whose steps I walk, and gladly share such knowledge as is mine with those who are to follow.

I will apply, for the benefit of the sick, all measures [that] are required, avoiding those twin traps of over-treatment and therapeutic nihilism.

I will remember that there is art to medicine as well as science, and that warmth, sympathy, and understanding may outweigh the surgeon's knife or the chemist's drug.

I will not be ashamed to say "I know not," nor will I fail to call in my colleagues when the skills of another are needed for a patient's recovery.

Continued on next page

I will respect the privacy of my patients, for their problems are not disclosed to me that the world may know. Most especially must I tread with care in matters of life and death. If it is given me to save a life, all thanks. But it may also be within my power to take a life; this awesome responsibility must be faced with great humbleness and awareness of my own frailty. Above all, I must not play at God.

I will remember that I do not treat a fever chart, a cancerous growth, but a sick human being, whose illness may affect the person's family and economic stability. My responsibility includes these related problems, if I am to care adequately for the sick.

I will prevent disease whenever I can, for prevention is preferable to cure.

I will remember that I remain a member of society, with special obligations to all my fellow human beings, those sound of mind and body as well as the infirm.

If I do not violate this oath, may I enjoy life and art, respected while I live and remembered with affection thereafter. May I always act so as to preserve the finest traditions of my calling and may I long experience the joy of healing those who seek my help.

Written in 1964 by Louis Lasagna, Academic Dean of the School of Medicine at Tufts University. Source: Nova Online. (n.d.). *The Hippocratic Oath: Modern version*. Retrieved May 29, 2009, from http://www.pbs.org/wgbh/nova/doctors/oath_modern.html

Paternalism

The attempt to control or influence another's decision regarding medical care. Paternalism does not honour the client's right to autonomy.

Assuming the responsibility of decision making for clients or directing their decisions in choosing treatments is called **paternalism**. Because the concept of paternalism may restrict a person's rights, it clashes with modern theories and philosophies.

Over the past several years, views on how far a health care professional should go in making decisions for—instead of with—the client have changed. Emphasis has shifted from what the professional believes to be best for the client to what the client believes to be best for him- or herself. This shift may result in moral dilemmas for physicians committed to beneficence when, for instance, a client refuses life-saving treatment. In most cases, however, health care professionals both respect and uphold clients' decisions. When, on occasion, they do not, significant stress and often litigation results.

Thinking It Through

Clients frequently ask health care professionals for advice based on their specific professional knowledge and expertise. For example, Jennifer, an asthmatic, may ask a respiratory therapist whether she should use her inhalers as often as prescribed.

1. Is it acceptable for a health care professional to give treatment advice to a client based on his or her own judgement and experience—for example, "If I were you, I would do this"?

2. Where do you draw the line between strongly suggesting the client follow your advice and allowing the client to make an independent choice?

TRUTHFULNESS

All clients have a right to the truth, and health care professionals, as discussed above, have a duty to provide it. Expecting that others will be truthful and honest is central to trust, even in our daily lives.

In the past, physicians would often choose to withhold "upsetting information" from a client, or family members would ask a physician to withhold such information (Case Example 9.6). The modern, client-focused (not physician-focused) approach to treatment requires physicians to keep the client fully and truthfully informed. Denying clients information or lying to them causes more harm than good in most situations.

Thinking It **Through**

People often justify untruthfulness by claiming they are sparing someone from being hurt.

1. How do you feel about friends you know have lied to you?

2. Do their intentions really matter?

Case Example 9.6

Ira, 86, has terminal lung cancer. He has other chronic health problems that have reduced both his quality and his enjoyment of life. Unsure how capable Ira is, mentally and physically, to deal with the news of his cancer, the physician tells Ira's family first. His wife and grown children do not want Ira to know, believing that it would be best that he enjoy some degree of quality in the last months of his life without having to face the stress related to the diagnosis. Ira worries

Continued on next page

excessively about his health. The doctor, against his better judgement, agrees to remain silent. Only days before he dies, Ira learns of the diagnosis of several months before. Bitter, he feels that had he known, he could have put his affairs in order, come to terms with dying, and better prepared his children for his death.

PARENTAL RIGHTS AND THE LAW

Paternalism and the legal system sometimes join forces when life-saving treatment is thought to be necessary yet is refused—for example, when parents make decisions for their minor children that the health care professional believes will compromise the health or life of the child, as in the case of Jehovah's Witness parents refusing a blood transfusion that would save their child's life. When a client is considered an adult, self-determination takes precedence over paternalistic intervention, even when the client's life is at stake. But when children are involved and parents reject medical intervention, the provincial or territorial courts almost always obtain legal custody for the child and allow the recommended treatment. Numerous cases have surfaced over the past few years involving children from newborns to teenagers (In the News: Rights of the Individual Versus Medical Advice).

In the **News** — **Rights of the Individual Versus Medical Advice**

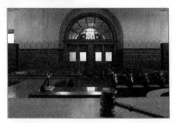

In 2006, a Manitoba adolescent, aged 14, refused a blood transfusion to treat severe intestinal bleeding resulting from Crohn's disease (a chronic, inflammatory disease of the gastrointestinal tract) because it breached her religious beliefs as a Jehovah's Witness. Her parents and family supported her decision. Manitoba's director of child and family services went to court and won an order authorizing doctors to perform the necessary treatment because the minor was in danger of serious harm. The Manitoba adolescent, now recovered, has challenged the law at the Supreme Court of Canada, asking to be considered a "mature teen," which would enable her to make her own decision if a similar situation were to arise again. The Supreme Court has reserved judgement in the case.

Sources: Canadian Broadcasting Corporation. (2006, September 7). Winnipeg girl in court to fight blood transfusions. *CBC News.* Retrieved May 29, 2009, from http://www.cbc.ca/canada/manitoba/story/2006/09/07/jw-crohns.html; Canadian Broadcasting Corporation. (2009, May 20). Top court reserves judgment in girl's blood transfusion. *CBC News.* Retrieved May 29, 2009, from http://www.cbc.ca/canada/story/2008/05/20/blood-transfusion.html

Photo credit: © iStockphoto.com/ftwitty.

Conflicts often arise among the principles of personal autonomy, the protection of minors, and the duty of the health care professional to preserve life.

1. Is there a right or a wrong position?

2. Should doctors stand aside and watch underage clients die for lack of intervention? Do you think the doctor would feel differently if he or she shared the client's religious beliefs?

All involved parties want what is best for the client, but what one considers best may differ from what another considers best. Values, cultural and religious beliefs, and ethical codes can conflict. Who is to say which path should be followed? Do parents not have the right to make decisions for their underage children? Do doctors not have a legal obligation to preserve life? For physicians, cases such as the blood transfusion one cited in the In the News box differ significantly from withdrawing life support for a terminally ill client. Jehovah's Witnesses do not want their children to die, nor do they refuse all medical treatments—only those involving blood products.

Clients who refuse a blood transfusion, even in the face of death, are following the divine command theory. Their religious beliefs dictate their course of action. Physicians, on the other hand, observe duty ethics; their duty is to treat the client. Some might argue for a teleological approach—treating the client saves the client's life and, in the end, benefits everyone involved. Could that outcome be argued, however, if the client is ostracized by his or her community for having had a blood transfusion and if the client feels wronged for having been forced to do something contrary to his or her religious beliefs? What do you think?

RIGHTS AND MENTAL COMPETENCE

Conflict with a client's autonomy frequently arises when a question of mental competence exists. Consider a person with anorexia nervosa, a devastating eating disorder that primarily affects young women, although both men and women of all ages are vulnerable. It is often caused by another physiological disorder, or vice versa. Conditions associated with anorexia include obsessive compulsive disorder, borderline personality disorder, bipolar disorder, post-traumatic stress disorder, and depression. The nature of these diseases often hinders the client's ability to make rational decisions.

Does a person whose illness skews his or her ability to make rational decisions have the right to self-determination? Concerns over such situations led psychiatrist Marian Verkerk to propose the concept of **compassionate interference**, which allows physicians to treat individuals against their will (Verkerk, 1999). Dr. Verkerk argues that treatment restores clients to a sound physical and mental state, allowing them then to make informed decisions.

As discussed, parental authority has been removed when parents or guardians refuse medical treatment deemed necessary to save a child's life. These cases can become more complex—for example, when the child in question also refuses treatment but is considered mentally unfit to make such a decision, as illustrated in the case below (In the News: When Can a Parent Refuse Treatment for a Child?).

In the **News**

When Can a Parent Refuse Treatment for a Child?

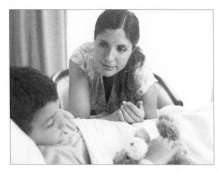

In 2004, an 8-year-old boy living in Hamilton, Ontario, was successfully treated for leukemia. The father described the treatments as "hell." The boy lost his hair, had sores all over his body, had to wear diapers, and couldn't keep food down. In 2008, the leukemia returned. This time, his father and stepmother refused further treatment, claiming they would rely on spiritual healing and the outcome determined by their Creator. The boy, then 11, claimed he did not want the treatment because he was unprepared to experience the overwhelming side effects again. The boy, who suffers from fetal alcohol syndrome and attends special education classes, was assessed as incompetent to make such a decision.

The court obtained statements from two of the country's top specialists in the field of leukemia, both of whom felt that treatment was Dillon's only hope and that a reasonable chance of a positive outcome existed. The boy was made a ward of the Children's Aid Society, and treatment was imposed.

Sources: CTV. (2008, May 10). Boy undergoing chemotherapy against his wishes. *CTV News*. Retrieved May 29, 2009, from http://toronto.ctv.ca/servlet/an/plocal/CTVNews/20080510/ unwanted_chemotherapy_080510/20080510/?hub=OttawaHome; Canadian Broadcasting Corporation. (2008, May 13). Forced chemo treatment of child "heavy-handed" decision: Bioethicists. *CBC News*. Retrieved May 29, 2009, from http://www.cbc.ca/health/story/ 2008/05/13/cas-chemo.html

Photo credit: © OJO Images/Fotosearch.

ETHICS AT WORK

All regulated health care professions have codes of ethics, as do many places of employment. Review the one belonging to your profession or organization. If none exists, you should consider recommending that one be implemented. Many ethical situations arise in the health care industry, and codes of ethics significantly help professionals make appropriate decisions.

CODE OF ETHICS

A formal statement of an organization's or profession's values regarding professional behaviour, a code of ethics provides guidance for ethical decision making, self-evaluation, and best practices policies. Most codes cover expectations related to professional conduct that, if violated, can result in loss of the person's professional licence, dismissal from employment, or legal action.

Special Boundaries and Relationships

With Clients

Personal relationships between clients and health care professionals in any discipline are, for the most part, prohibited while the formal relationship remains and, sometimes, even for a period of time after the professional relationship ends. Codes of ethics for physicians clearly outline these boundaries. Doctors may not establish personal relationships with clients under their care. In most circumstances, a physician may not date a former client for one year after the termination of the client–physician relationship. Most other health care professions take a similar, though often not as strict, stand on developing personal relationships with clients. For example, no formal objection exists to a physiotherapist starting a relationship with a former client several weeks after their professional relationship has ended.

Thinking It **Through**

In some situations, dating or developing an intimate relationship with a former client never becomes ethical (e.g., between a psychiatrist and former client). Some physicians working in small, remote communities where social contacts are limited have challenged this guideline.

Continued on next page

In a community with only one physician, would you consider this "rule" reasonable? If the physician provides care for most of the community's residents, how would he or she establish any social relationships or activities?

Often, especially in small centres, a client admitted to hospital knows many of the staff members. Depending on the nature of the relationship, this may or may not cause concern. If the health care professional feels uncomfortable caring for a particular client, or the other way around, however, it would be in the best interests of both to have someone else assume that client's care.

Thinking It Through

In the workplace setting, you will meet a wide range of people, some of whom you are drawn to and feel a natural desire to want to develop a friendship with.

1. Is it ethical for a health care professional to exchange phone numbers with a client with the intent of dating after the client is discharged?

2. Does it make a difference if the exchange of phone numbers is for the purpose of developing a platonic friendship?

With Colleagues

Inevitably, you will develop friendships in the workplace. Unless these friendships interfere with how you do your job, this is not considered unethical. However, you must remain impartial and not choose favourites among the staff. Developing alliances by forming cliques at the expense of others is both unprofessional and destructive. Tight-knit groups in the workplace make it difficult for new staff members to integrate and feel welcome. Starting a new job is difficult enough. A warm and inviting environment goes a long way toward helping new employees fit in and begin to function competently as a member of the health care team.

Personal business has no role in the workplace, either. Discussing last night's party, tomorrow's trip, or someone's recent breakup remains inappropriate in any work environment.

In the Hospital Setting

Health care professionals employed in a hospital setting are expected to carry out their duties in a professional, legal, and ethical manner. All health care facilities have procedures, policies, and guidelines governing ethical conduct. As well, employers expect health care professionals to uphold the ethical codes of their individual professions. Although members of the health care team should support each other, overstepping certain boundaries can breach ethical conduct (e.g., moving a colleague's family member up a wait list).

Health care professionals also have an obligation to report fellow health care professionals' misconduct or incompetence, whether regarding their job performance or a violation of the principles of confidentiality. Most health care environments develop procedures outlining what to report and whom to report it to. Ethical issues unresolved at a lower level, in most facilities, will be reported to an ethics committee.

Rationale for Boundaries

Trust

A health care professional providing medical services for a client does so within a therapeutic relationship. Clients trust the health care professional to perform his or her professional services impartially and competently. Not only is changing the nature of that relationship ethically and morally wrong; it can also interfere with the care and compromise the ability of the health care professional to fulfill his or her professional duties. The higher the professional's level of responsibility (e.g., a physician versus a physiotherapist, respiratory therapist, or medical secretary), the more damaging this can be.

Vulnerability

The client occupies the vulnerable position within the client–health care professional relationship. As a result of this vulnerability, the client may exhibit sick role behaviour (see Chapter 1) and feel dependent.

Balance of Power and Transference

In a physician–client relationship, decisions made by the physician can have a significant impact on the client's health and recovery. Along with feeling vulnerable, the client may be in awe of the physician and misread feelings for him or her. Clients somewhat commonly feel a sense of "falling in love" with physicians or other health care professionals. The health care professional has a responsibility to recognize the relevant signs and to ensure the relationship remains formal. In some cases, physicians have to stop providing care for the client.

All health care professionals dealing with clients should be aware of the possibility of such situations. Clients have a right to equitable and fair care—and to trust that they receive it. Any personal ties with a client, therefore, have the potential to interfere with the care of that client or others, to interfere with a trusting relationship, and to put the client in a vulnerable position.

Accepting Gifts

Clients often give gifts to health care professionals who have cared for them, usually as an expression of gratitude. Little literature is available about the ethics of accepting gifts. A box of chocolates for the nursing station when a client leaves the hospital, some flowers sent to the office, or a card with a small ornament are examples of acceptable gifts. Anything more is inappropriate and may place the health care professional in a difficult position because the client may expect favouritism, such as access to special treatment or an appointment whenever he or she wants it. Some health care professionals make it a policy not to accept anything—ever. If your employer has guidelines about accepting gifts, follow them.

Seasonal gifts may be an exception. During the holidays, clients often give health care professionals and their office staff gifts, such as home baking, wine, or other tokens of appreciation—usually with no strings attached. Some people get a true sense of satisfaction from the opportunity to express gratitude. Common sense and familiarity with the client are the best guidelines when accepting seasonal gifts.

Gifts may also be exchanged between health care professionals, particularly during the holiday season. Physicians often send chocolates or fruit baskets to client care units in hospitals or long-term care facilities they are affiliated with. In the office setting, health care professionals may host a staff dinner or get-together or gift staff members with a holiday bonus as a way of showing appreciation for their contributions as members of the health care team.

The Ethics Committee

An ethics committee consists of a group of people—often volunteers—who listen to, evaluate, and make recommendations about acts perceived as unethical. Members of such committees usually come from a variety of backgrounds and may include doctors, nurses, social workers, physiotherapists, lawyers, ethicists, and members of the public. Public members do not require special qualifications other than the ability to listen and assist with making fair and unbiased decisions. Members remain on the committee for designated time frames.

Aside from evaluating unethical acts, ethics committees may provide health care professionals with guidance in making controversial medical decisions and compile research for policy development within the facility. In the health care profession, decisions are often neither unanimous nor easy. All matters discussed and reviewed by an ethics committee remain strictly confidential.

END-OF-LIFE ISSUES

End-of-life issues that raise ethical concerns include clients' wishing to withdraw life-saving measures, issuing do-not-resuscitate (DNR) orders, and requesting supportive or palliative care in the face of a terminal illness.

EUTHANASIA

The purpose of euthanasia (also called "aid in dying") is to deliberately end a life in order to relieve pain and suffering due to an incurable disease. Various categories of euthanasia exist. **Voluntary euthanasia** occurs when a person causes the death of another with the dying person's consent—often in the form of a living will or advance directive (see page 346). **Involuntary euthanasia** occurs when a person causes the death of another without the dying person's consent. **Active euthanasia** refers to someone taking deliberate steps to end another's life (e.g., with a lethal injection). **Passive euthanasia** refers to the process of allowing a person to die by removing life support or other life-sustaining treatment. In the case of **physician-assisted suicide**, the doctor provides the client with the means to end his or her own life; the client, however, carries out the act.

With the exception of passive euthanasia, the act of ending or assisting to end a person's life is illegal in most countries, including Canada. Euthanasia, a highly controversial concept, has both legal and ethical implications. The act conflicts with the moral values of most societies, which value the sanctity of life and the duty of the health care professional to save or preserve life. On the other hand, allowing euthanasia respects the autonomy of the person who wishes to die.

The possibility of legalizing euthanasia raises fears of misuse of the process—for example, ending Aunt Sally's life to inherit her money or putting Dad to sleep because he is too difficult to care for. Euthanasia has also been proposed to end lifelong suffering, even when death is not eminent (In the News: The Latimer Tragedy).

In the **News**   **The Latimer Tragedy**

A noteworthy case of involuntary active euthanasia, with ramifications that persist today, is that of Robert Latimer, a Saskatchewan farmer who killed his daughter, Tracy, in 1993 by placing her in a car and rerouting exhaust fumes to euthanize her. Tracy, a 40-pound, 12-year-old quadriplegic with cerebral palsy, functioned at the level of a 3-month-old. According to most reports, she suffered constant and severe pain. Her father could not bear to see her life continue

Continued on next page

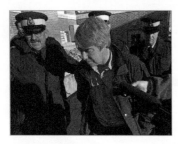

indefinitely in this manner. Convicted of second-degree murder, Mr. Latimer went to jail. In 2008, he received day parole and continues to protest his conviction.

Source: Canadian Broadcasting Corporation. (2008, March 17). "Compassionate homicide": The law and Robert Latimer. *CBC Archives*. Retrieved May 29, 2009, from http://www.cbc.ca/news/background/latimer/

Photo credit: THE CANADIAN PRESS. 1997 (str-Kevin Frayer).

Debate about the ethics in the Latimer case and the severity of the sentence Mr. Latimer received continues to this day. At Mr. Latimer's second trial, ordered because of jury interference in the first trial, the jury upheld the charge of second-degree murder but recommended Mr. Latimer be eligible for parole after one year. In this trial, Justice Ted Noble tried to distinguish between murder and mercy killing. He called Tracy Latimer's murder a "rare act of homicide that was committed for caring and altruistic reasons. That is why for want of a better term, this is called compassionate homicide" (Canadian Broadcasting Corporation, 2008). Does Robert Latimer present a danger to society? Most would say no. However, in 1998, the Saskatchewan Court of Appeal overturned Judge Noble's ruling, imposing the mandatory minimum sentence: 25 years, with no parole for 10 years. Latimer's first bid for parole in 2007 was denied because he maintained his belief that he killed Tracy for her benefit and would not express remorse. Groups championing the rights of the disabled argued that showing leniency would endanger disabled persons and rate them as second-class citizens. Canadians with disabilities continue to campaign for protection of what they deem a fundamental human right—the right to life (Canadian Broadcasting Corporation, 2008).

Another widely known case is that of British Columbia resident Susan Rodriguez, who suffered from amyotrophic lateral sclerosis (ALS—also called Lou Gehrig's disease). For months, Ms. Rodriguez petitioned the courts for permission to die legally with medical assistance. The courts refused (*Rodriguez v. British Columbia*, 1993). In the end, she terminated her own life in 1994 with physician assistance. The physician was never named or charged. See the Web Resources list at the end of this chapter for a link to videos of Susan Rodriguez petitioning the courts.

In another case, Nancy B. developed Guillain-Barré syndrome, which left her incapable of movement, including breathing, although her mental capacities remained. She petitioned the Superior Court of Quebec to have her respirator turned off. The court upheld Nancy B.'s right to consent or withhold consent to any medical intervention (*N.B. v. Hôtel-Dieu de Québec*, 1992).

Some of the most complicated cases involve individuals in a vegetative state who are kept alive by respirators, feeding tubes, or both. Often the family cannot agree on a course of action—some family members want life-sustaining measures withdrawn, and others want them continued. Depending on the situation, after the withdrawal of life-sustaining measures, death can take days to occur or can occur almost immediately (In the News: Who Has the Right to Decide?).

Thinking It **Through**

The cases of Susan Rodriguez and Nancy B. illustrate two individuals wanting the right to die—one being refused this right; the other being granted it.

1. Why do you think the courts ruled differently?

2. Should the person or persons who assisted Ms. Rodriguez to die face legal action?

In the **News**   **Who Has the Right to Decide?**

In 1990, an American woman, Terri Schiavo, was declared brain dead after her heart stopped beating temporarily, depriving her of oxygen. Finally convinced that she would not recover, in 1998, her husband, Michael, petitioned to have Terri's feeding tube removed. Michael held that removing the feeding tube was in keeping with Terri's wishes, thus respecting her right to autonomy. Her parents, still believing their daughter may recover, claimed that Terri would not want life-saving interventions terminated. A lengthy legal battle ensued. Terri's parents believed that their daughter responded 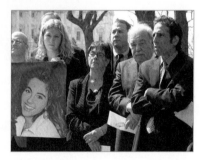 to them and that she was not, in fact, brain dead. After several court decisions alternately allowing the tube to be removed and reinserted, the feeding tube was removed one last time when the parents' final appeal was denied. It took Terri 13 days to die. According to a CTV news report on March 31, 2005, the Vatican denounced Terri's "arbitrarily hastened" passing as a violation of principles of Christianity and civilization.

Sources: Canadian Broadcasting Corporation. (2005, March 31). Schiavo timeline. *CBC News*. Retrieved May 29, 2009, from http://www.cbc.ca/news/background/schiavo/; CTV.ca. (2005, March 31). After long struggle, Terri Schiavo dies at 41. *CTV News*. Retrieved May 29, 2009, from http://www.ctv.ca/servlet/ArticleNews/story/CTVNews/1112278242558_9/?hub=World

Photo credit: THE CANADIAN PRESS. Photo by Olivier Douliery/ABACAUSA.COM.

THE RIGHT TO DIE

People suffering from a poor quality of life as a result of illness, usually a terminal illness, may request the right to die (i.e., passive euthanasia). As discussed earlier, mentally competent adult clients have the right to refuse medical treatment, to request a DNR order, or to ask for only comfort measures in the face of a serious, possibly terminal, illness.

Older people and those with debilitating diseases commonly request that they not be resuscitated (through a DNR order) if they suffer a cardiac arrest (i.e., heart attack). These people are not pursuing euthanasia; they simply do not want any intervention if a major health event occurs. Health care professionals are legally bound to honour such requests, which can be difficult for those who believe that active measures should be taken at all costs. Importantly, a person can reverse his or her DNR request at any time.

Thinking It Through

Currently hospitalized, Pierre suffers a cardiac arrest. His nurse, Nancy, is in his room at the time and knows that he has a DNR order because he was constantly reminding the staff of it. However, because of Nancy's religious beliefs, she feels that saving a person's life takes precedence over everything else. Not resuscitating Pierre is a difficult choice for her to make, but resuscitating him would violate the client's personal request and, thus, his right to autonomy. What Should Nancy do?

An **advance directive**, also called a *living will* or *treatment directive*, specifies the nature and level of treatment a person would want to receive in the event that he or she becomes unable to make those decisions at a later time. People prepare advance directives so as to ensure their wishes are known and honoured by family and loved ones and carried out by medical caregivers. Advance directives that appoint a power of attorney for personal care are most likely to result in the person's instructions being followed.

A **values history form** is a comprehensive document that guides people in thinking about treatment options they would or would not want in the event that they were to become unable to make decisions about their own health care. People can detail their feelings, thoughts, and values as they relate to medical interventions. The form may also assist loved ones who might have to make decisions on the person's behalf, as well as clarify the person's choices if disagreements among loved ones occur (Case Example 9.7).

Case Example 9.7

Sam, a 67-year-old who recently suffered a severe stroke, created an advance directive expressing his wish to receive no active intervention if he has another stroke. However, concerned that another stroke may leave him unable to communicate and on a respirator, he begins to have doubts about his decision, fearful that if he has a change of heart, he would be unable to communicate it. (Many people who have decided against intervention change their minds when actually facing death.) Some family members know of his recent second thoughts about his advance directive. Sam decides to complete a values history form to clarify his feelings and thoughts about medical intervention. This form *might* help Sam's family if they ever have to make treatment decisions for him.

A client in hospital can request varying levels of care in the event of a life-threatening incident, ranging from comfort measures only to active treatment but no cardiopulmonary resuscitation (CPR) to full and active treatment (e.g., every possible intervention to preserve the person's life). Rating systems vary among agencies, but "comfort" or "supportive" measures usually include pain control and any other intervention to prevent suffering, whereas "active" treatment may refer simply to, for example, the administration of an IV for hydration and pain medication but no antibiotics or the use of any and all medications that will sustain life and end the crisis. Some individuals refuse their daily medications (e.g., antihypertensive medication, diuretics) in an attempt to accelerate their demise. Such refusal is perfectly legal but may pose moral questions for those involved in the individual's care.

PALLIATIVE CARE

In the mid-twentieth century, people with terminal illnesses were cared for in the hospital, where the focus remained on actively intervening to preserve life. In the early 1970s, hospitals in Montreal and Winnipeg introduced hospital-based palliative care. Since that time, palliative care programs have developed within communities and have begun to be offered in the home. The philosophy and ethics of end-of-life care have shifted from preserving life at all costs to controlling symptoms and honouring the client's wishes.

Today, **palliative care**, an increasingly important component of medical care in Canada, addresses the physical and emotional needs of those who are dying. Whether delivered in a hospital, in a hospice, or at home, palliative care can aid any person at any age and at any stage of a life-threatening illness. Teams of experts work with clients and their families to manage physical discomfort and psychological distress and to meet spiritual needs. Palliative care offers terminally ill people an alternative to facing death alone and an end to the fear of a painful death that strips them of human dignity. Many consider palliative care an important alternative for those who might consider ending their lives by other means.

ALLOCATION OF RESOURCES

The term *allocation of resources* refers to who gets what, when, and for what reason. Rising health care costs, expensive technologies, and limited access to many services have made the allocation of resources an increasing concern in the health care industry. And limited resources means that "Who gets what?" becomes a huge ethical problem. A brief discussion of select limited resources follows, with the intent of promoting thought and discussion.

ORGAN TRANSPLANTATION

The advancements that led to the ability to transplant organs, a scarce resource, have introduced several ethical issues. Consider Case Example 9.8.

In Case Example 9.8, Olga has been unable to overcome the disease of alcoholism. Although she has managed to give up drinking for limited periods of

Case Example 9.8

The transplant team at a large hospital has just received word that a liver has become available. The list of approved critical candidates includes both Joe and Olga. Joe, despite living a very healthy lifestyle, suffers from an autoimmune disease that has destroyed his liver. Olga, an alcoholic, has advanced liver disease and generally very poor health. Her history suggests that she remains at high risk for returning to drinking—a setback that would surely damage the new liver should she receive one. All other things being equal (age, family situation, finances), which candidate do you think should get the liver? Should Olga be considered a less desirable candidate because of her disease than Joe?

time, her ability to maintain sobriety remains questionable. A return to drinking would sharply decrease her chances of maintaining even reasonable health with a transplanted liver. Should she therefore be denied a chance at a new life? Joe, on the other hand, lives a healthy lifestyle yet has contracted a disease typically considered less preventable than alcoholism. But what if, as is debated in modern medicine, alcoholism were more commonly considered a disease, rather than a moral failing? Would Olga then be in a more favourable position to compete for the liver? Would she be on equal footing with Joe?

Other considerations from a medical perspective encourage the following questions: Who would be more likely to see significant improvements in his or her health with the new liver? What damage has alcoholism done to Olga's over-all health? Alcoholics tend to have lower success rates with transplantation since their general health is usually poorer. A return to drinking would interfere with compliance with the necessary post-transplant treatment regime, which requires taking immunosuppressant drugs. Nonetheless, do any of these factors provide a solid reason to deny Olga?

FINANCES AND RESOURCES

In Canada, the demand for health care resources—including finances, health care professionals, and medical services such as diagnostic tests and hospital beds—sometimes exceeds supply. The allocation of resources in health care presents an ethical problem because it raises questions about fairness and justness. Priorities should be based on need, but how does a person, organization, or government assess need?

Because of limited funds for health care services across Canada, the provincial and territorial governments allocate funds to communities, regional health authorities, hospitals, and other organizations, allowing each to set priorities and to make decisions about how best to meet the health care needs of the populations they serve. If funds increase, however, who gets the surplus? If funds decrease, which services are maintained and which are sacrificed? How can someone make a decision, for example, to fund expensive treatment for a small number of autistic children if that same amount of money might be spent on cancer treatment that could save hundreds of lives?

All levels of government and an army of health care professionals collaborate to implement strategies they believe will be the most cost-effective. The recent thrust toward preventive care has directed funding toward raising awareness of the importance of, for example, periodic physical examinations, breast screening and Pap smears for women, immunizations for children, colon cancer home tests, and a healthy lifestyle (e.g., a proper diet, regular physical activity, and avoidance of self-imposed risk behaviours such as smoking). The healthier the Canadian population is, the fewer health care dollars ultimately need to be spent. Although many consider immunizations among the most important advances in preventive care, others argue that vaccines pose more risks than do diseases such as polio, measles, mumps, typhoid, and rubella, suggesting that immunizations have caused autism in some Canadian children (no definitive proof of this exists).

Many groups compete for health care dollars—some for treatments for rare conditions that would empty the health care pot of millions of dollars. Teleological theorists, however, would suggest that funds should go to those services that meet the needs of the most people. Most Canadians take the stand that treatment should be available to all Canadians and that governments should ensure such universal availability without imposing financial hardship on an individual or family. The sentiments of Canadians, as summarized in the Romanow Report, are outlined in Box 9.2.

Box 9.2   Canadians' Views on Health Care

The Romanow Commission found that most Canadians shared the following basic beliefs and concerns about health care:

- The poorest in society should have access to health care.

- Individual Canadians should not be bankrupted by the cost of acquiring needed health care services.

- Need should be taken into account in determining what medical services should be covered by public health insurance.

- Both the federal government and provincial and territorial governments must play a role in reforming the health care system.

Source: Romanow, R. (2002). Building on values: The future of health care in Canada. Retrieved May 29, 2009, from http://www.cbc.ca/healthcare/final_report.pdf

---

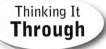

Thinking It
Through

Thousands of Canadians suffer from relatively rare conditions that are incurable but that can be treated with some success. These treatments, however, are often extremely expensive and do not fall within the definition of "medically necessary."

1. Is it ethical to spend a large amount of money on a few individuals when that money could be used to improve health care services for a much larger group?

2. Does each life not deserve the same consideration?

New technologies have introduced treatment modalities that preserve and prolong life, and Canadians feel a sense of entitlement to these technologies. However, funds are limited; if every life-saving or treatment measure were offered to every person in need, the health care system would collapse. For example, significant (and costly) advancements have been made in sustaining life for very premature babies; however, these infants often have little hope of recovery or a satisfactory quality of life if they do recover (Case Example 9.9). With health care costs rising, Canadians may ultimately be asked to consider the expense of their choices.

Case Example 9.9

Raja delivered a baby, Damian, at 23 weeks gestation. Damian was transported to the nearest neonatal intensive care unit. Three days later, the doctors told Raja that her baby had a 30% chance of survival and that if he did survive, he would likely be blind, require multiple heart surgeries, suffer from a seizure disorder, and have cerebral palsy. They asked whether she wanted them to continue treatment to attempt to save the baby's life. The cost to the health care system would be enormous, and the quality of life the baby would have, questionable. Left to make her very difficult decision, Raja had to consider the small margin of hope that her son would live and, if he did survive, the complications he would have to endure. The last thing on her mind was the expense of the treatments—they were covered by the health care system.

NORTHERN ACCESS TO HEALTH CARE

Providing health care resources for the population of Canada's northern communities is very costly. Remote Aboriginal reserves and villages with few resources result in a large percentage of available health care dollars being spent on transportation costs to larger centres. (Such services are covered under provincial and territorial health plans in accordance with the principles of the *Canada Health Act.*) Canada's Inuit population in the Arctic especially lacks adequate health care (Box 9.3). Is it moral or ethical that this portion of Canada's population endures conditions that Canadians in more southern, populated communities would consider unacceptable?

Box 9.3   The Stark Reality in the Far North

At a First Nations Summit, Jose Kusugak of the Inuit Tapiriit Kanatami summarized the special problems facing the 45,000 Inuit who live mainly in the country's far north as follows:

- Clients with serious illnesses must wait 8 to 12 hours for a flight to see a physician in the south.

- Only about 40% of Inuit living in the Arctic get to see a doctor throughout the year, compared with 70% of other Canadians.

- The average food basket, which Statistics Canada measures to determine the cost of living, costs $135 in the south and $327 in the north, where incomes are far lower. As a result, northern families find it much harder to eat a healthy diet.

- Inuit suicide rates are six times higher than the national average.

Sources: Crisis Intervention and Suicide Prevention Centre of British Columbia. (2008). *Key suicide statistics*. Retrieved May 29, 2009, from http://www.crisiscentre.bc.ca/learn/stats.php; Inuit Tapiriit Kanatami. (2004). *Inuit youth experiencing alarming suicide rates*. Retrieved May 29, 2009, from http://www.itk.ca/media-centre/media-releases/inuit-youth-experiencing-alarming-suicide-rates; World Health Organization. (2007). *Health of indigenous peoples*. Fact sheet No 326. Retrieved May 29, 2009, from http://www.who.int/mediacentre/factsheets/fs326/en/index.html

OTHER ETHICAL ISSUES IN HEALTH CARE

ABORTION

One of the most longstanding and controversial issues in health care, abortion has remained without restrictions in Canada since 1988, when the Supreme Court of Canada declared that the law could not forbid abortion because doing so would violate Section 7 of the Charter. Moreover, this court decision held that the then current restrictions on access to abortion were unfair and unreasonable. Section 7 states that "everyone has the right to life, liberty and the security of the person and the right not to be deprived thereof except in accordance with the principles of fundamental justice" (*Canadian Charter of Rights and Freedoms*, 1982).

In Canada, abortions remain legal to the point of "viability" (defined as a fetus weighing more than 500 grams or having reached more than 20 weeks gestation) (Canadian Medical Association, 1988). Second-trimester abortions are allowed only under certain circumstances, usually when the mother's life is at risk. Third-trimester abortions may also be performed under such circumstances; however, new technologies have given most babies born at that stage a reasonable chance of survival. Babies born after 28 weeks gestation receive the best chance of achieving a healthy life.

Access to and coverage for abortion vary among provinces and territories. For instance, Nova Scotia provides limited funding and New Brunswick provides no funding for abortions obtained in clinics. Prince Edward Island offers no abortion facilities at all. In early 2008, Quebec decided to fund abortions without limitations.

Since health care professionals are not obliged to perform abortions, many will opt not to because of religious or moral beliefs, providing clients some limitations on access. Canadians in northern and other remote regions usually must travel long distances at their own expense to access abortion services.

The moral and ethical issues around abortion concern two main issues: the right of the fetus to life and the right of women to make decisions that involve their own bodies. These issues also include philosophical, religious, and political components.

Pro-life groups believe that personhood (i.e., the state of being considered a person) begins at conception—the moment the sperm meets the ovum. From a spiritual perspective, some believe that the soul enters the body at this point. Pro-lifers consider any deliberate interference that threatens the life of this "person" murder, believing that the fetus shares the same rights as all other humans, including the right to life.

Pro-choice groups argue that the mother has the choice to carry the baby to term or to end the pregnancy, maintaining that abortion is a constitutional right and that, therefore, safe and timely access in hospitals and clinics must be guaranteed. Views among pro-choice groups vary as to when the fetus becomes a person with rights. People who, for example, believe that personhood does not begin until the start of the second trimester or later assert that an abortion occurring prior to 13 weeks is both moral and ethical if it reflects the wishes of the pregnant woman.

The debate over whether abortion is right or wrong, ethical or unethical, will continue. The argument comes down to personal, moral, religious, and cultural values and beliefs.

GENETIC TESTING

Through genetic testing—the examination of one's deoxyribonucleic acid (DNA)—people can learn whether they carry any genes that put them at a higher risk for disease, such as certain types of cancer. Similarly, carrier testing determines whether the potential exists to pass on a genetic disease (e.g., sickle cell anemia) to offspring. A couple who undergo such tests and have positive results then must weigh the severity of the potential disease and the chances of its occurrence when deciding whether to bear children.

Prenatal diagnostic screening can determine a fetus's risk for certain genetic disorders, aid in earlier diagnosis of fetal abnormalities, and provide prospective parents with important information for making informed decisions about a pregnancy.

Genetic testing raises a number of moral and ethical questions, however. For instance, if an insurance company obtained records showing that a prospective client carried a gene that put him or her at risk of developing cancer, would that person be considered uninsurable? Would an employer with access to similar information decide against hiring that person?

What the individual does with the information obtained raises further issues. For example, a woman who learns she has the breast cancer gene might elect to have her breasts and ovaries removed.

Canadians are encouraged to think carefully (i.e., to ask what the benefit is in knowing) before having genetic testing for presumed or established conditions. For example, would it help a person to know that he or she may develop Huntington's disease, an incurable neurological disorder? Such knowledge might provide relief from uncertainty and give a person an opportunity to get his or her affairs in order. On the other hand, the anxiety produced from living with the risk for an incurable disease can be overwhelming.

Thinking It **Through**

Assume that several members of your family have suffered from Alzheimer's disease. A genetic test will tell you whether you carry the inherited gene, which would increase the likelihood of your developing the disease.

1. Would you want to know if you carried the gene?
2. What advantages and disadvantages exist of either knowing or not knowing?

Hemochromatosis
A condition that causes the body to absorb and store excessive amounts of iron and that, if untreated, can cause the major body organs to fail.

Although demand for genetic testing in Canada is growing, resources are limited, and individuals who turn to private laboratories (e.g., in the United States) surrender the advantage of receiving counsel from their doctors. Results can be indefinite, stressful, damaging to family relationships, and harmful to careers. Genetic tests covered under public insurance in Canada include those for breast and ovarian cancer, colon cancer, **hemochromatosis**, high cholesterol, and Alzheimer's disease.

Provincial and territorial governments have questioned the cost-effectiveness of genetic testing (i.e., allocation of resources) and have agreed that the cost-effectiveness depends on the test. For example, genetic testing for colon cancer is probably cost-effective since individuals who test positive for a colon cancer gene can undergo regular screening (usually via colonoscopy) that can diagnose cancer in its early stages. Testing for lesser-known conditions is sometimes considered expensive and unlikely to save the health care system money in the long run.

Expert genetic counselling accompanies genetic testing in some Canadian jurisdictions, but not all. Genetic counselling aims to provide individuals with an understanding of the implications of a positive test, both for themselves and for their relatives, and to ensure individuals make an informed choice about taking the test.

SUMMARY

❖ Ethics in health care is a controversial, emotional, and often abstract topic. Health care professionals must function with the highest ethical, moral, and professional standards and must support their clients in their decisions regardless of the health care professionals' personal views.

❖ Understanding your own moral and ethical beliefs, your values, and your method of making ethical decisions will help you to understand your responses to ethical problems encountered in your professional role. Four ethical theories (teleological theory, deontological theory, virtue ethics, divine command) define how most people make ethical decisions, providing some explanation for decisions that individuals make about their own health or the health of those they love.

❖ Six principles (beneficence and nonmaleficence, respect, autonomy, truthfulness, fidelity, and justice) provide the foundation for ethics in health care. Beneficence—doing what is right and good for the client—dates back as far as the practice of medicine itself and figures in the Hippocratic Oath. Establishing a trusting relationship with clients and being respectful, honest, and truthful allows the client to make his or her own decisions. This approach also supports the principle of autonomy, or the client's right to self-determination. In most circumstances, paternalism is no longer acceptable in health care. Clients retain the right to have active treatment withdrawn, to refuse treatment, and to die with dignity.

❖ Advance directives (also called *living wills*) help to ensure that clients' wishes are honoured when they can no longer make their wishes known.

❖ Health care professionals must establish and maintain therapeutic and respectful relationships with their clients. The balance of power that exists between a health care professional and a client puts the client in a vulnerable position in which feelings can be misinterpreted. Health care professionals faced with a relationship issue must respect the codes of ethics of their profession, their employer, or both.

❖ Many areas of health care (e.g., abortion, the right to die, genetic testing) cause controversy in the application of morals, values, and ethics. For the most part, no right or wrong answers exist—only what beliefs and values dictate. It is essential for health care professionals to maintain an open mind, respect the rights of others to make their own decisions, and recognize that this can be achieved without compromising one's own beliefs and values.

REVIEW QUESTIONS

1. What is the difference between morals and values?

2. What is an ethical theory?

3. How do deontological and teleological ethical theories differ?

4. How are paternalism and the principle of autonomy in opposition to each other?

5. Is role fidelity the same thing as functioning within one's scope of practice? Explain.

6. What is meant by the balance of power between a health care professional and a client?

7. Explain the difference between a values history form and an advance directive.

8. How can palliative care provide an alternative for someone who is terminally ill and contemplating euthanasia or who is seeking physician-assisted suicide?

9. What is meant by the "allocation of health resources," and why does it present an ethical problem?

10. How would you define "personhood"?

DISCUSSION QUESTIONS

1. In April 2009, a young Canadian couple removed their baby from life support in order to save another baby in the same hospital who was in dire need of a heart. The first baby was born with a brain malformation that prevented her from being able to breathe without a respirator and that was deemed "incompatible with life." The parents stated that they would take comfort knowing their daughter's organs would save the life of another child. Once off the respirator, however, the baby continued to breathe on her own, putting the heart donation on hold. Do you think that the parents acted ethically? Should a family be allowed to select an organ recipient? Should the family have made the decision to remove their baby from life support based solely on wanting to make her heart available to someone else? Does the principle of double effect apply here?

2. Recently, doctors have begun interviewing potential clients and "cherry-picking" those they want in their practices, often choosing younger, healthier individuals who will require less time, be easier to treat, and be less demanding. The Canadian Medical Association is currently reviewing this process. Do you think a client-selection process is moral or ethical? Support your view.

3. Review some of the videos of Sue Rodriguez as she struggled for the legal right to die. Taking into account your own views on euthanasia, would you support her request? Consider the principles of autonomy, beneficence, justice, and fidelity in justifying your decision.

4. Dr. Rogers was in the ER when a woman who was badly injured in a car accident was admitted. She was bleeding profusely; the health care team would have to act fast to save her life. Dr. Rogers ordered five units of blood. As Dr. Rogers started the IV, a student nurse who had been searching the woman's wallet for her name and a contact person said, "Dr. Rogers, her name is Berta Granger . . . and here is a Jehovah's Witness card that says no transfusions for any reason." Dr. Rogers shrugged. "Is there a next of kin?" "No," relayed the student nurse, "I don't see a contact." "I don't have time to wait," said Dr. Rogers. "Hang the first unit . . . and let's get this lady to the OR." The woman received 15 units of blood, and the doctors saved her life. She later sued the hospital.

Assuming that you were a member of that health care team, what would you have done? Did the doctor have the right to make the decision to give the woman the blood? Consider the client's rights,

DISCUSSION QUESTIONS

the principle of informed consent, the duty of the doctor and the nurses to preserve life, and the fact that the situation was an emergency (i.e., the client was unconscious and critically ill). Discuss your findings with another student or in small groups. When you have completed your discussions, read the article about *Malette v. Shulman et al.*, cited in Web Resources below. Compare the rationale you used to justify your decision with the thoughts outlined in the article.

5.   In 2009, the province of Quebec announced that the provincial health plan would cover the cost of three in vitro fertilization (IVF) treatments. The cost of one treatment ranges from $6000 to $10,000, and the success rate is limited (about 40%), with an average of three treatments needed before a woman becomes pregnant. Couples in Quebec also can claim 50% of the cost of subsequent treatments as a tax credit. Currently, Quebec is the only jurisdiction to provide such comprehensive coverage for IVF, although other jurisdictions are reviewing their policies on the issue.

a.   Do you think Canadians have a right (i.e., an entitlement) to IVF treatments at the expense of their provincial or territorial health plan if they are unable to conceive otherwise?

b.   Is infertility a medical condition? If so, would IVF be considered a "medically necessary" treatment option for people suffering from such a condition? In your discussion, consider the following: Jacob and his wife, Maja, are 36 and 34 years of age, respectively. They have tried unsuccessfully for five years to have children. Jacob was diagnosed with a low sperm count as a result of his long-term diabetes. Should their provincial or territorial government cover the cost of IVF? Why or why not? What if Jacob was 45 and Maja was 55 years of age?

WEB RESOURCES

Canadian Medical Association: Allocation of Health Resources
http://www.cma.ca/index.cfm/ci_id/53574/la_id/1.htms

Founded in 1867 and incorporated in 1909, the Canadian Medical Association (CMA) is a national, voluntary association of physicians advocating on behalf of its members and the public for access to high-quality health care. This Web page provides information about a values-based process for the allocation of health care resources.

Creating a Code of Ethics for Your Organization
http://www.ethicsweb.ca/codes/

This Web page provides in-depth information on codes of ethics, including reasons to have a code of ethics and samples of codes of ethics. It also provides links to relevant essays and speeches.

Sue Rodriguez and the Right-to-Die Debate
http://archives.cbc.ca/politics/rights_freedoms/topics/1135/

After losing in both the British Columbia Supreme Court and the Court of Appeal, Sue Rodriguez took her case to the Supreme Court of Canada, where she asked the judge to grant her the right to assisted suicide. In this video, Rodriguez's lawyer, Chris Considine, once again pleads Rodriguez's case.

Malette v. Shulman et al.
http://aix1.uottawa.ca/~srodgers/rtf/malette.rtf

This document describes the case of a Jehovah's Witness member who received blood against her will in Kirkland Lake, Ontario, in 1979. The case went to court, and the plaintiff was awarded damages against the physician for battery related to physical and emotional suffering.

WEB RESOURCES

"Compassionate Homicide": The Law and Robert Latimer

http://www.cbc.ca/news/background/latimer/

This article describes the case of Robert Latimer, who in 1993 killed his 12-year-old quadriplegic daughter because he could not bear to watch her suffer from a severe form of cerebral palsy. It looks at the rationales and controversies of the case and also provides a historical timeline.

Values History Form

http://myersandporter.com/14pg.html

The law firm Myers & Porter LLC has created this form to assist people in thinking about and documenting what is important to them about their health, with the goal of helping loved ones make health care decisions for them in the event that they are unable to make decisions for themselves.

ADDITIONAL RESOURCES

Edge, R.S., & Groves, J.R. (2005). *The ethics of health care: A guide to clinical practice* (3rd ed.). New York: Thomson Delmar Learning.

Purtilo, R. (2005). *Ethical dimensions in the health professions* (4th ed.). Philadelphia: W.B. Saunders.

REFERENCES

Alberta Health Services. (n.d.). *What is ethics?* Retrieved May 29, 2009, from http://www.capitalhealth.ca/HospitalsandHealthFacilities/Hospitals/UniversityofAlbertaHospital/AboutUs/ClinicalEthicsCommittee/What_Is_ethics.htm

Canadian Broadcasting Corporation. (2008, March 17). "Compassionate homicide": The law and Robert Latimer. *CBC News.* Retrieved May 29, 2009, from http://www.cbc.ca/news/background/latimer/

Canadian Charter of Rights and Freedoms (1982).

Canadian Medical Association. (1988). *Induced abortion.* CMA Policy. Retrieved May 29, 2009, from http://policybase.cma.ca/PolicyPDF/PD88-06.pdf

Flood, C., & Epps, T. (2002). *Can a patient's bill of rights address concerns about waiting lists.* A draft working paper, Health Law Group, Faculty of Law, University of Toronto. Retrieved May 29, 2009, from http://www.irpp.org/events/archive/oct01/flood.pdf

Gert, B. (2008). The definition of morality. *Stanford Encyclopedia of Philosophy.* Retrieved May 29, 2009, from http://plato.stanford.edu/entries/morality-definition/

Legislative Assembly of New Brunswick. (2003). *Health Charter of Rights and Responsibilities Act.* Retrieved May 29, 2009, from http://www.gnb.ca/legis/bill/editform-e.asp?ID=208&legi=54&num=5

N.B. v. Hôtel-Dieu de Québec, Q.J. No. 1 (1992).

Online Ethics Center for Engineering. (2006). Chapter 2: What is ethics? *Section I—A guide to teaching the ethical dimensions of science.* Retrieved May 29, 2009, from http://onlineethics.org/CMS/edu/precol/scienceclass/sectone/chapt2.aspx

Rodriguez v. British Columbia (Attorney General), 3 S.C.R. 519 (1993).

Sheldon Chumir Foundation for Ethics in Leadership. (n.d.). *What is ethics?* Retrieved May 29, 2009, from http://www.chumirethicsfoundation.ca/main/page.php?page_id=19

Verkerk, M. (1999). A care perspective on coercion and autonomy. *Bioethics, 13,* 358–368.

Current Issues and Future Trends in Health Care in Canada

Learning Outcomes

1. Detail the main health care problems facing Canadians today.

2. Discuss the state of mental health and mental health services in Canada.

3. Summarize the reasons for Canada's aging population.

4. Detail the impact of an aging population on health care.

5. Discuss how Canada is dealing with the current shortage of human health resources.

6. Explain the problems facing home care services in Canada.

7. Summarize the main barriers to accessing health care services.

8. Identify the five major services that Canadians wait the longest to access.

9. Understand the impact electronic health records will have on health care.

10. Discuss measures underway to implement electronic health records across Canada.

11. Discuss future initiatives for the health care system.

KEY TERMS

Disease burden, p. 364

Electronic health record
(EHR), p. 398

Electronic medical record
(EMR), p. 398

Forensic psychiatric
hospitals, p. 369

Interoperable EHR, p. 400

Orphan patient, p. 379

Reserve, p. 395

Consider the following stories. What do they suggest to you about the current state of health care in Canada?

> *Homeless and mentally ill, Lucy often does not take her medications, causing her to be in and out of psychotic episodes. She has no doctor and little support, and, most days, she appears incapable of making any effort to help herself. She wanders from shelter to shelter. When out of money, she sometimes sits in front of a store begging. Other times, she wanders aimlessly, unaware of who or where she is. Provinces and territories often have no coordinated plan of care to deal with Lucy and others like her.*
>
> *Experiencing chest pain, Helga went to an emergency room (ER). She waited two hours to be seen, despite being triaged as urgent. She had a cardiac arrest and died 10 minutes after being admitted to an examination room.*
>
> *At 78 years of age, Merle has congestive heart failure, debilitating osteoarthritis, hypertension, diabetes, and chronic pain. She requires home care but qualifies for only two hours per day and needs more.*
>
> *Hakeem, a new immigrant to Canada, is 23, works part-time, and needs medication for asthma. He has no drug plan and does not qualify for provincial drug coverage, so most of the time, he goes without his medication. As well, he has no family doctor despite trying for a year to get one.*
>
> *Nigel needed a hip replacement. Thirteen months passed from the time his family doctor made an appointment with the orthopedic surgeon until the time Nigel had his surgery. By that point, he had had to stop working, had gone on disability, and had become addicted to painkillers.*

These stories illustrate the major issues facing the Canadian health care system:

- Care for mentally ill people is underfunded and often poorly coordinated. The enduring stigma attached to mental illness often results in discrimination against those affected.

- Access to emergency services remains inadequate, resulting in long waits with sometimes fatal results.

- Home care remains underfunded—many Canadians cannot pay for the services they need; many others cannot get the services they need because of lack of availability.

- Thousands of Canadians have no drug benefits, do not qualify for government assistance, and cannot afford to buy the drugs they need.

- Human health resources are in short supply.

- Core services, such as elective hip replacements, have long wait times, although a person who breaks a hip usually has surgery within 48 hours.

Despite numerous positive things about Canadian health care, many would say our health care system itself requires emergency care. Health care in Canada is in transition, struggling to adapt to changing demographics and changing economic realities. It is also striving to overcome a number of problems caused by erroneous predictions and poor planning.

Two major reports evaluating the issues in Canada's health care system—the Romanow Report (*Building on Values: The Future of Health Care in Canada*) and the Kirby Report (*The Health of Canadians—The Federal Role*)—identified the problems illustrated in the stories above and concluded that the most significant issue facing the health care system was underfunding, causing far-reaching problems. These reports are addressed further in Chapter 3.

This chapter will discuss the current issues in health care, their probable causes, and the measures that have been taken to deal with them. It will also look at the establishment of electronic communication systems across Canada—both the benefits they will provide and the challenges they present.

MENTAL HEALTH

In Canada, mental health falls primarily under the jurisdiction of the provincial and territorial governments, which collaborate with Health Canada and the Public Health Agency of Canada to plan strategies and interventions aimed at caring for mentally ill people.

The Romanow Report described mental health as the "orphan child of health care" and called for sweeping changes to address and treat mental illness in Canada (Romanow, 2002). Mental health services are, in most regions, inadequately covered under provincial and territorial plans. Adding to this problem is an alarming shortage of psychiatrists, particularly in rural regions. Other health care professionals who provide counselling, support, and direction for people with emotional or mental illnesses operate, for the most part, outside of provincial and territorial health insurance plans. Although family doctors may provide counselling or psychotherapy that is funded by provincial and territorial health plans, most jurisdictions limit the number of counselling hours physicians can charge the province or territory for. Furthermore, many family doctors, stretched to their limits handling physical complaints, choose not to offer counselling because of its time-consuming nature; many also believe significant mental health issues are best left to a specialist or other professionals trained in the field.

The number of mentally ill people in Canada is growing, with mental illness directly or indirectly affecting every Canadian. Roughly 20% of Canadians will experience mental illness at some point in their lives. An estimated 4000 Canadians commit suicide annually. Suicide rates among Canada's Aboriginal population are two to three times higher than the Canadian average, with youth rates even worse. The primary causes of hospitalization for mental illness include anxiety disorders, bipolar disorder, schizophrenia, major depression, personality disorders, eating disorders, and suicidal tendencies (Health Canada, 2002).

Disease burden
The impact of a health problem, measured by financial cost, mortality, morbidity, or other indicators.

By 2020, various forms of depression are expected to create the biggest **disease burden** in developed countries, including Canada (Kanchier, 2006; National Alliance on Mental Illness, 2009). Stressors such as hectic lifestyles and lack of leisure time contribute to this growing trend. Mental illness has become the fastest-growing category of disability insurance claims in Canada.

Until the mid-1960s, large psychiatric facilities managed the care of the mentally ill. Overcrowded, underfunded, and understaffed, these facilities offered questionable care. In the mid-1960s, a move to decentralize mental health care occurred, resulting in the closure of psychiatric institutions. Those who required institutionalized care were moved to smaller units in general hospitals; those deemed able to manage more independently were introduced into the community. The objective of this change was to provide mentally ill persons with more individualized care in an environment that would aid the progress toward independent living. However, community supports and services were never fully implemented. Many current initiatives remain poorly organized and underfunded and lack coordinated support and adequate numbers of properly trained health care professionals.

THE STIGMA OF MENTAL ILLNESS

Unfortunately, people with mental illnesses often do not have the understanding and support of those around them. Despite some progress over recent years, persons suffering from any form of mental illness are often avoided, snubbed, and treated differently from people with only physical complaints. Many falsely believe that sufferers of mental illness bear the fault for their illness because of an inability to cope. Others fear that the mentally ill present a danger. (While this may prove true in a few cases, such cases are the exception.) As a result of society's beliefs about and behaviour toward the mentally ill, those afflicted with mental illness rarely discuss it and sometimes hesitate to seek treatment. Some cultures actively hide mentally ill family members. Not many people admit to suffering depression; fewer still admit to taking medication for it. However, most people would have no qualms about saying, "Yes, I have pneumonia, and I'm taking antibiotics."

The Canadian government has made it a priority to educate the public about both mental illness and mental health. Change will take time, but, with a firm commitment by the various levels of government and a public willing to learn, attitudes will begin to shift.

Thinking It Through

Many Canadians are reluctant to admit to suffering from depression or another mental illness.

1. Would you be more likely to keep quiet about an emotional or mental illness than a physical disorder?

2. In your opinion, why does a stigma remain attached to mental illness?

HOMELESSNESS

A large number of homeless people in Canada suffer from mental illness, alcoholism, or drug addiction, or a combination of these afflictions. Gathering accurate figures about how many people are homeless in Canada remains a difficult task; however, estimates suggest that 10,000 people in Canada sleep on the street or in homeless shelters on any given night and that 35% of visits homeless people make to emergency departments are related to mental and behavioural disorders (Canadian Institute for Health Information [CIHI], 2007a). Street counts indicate that the number of homeless people has increased at an alarming rate (e.g., by 740% in Calgary and 235% in Vancouver between 1994 and 2006) (NationTalk, 2008). Homeless people report high stress levels, low self-esteem, and little or no social support. They also often experience depression, suicide attempts, and poor physical health. It is, however, hard to determine which comes first. Being homeless and living in poverty can result in depressive illnesses, which can lead to alcohol or substance abuse and evolve into even more serious mental health problems. At the same time, many individuals with diagnosed mental health problems, inadequate care, and little or no support end up homeless.

Individual communities bear most of the burden of looking after the homeless—some programs receive government funding; others rely entirely on volunteers. Vancouver, for instance, has a triage centre that offers numerous services (e.g., shelter, affordable housing, addiction and counselling referrals) to mentally incapacitated individuals who are homeless. The centre reports a 63% decrease in admissions to emergency shelters because of the services they provide (Canadian Broadcasting Corporation, 2007). Funding for this shelter comes in part from the federal government's National Homelessness Initiative.

Legal Issues

In some jurisdictions (e.g., Ontario), any encounter a person has with the police results in a police record, largely affecting people with mental illness. Police records differ from criminal records, which list an individual's convictions. A police record may contain information about something as harmless as a person's transfer to a hospital by the police—no charges need to be laid and no actual wrongdoing needs to occur. The release of a police record requires the written consent of the person involved, but he or she may be unaware of the information in the file. Prospective employers sometimes request a police check, which can prove problematic for the applicant. This practice is under investigation (Canadian Mental Health Association, n.d.b).

In 1997, 7% of male offenders entering the federal correctional system were diagnosed with a mental health problem. By 2007, this figure had jumped to over 12%. A similar rate of increase has been seen in women offenders. According to the Canadian Mental Health Association (n.d.a), the number of individuals with mental illnesses who interact with the justice system is increasing at a rate of 10% per year, primarily for more minor offences.

In 2009, Canada's public safety minister estimated that, overall, 20% of federal inmates, many incarcerated for nonviolent (i.e., less serious) crimes, such as disorderly conduct or trespassing, suffered from "significant" mental health problems (Brennan, 2009). The Canadian Mental Health Association (CMHA) (2005) suggests that this percentage directly relates to the lack of both treatment and community support, which would likely keep significant numbers of mentally ill people out of the penal system. Incarceration may provide inmates with a roof over their heads, but while incarcerated, mentally ill people receive only limited treatment, and, for the most part, correctional staff are not trained to recognize or deal with mental health disorders. Sadly, suicide remains the leading cause of death in Canada's correctional facilities (Canadian Mental Health Association, n.d.a) (In the News: The Consequences of Inadequate Mental Health Care in Prisons).

In the **News** The Consequences of Inadequate Mental Health Care in Prisons

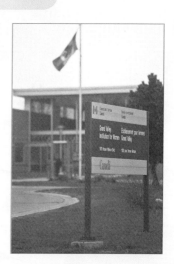

On October 19, 2007, 19-year-old Ashley Smith of New Brunswick was found unconscious in her segregation cell at the Grand Valley Institution for Women in Kitchener, Ontario, after attempting to strangle herself. She died in hospital shortly thereafter. Ashley's history showed that she had been involved with the court, correctional, and health care systems since she was 13 years old and had tried to harm herself on previous occasions. Reports revealed that despite her mental health issues, Ashley had not had a psychological assessment during her 11 and a half months in federal custody, nor had she had access to adequate mental health services. Guards watching Ashley trying to strangle herself had reportedly been instructed not to intervene as long as she was still breathing because these attempts were frequent—a decision that proved fatal. Reports that surfaced later showed that Ashley was scheduled for transfer to a psychiatric hospital, but no beds had become available. It was concluded that Ashley's death was both tragic and preventable and that it continued a "disturbing and well-documented pattern of deaths in custody" (Office of the Correctional Investigator, 2009).

Sources: Canadian Broadcasting Corporation. (2008, June 24). Death of Moncton girl preventable, prison ombudsman says. *CBC News*. Retrieved May 29, 2009, from http://www.prisonjustice. ca/starkravenarticles/ashley_smith_CI_0708.html; Office of the Correctional Investigator. (2009, March 3). Backgrounder: "A preventable death." Retrieved September 25, 2009, from http://www.oci-bec.gc.ca/rpt/oth-aut/oth-aut20080620info-eng.aspx; Brennan, R.J. (2009, March 7). Mental illness rife in prisons. *The Toronto Star*. Retrieved May 29, 2009, from http://mentalhealthfamilyguide.ca/news.php?id=70

Photo credit: THE CANADIAN PRESS/Geoff Robins.

In May 2009, the Alberta government opened 60 new mental health and addiction treatment beds in the southern and central regions of the province with the aims of improving health care services to Albertans with drug, alcohol, or mental problems and decreasing the frequency of mentally ill individuals' getting into trouble with the law. The province also transferred responsibility for treatment inside correctional facilities from the Department of the Solicitor General to Alberta Health and Wellness so that those with mental health or addiction problems can better receive proper health care (Canadian Broadcasting Corporation, 2009).

In 2009, the Canadian Mental Health Association began pushing for the development of a national mental health strategy to protect youth living with a mental illness in the criminal justice system. The CMHA will work with such organizations as the Mental Health Commission of Canada and the Correctional Service of Canada to make this become a reality (Canadian Mental Health Association, 2009).

EMPLOYMENT ISSUES

In general, individuals diagnosed with mental illnesses suffer higher levels of unemployment than do people without such diagnoses; those who are employed but do not receive proper treatment or do not respond well to treatment often work less productively. The economic impact resulting from lost time at work for mental health reasons is considerable. For example, lost productivity due to short- and long-term disability for mental health reasons and early death costs Canadian businesses and employees an estimated $8 billion per year (Here to Help, 2006).

A study done in Ontario (home to 37% of Canada's population) showed that 8.4% of the workforce experienced some type of work-related mental health problem (e.g., depression, anxiety disorders) over a 30-day period. The most affected groups include professionals, middle managers, and unskilled workers (Dewa et al., 2004). More than 30% of Canadians report that most days at work are stressful or very stressful (Statistics Canada, 2007). Some workplaces have taken steps to reduce occupational stress by providing support and preventive strategies, such as flexible working hours, work-at-home days, access to counselling, "sleep rooms," exercise facilities, and measures to improve job satisfaction.

Thinking It
Through

You are suffering from extreme stress and depression. Your family doctor has recommended that you take time off from work, which would mean that you would have to inform the company physician and the company nurse (who is both a friend of your family's and related to your boss) about the nature of your problem. Your alternative is to remain at work and to try to cope through counselling and medication. What would you do?

CURRENT SERVICES

Currently, mental health care is offered in tertiary care psychiatric hospitals, **forensic psychiatric hospitals** and clinics, community mental health centres, correctional facilities, adolescent assessment and treatment facilities, alcohol and drug treatment programs, and long-term care facilities. As well, in most jurisdictions, acute care hospitals offer mental health care to varying degrees, usually in a wing or a nursing unit devoted to that specialty, and often in secure units (units with controlled access and exits). As well, many acute care hospitals support psychiatric outpatient clinics.

In each province and territory, a mental health organization contributes significantly to the care of the mentally ill and provides public education about mental illness and mental health. These organizations depend heavily on a dedicated team of volunteers to deliver and maintain their community programs. As well, organizations such as the United Way fund some services for those unable to pay. However, many services remain accessible only to those who can afford them, leaving the most disadvantaged with little assistance.

Despite the system's problems, most believe that the move away from institutionalized care was a sound one. Evidence shows that with adequate funding, sufficient numbers of well-trained health care professionals, and community support, people with mental illness can achieve productive lives in the community setting. Mental health services, however, must remain available to those in need for their entire lifespans and have the flexibility to meet changing requirements. Acutely aware of the need to increase mental health services, the provinces and territories are currently implementing policies to improve access to and quality of sustainable care and services.

THE FUTURE OF MENTAL HEALTH

Out of the Shadows at Last, the final report resulting from Senator Michael Kirby and the Standing Senate Committee on Social Affairs, Science and Technology's investigation into the state of mental health services in Canada, made the following recommendations for renewing efforts to improve services for the mentally ill (Kirby & Keon, 2006, p. 6):

- Choice: Providing access to a wide range of publicly funded services and supports (e.g., assessment, counselling, support with decision making) that offer people living with mental illness the opportunity to choose those that will benefit them most.

- Community: Making mental health services and supports available in the communities where affected individuals live and providing clear direction (in terms of both location and scope) to the services offered.

Forensic psychiatric hospitals
Hospitals that serve individuals referred by the Canadian courts for treatment and assessment and that provide treatment and support for individuals requiring a secure inpatient facility due to their risk of harm to self and/or others.

- Integration: Ensuring seamless integration of services and supports across all levels of government and within communities, including both public and private initiatives and both professional and nonprofessional (e.g., volunteers) care providers.

The report recommended the creation of a Mental Health Transition Fund, through which the federal government would provide continual funding to provincial governments to support community-based mental health services. As well, the report advised that $2.25 billion over 10 years go toward addressing the problem of housing shortages for the mentally ill. Senator Kirby also proposed that extra funding be delivered to the territories and Prince Edward Island to deal with concerns unique to remote and nonurban communities.

As well, the report endorsed the creation of the Mental Health Commission of Canada, a concept originally proposed by the Standing Senate Committee on Social Affairs, Science and Technology in November 2005. In March 2007, the federal government confirmed that it would provide funding for the commission, and that same year, the commission was formally established as a nonprofit corporation. All provinces and territories except Quebec supported its creation.

The commission wasted no time drawing up its agenda, creating clearly defined objectives, and implementing a 10-year plan to raise public awareness about mental illness and to promote a better understanding of mental illness among the general public. The commission aims to develop the following:

- An anti-stigma campaign—the Canadian Mental Health Association proposed that the commission specifically target population groups and organizations, first responders, police, and the mental health system itself (Mental Health Commission of Canada, 2007)
- A national strategy for mental health
- A knowledge exchange centre (Mental Health Commission of Canada, n.d.)

The commission acknowledged that developing a national strategy for mental health presents challenges. Services offered across the country are uneven, and opinions vary as to which strategies are best and how they should be implemented. Current political views and policies will have to undergo revision to ensure consistency, cohesiveness, and effectiveness.

To aid knowledge exchange, the commission proposes a formal environment in which organizations and other stakeholders across Canada can share information and best practices policies, strategize, and stay connected. Identifying those most in need of immediate support and medical care—at the top of the list, homeless mentally ill people—is a priority.

In February 2008, the federal government committed $110 million to the commission for research to help homeless people living with mental disorders. Five projects funded by the commission are underway in Vancouver, Winnipeg, Toronto, Montreal, and Moncton. These projects, diverse in nature but all focused on homelessness and mental health, aim to analyze and improve on changes made to mental health services as far back as the 1960s.

CANADA'S AGING POPULATION

In 2005, Canada ranked near the top among the G7 countries for its population's longevity; Japan placed first (Figure 10.1). In world ranking, however, Canada fell much lower on the scale—around tenth, coming behind such other countries as Sweden, Switzerland, and Australia. The small country of Andorra (near France) ranked at the top, with a longevity of 83.5 years.

Recent data for G7 countries indicate that Japan still has the highest life expectancy at birth (82 years), while the United States has the lowest (77.9 years).

Figure 10.1   Life Expectancy at Birth, G7 Countries, 2005 (years)

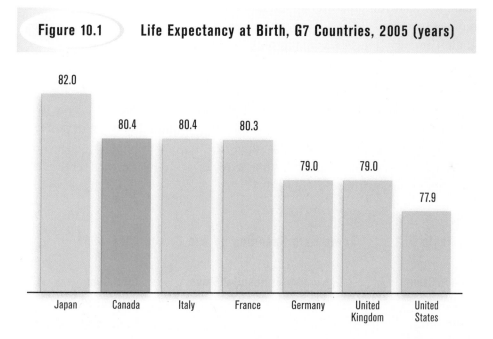

Sources: Life expectancy at birth from OECD Health Data, http://www.oecd.org/health/healthdata. Organisation for Economic Co-operation and Development (OECD). *OECD Health data 2007, Selected data. OECD Statistics.* Available from: http://www.oecd.org/statsportal/0,3352,en_2825_293564_1_1_1_1_,00.html [cited March 5, 2008]. Indicators of Well-being in Canada Web site. http://www4.hrsdc.gc.ca/h.4m.2@-eng.jsp. Human Resources and Skills Development Canada, 2008. Reproduced with the permission of the Minister of Public Works and Government Services Canada, 2008.

Canada has the second highest life expectancy at birth (80.4 years) (Human Resources and Skills Development Canada, 2009).

The high number of older Canadians affects almost every area of health care. According to Statistics Canada, as of July 1, 2008, the median age of Canada's population was 39.4 years. The report states that nearly one Canadian out of seven (13.7%) is aged 65 or over, and 16.8% of the population is 15 years of age or less. Estimates suggest that, by 2026, one in five Canadians will have reached age 65. Quebec, New Brunswick, Prince Edward Island, Nova Scotia, and Newfoundland and Labrador have an average age higher than the national average and also have the highest ratio of older residents (i.e., those over 65 years of age) in Canada. The median age in Newfoundland and Labrador is 42.5 years—the highest in the country. Newfoundland and Labrador also has the lowest proportion of youth (i.e., those under 15 years) in the country, at 15%. Manitoba, Alberta, and Saskatchewan boast the youngest median age, with the highest proportions of younger Canadians (averaging 19%). The median age of Alberta's population, 35.7 years, is notably the lowest in Canada; the province also lays claim to the lowest proportion of older Canadians (10.4%). Atlantic Canada has more older Canadians and a lower ratio of youth because of the high rate of migration among younger Canadians to the west (Statistics Canada, 2009).

Longevity and Birth Rates

Advances in medical science and clinical practice have resulted in people living longer—some with good health, but many others with multiple health problems requiring medical intervention and support. Contrary to popular belief, however, older adults are not the principle users of acute health care services and facilities, as demonstrated in Table 10.1.

Table 10.1   Acute Care Spending by Age Group, 2004–2005

Age Group	Number of Hospital Stays	Total Cost
75–85	342,358	$3,426,519,733
65–74	307,098	$3,005,007,974
45–64	495,034	$4,161,344,395
15–44	710,252	$3,396,307,083

Source: Canadian Institute for Health Information. (2008). *The cost of acute care hospital stays by medical condition in Canada, 2004–2005.* Ottawa: CIHI. Appendices D-4, D-5, D-6, D-7. Retrieved May 29, 2009, from http://secure.cihi.ca/cihiweb/products/nhex_acutecare07_e.pdf

Baby boomers comprise those born between 1945 and 1963. During those years, approximately 28 births happened in Canada per 1000 people. The boomer phenomenon set the stage for the large number of aging Canadians that we have today. By 1970, the birth rate had dropped to 17 births per 1000 (UNICEF, 2004).

In April 2004, Statistics Canada announced that the birth rate, as measured in 2002, had dropped to 10.5 live births for every 1000 people, the lowest since vital statistics began to be produced nationally in 1921. The rate represented a drop of 25.4% over the previous 10 years alone. Canada's population continues to grow, however. On April 1, 2008, the population was estimated at 33,223,800, up by 80,200 from January 1, 2008, an increase of 0.24%, marking the strongest first-quarter growth rate since 2002. Despite increases in birth rates and immigration, Canada still faces a dramatic rise in the number of older Canadians (Statistics Canada, 2008a).

IMMIGRATION AND CULTURE

Approximately one-quarter of Canada's older adult population was born outside Canada. These individuals remain more dependent on relatives than on the health care system. Because of cultural and religious beliefs, many immigrants try to care for their aged family members at home. For example, only 8% of the older Vietnamese Canadian population lives away from their families in contrast to 29% of the general older adult population (Statistics Canada, 2001). In 2009, Canada welcomed between 240,000 and 265,000 new immigrants, around the same number welcomed in 2008, although other countries, such as Australia and Great Britain, are decreasing their immigrant numbers (Citizenship and Immigration Canada, 2008). Accepting this many immigrants strengthens Canada's economy but has little effect on age-related demographics. Some have suggested trying to alter immigration patterns to change the demographics of an aging population; however, simulations have shown that whatever the benefits of immigration to Canada's economy, age filtering cannot relieve the country of the challenges of an aging population. The number of young immigrants accepted would have to be far too large to be even remotely practical. It is perhaps more important that Canadians be encouraged to save adequately for retirement and that government deliver both pensions and health care in an efficient and cost-saving manner.

ASSOCIATED CONCERNS

As Canadians retire, they take with them a vast amount of information, wisdom, and experience that guide workplace decisions. As well, having more retired Canadians means higher government spending for pensions. At the same time, concerns arise about how to sustain the health and wellness of our aging population while retaining the resources to care for the rest of the population.

Lower Taxation Base

Fewer working-age Canadians will result in a smaller workforce; with this comes a reduction in tax dollars for all levels of government. Although older Canadians have worked hard throughout their lives and contributed their fair share to the economy, as they retire, government taxation revenue will suffer significant reductions. This means the government will have less money to spend on health care and social programs, such as the old-age pension. Canada's younger population is rightfully concerned about what social benefits will remain for them when they retire.

Loss of a Skilled Workforce

Over the past 10 years, many Canadians have retired at an earlier age, and a large number of Canadians—roughly 3.8 million—are expected to retire over the next 5 to 10 years (Human Resources and Skills Development Canada, 2007). The exit of so many people from the workforce will affect all sectors of society including health care, where shortages of professionals, particularly doctors and nurses, have already incurred problems.

Physicians' Time

Caring for older adults requires special skills, time, and money. Although older adults do not appear to overuse physician time in terms of the number of visits, physicians state that an office visit from an older client takes more time than one from a younger person. Rarely do older adults have just one problem to be addressed. A person's main complaint may be joint pain or indigestion, but isolating and dealing with a single complaint is difficult. When multiple problems exist, the doctor usually has to address related complaints or several different ones during the same office visit, reducing his or her time for other clients in the practice. For this reason, younger doctors often interview prospective clients and try to "select" a healthy population base for their practice.

As discussed in Chapter 7, Canada is suffering an acute shortage of specialists to care for older Canadians (geriatricians). In 2008, an estimated 216 geriatricians were in place to care for approximately 4.3 million older Canadians, a ratio of 1 to 19,907. Although most jurisdictions are attempting to attract more physicians to this specialty, doing so is proving to be an uphill battle. Doctors are in short supply in general, and geriatrics does not boast a wide appeal. The fact that compensation for geriatricians typically falls below that for physicians in other specialties does not help.

To address the problem, primary care physicians could be provided with more training in geriatrics, and more clinics dedicated to caring for older adults could be introduced. Primary health care reform initiatives already in place (e.g., a team approach to care) may also prove helpful. For example, a dietitian could teach an individual how to manage high cholesterol levels; a pharmacist could provide advice about a person's multiple medications; and a social worker could provide support for socioeconomic problems (Steed, 2008).

Acute Care Hospital Beds

An aging population means that more individuals require extended care, which typically takes place in a long-term care facility or at home with the aid of home care services. Older individuals admitted to hospital frequently find that because of their medical condition, they cannot return home and live independently. Hospital beds are thus often occupied by individuals not requiring active treatment. The issue of finding space and providing care to individuals in transition between the hospital and a nursing home is ongoing.

According to a recent Canadian Institute for Health Information (CIHI) report, in 2007–8, with the exception of Quebec, Canadians over the age of 75 occupied 35% of acute care beds. Of these individuals, 85% entered the hospital through the emergency department from long-term care facilities. Conditions typically associated with advanced years (e.g., cardio-respiratory problems, circulatory problems, and trauma) accounted for most of these admissions. Other older Canadians were admitted to acute care beds from home and were waiting for admission to alternative care facilities such as nursing homes. Although most jurisdictions have made improvements in the availability of long-term care or alternative care beds, a shortage remains, which, in turn, contributes to the shortage of acute care beds and backups in emergency rooms, where people requiring acute-level care must wait for admission (CIHI, 2008b). Older Canadians unnecessarily occupying acute care beds are sometimes referred to as "bed blockers" (Steed, 2008).

The Cost of Medical and Surgical Intervention

Meeting the health care needs of older adults is often expensive. Canadians are living longer with multiple health problems requiring medical intervention, surgery, or both. Those admitted to hospital tend to stay longer than do younger clients, often occupying acute care beds while waiting for space in long-term care facilities.

PREDICTIONS FOR THE FUTURE

Concerns about the burden of an older population may be blown out of proportion. According to Morris Barer, a health economist at the University of British

Columbia, the aging of the population will occur on a relatively gradual slope, causing less of an impact than most people predict (Canadian Health Services Research Foundation, 2001).

Other issues confronting the health care system, such as the shortage of health care professionals and the lack of finances, are more acute. Careful planning now (e.g., implementing team-based strategies to manage those with chronic diseases and disabilities associated with aging) can ease the situation.

Thinking It Through

Popular belief suggests that Canada's increasing percentage of seniors puts a burden on society, including the health care system.

Do you share this belief? Why or why not?

HUMAN HEALTH RESOURCES

Human health resources include everyone working in the health care field, and, unfortunately, shortages in human health resources exist in almost all areas of health care—from doctors and nurses to dentists, laboratory technologists, physiotherapists, diagnostic test technicians, psychologists, chiropractors, and midwives. (See Web Resources at the end of this chapter for a link to view Health Canada reports on human health resource strategies.)

SHORTAGE OF NURSES

In the late 1980s and early 1990s, funding constraints resulted in numerous cutbacks in health care services. Some hospitals closed beds, while other hospitals just closed. Still other hospitals downsized by decreasing services and merging with other facilities, resulting in fewer jobs for nurses. Hospitals cut nursing positions and imposed hiring freezes. In response, colleges and universities decreased their enrolment in nursing programs. Nurses who did graduate often moved out-of-country or went on to practise other professions, as did nurses who had lost their jobs due to downsizing. The uninviting job market made it difficult for universities and colleges to fill the limited seats in nursing programs.

When the looming nursing shortage became apparent, nursing schools increased the number of seats they offered to students. By the year 2000, because jobs for nurses were opening up again, an interest in nursing resurfaced, as evidenced by increased applications to nursing programs at both the college and university levels. Application numbers have remained steady since. Most jurisdictions have developed their own strategies both to recruit new nurses and to encourage existing nurses to stay in the profession. According to Lunau (2008), the average age of Canada's nurses is 45, with many looking to retire within the next 10 years, meaning that the provinces and territories must continue efforts to recruit nurses at all levels.

To help address the current nursing shortage, governments across Canada have invested millions of dollars in nursing programs at colleges and universities. As well, some provinces (e.g., British Columbia and Ontario) have implemented condensed programs to "fast-track" the graduation of nurses prepared at the degree level.

Working Conditions

Many nurses working in the field continue to encounter stressful work situations, long hours, and tremendous levels of responsibility. Today's clients are often older and sicker and require more time because of their complex care needs. For the nurses, this means they must prioritize and give only essential care.

Providing clients with the type and quality of care that they require is sometimes difficult, and, because of a heavy workload and the need to prioritize, nurses often go home at the end of a shift feeling as though they did not achieve the best care for all of their clients. The constant stress that results, coupled with the level of responsibility of nurses, contributes to burnout. A large number of nurses (7 out of 10) leave their jobs every year for one of the following reasons: retirement, lack of respect and support, and the physical and psychological demands of the job (CIHI, 2008c; Health Canada, 2007b).

Contract and Part-Time Positions

Since the early 2000s, the job market for nurses has improved dramatically. In fact, most hospitals cannot fill all of their available nursing positions, to the point that, at times, beds must be closed and surgeries cancelled because of insufficient numbers of nurses.

In Canada, only 55% of nurses work full-time. The other 45% are hired on a contract basis or work part-time, sometimes for two or more employers. This latter situation causes stress because of the lack of security, benefits (often), and workplace stability. Although nurses who work part-time often get full-time hours, this situation, too, produces stress. Unpredictable working schedules make planning non–work-related activities (e.g., with family or friends) almost impossible. Many nurses who work in "casual" positions, for example, are repeatedly called into work at odd hours and during their days off (Lunau, 2008). The hours remain long, the work intense, and the responsibility sometimes overwhelming. Many nurses simply choose not to work under these conditions.

An Aging Workforce

As in many professions, the average age of nurses continues to rise; currently, the largest group of nurses has reached retirement age. In 2007, the average age of Canadian registered nurses was 45.1 years, and nearly one-quarter of practising nurses had surpassed the age of 50 (CIHI, 2008a). The number of nurses graduating is not keeping up with the number retiring. Some jurisdictions offer older nurses incentives to stay in the workforce, such as select positions and reduced hours, with limited success.

STRATEGIES TO INCREASE NURSING SKILLS

Over the past several years, changes have been made to nursing education, and strategies have been implemented to meet the increasing and varied demands for skilled nursing services. These changes have resulted in nurses possessing a mix of skills and competencies.

Bachelor Degree Initiatives

All jurisdictions across Canada have eliminated (or are in the process of eliminating) diploma programs for registered nurses in favour of degree programs; graduates receive a bachelor of science in nursing (BScN). Alberta's RN diploma programs will be phased out in 2010. Programs in Quebec, the Northwest Territories, and Nunavut are currently in transition.

Nurses' being prepared at the degree (or baccalaureate) level fulfills a long-standing commitment by the Canadian Nurses Association to have a degree as the minimum criteria for entry to practice for the registered nurse. Perceived advantages of requiring registered nurses to be educated at the degree level include making nursing more attractive to potential students and improving the knowledge base of graduates—in turn, enhancing the quality of care.

Licensed Practical Nurses

Licensed practical nurses (LPNs) are closing the gap left by the diploma-prepared RN. Educational programs for LPNs, personal support workers, and the equivalent have been lengthened in most jurisdictions to prepare people entering these professions to assume a broader scope of practice, including much of the responsibility formerly assumed by diploma-prepared registered nurses. For example, LPNs (called *registered practical nurses* in Ontario) give medications, assume charge positions, look after IVs, and do dressings.

Advanced Educational Opportunities

Nurses can now advance to other levels within their profession, becoming nurse practitioners or qualifying for other designations. Other classes of nurses in the extended class (i.e., those with advanced skills) are also recognized—for example, clinical specialist radiation therapist, anaesthesia assistant, and surgical first assist. In Quebec, the scope of practice of specialized registered nurses allows them to monitor clients with chronic diseases, adjust medications, and order diagnostic tests. It is hoped that these measures will address gaps in the health care continuum, particularly related to physician shortages.

Strategies have also been undertaken to allow foreign graduates entry to practice. Many facilities are using a prior learning assessment tool to assess the competencies of internationally trained nurses. (Such strategies are in the works for other health-related disciplines also.)

Physician Assistants

Newcomers to the health care field, physician assistants receive training through degree programs, offered, for example, at the University of Manitoba and McMaster University (Hamilton, Ontario). The first set of graduates in this field will emerge in 2010. The university programs include clinical rotations, allowing students to apply the skills learned in class.

Nursing associations question the role of the physician assistant as it compares with that of the nurse practitioner; however, it is hoped that the two roles will complement one another and work together to ease the burden of care for physicians, thus helping to lessen the impact of Canada's physician shortage.

SHORTAGE OF DOCTORS

In 2007, 4.8 million Canadians were without a family doctor (Statistics Canada, 2008b)—marking a dramatic increase from the 1.2 million Canadians without a doctor in 2003 (Statistics Canada, 2004). The number of **orphan patients** continues to rise. The doctor shortage has affected every aspect of health care and all specialties—from family medicine to pathology.

Orphan patient
A person without a family doctor.

Why the Shortage?

In the early 1990s, stakeholders and health care policy advisors in both the federal and provincial and territorial levels of government determined that Canada had too many practising physicians in relation to the national population growth. To address this trend, the federal government commissioned the Barer-Stoddard Report, whose results were released in 1991. As well as looking at the physician supply, the report studied the causes of accelerating health care costs and made recommendations to deal with increasing health expenditures. The report claimed that an excess of human health resources (most notably, doctors) usurped a huge chunk of the health care budget. Consequently, the report recommended a decrease in the number of doctors graduating from Canada's medical schools and a limit to the number of foreign physicians allowed to practise in the country.

In 1993, medical schools across the country began to decrease enrolment by 10% to 20%. Some universities decreased enrolment abruptly, while others, including schools in Alberta and Quebec, phased in the decrease. This reduction in seats remained in effect for the next 10 years.

Steps were also taken to restrict the number of foreign doctors practising in the country. International physicians were given no guarantee of acceptance into medical practice if they immigrated to Canada. As well, fewer foreign medical students received visas to complete training in Canada.

Another measure resulted in older physicians being offered retirement incentives and included a proposal to "buy" practices. Although this approach had little impact, interestingly, in 1997, British Columbia initiated a failed attempt to implement a mandatory retirement age of 75 for doctors. (By that age, most physicians retire without coercion!) Most jurisdictions across Canada have since passed legislation ending mandatory retirement, although many provinces and territories introduced provisions to allow mandatory retirement for jobs in which physical ability plays a significant role, such as firefighting and police work.

Women in Medicine

The proportion of women accepted into medical schools increased from 13% in 1981 to nearly 60% in 2008, with the majority choosing to practise family medicine (CanWest News Service, 2008; Gulli & Lunau, 2008). Of doctors under the age of 35, 52% are women. Estimates suggest that, by 2015, 40% of doctors will be female.

Female physicians typically cease practising medicine for periods to have children and to spend time with their families. Those who return to their practice often choose to do so on a part-time basis. Although they have a right to do this, the fact remains that this trend affects the number of hours physicians are available to see patients.

Thinking It Through

Medical schools across Canada have admitted increasing numbers of women. Many female physicians want to have families and to spend time with them, meaning that they must reduce their workload, their hours, or both.

1. Do you think female physicians have a right to work fewer hours or to take on a smaller client load?

2. Should medical schools seek a more even balance in the male-to-female ratio?

Lifestyle Changes

Younger physicians of both genders—in family medicine as well as in other spe-cialties—are less apt to put in the hours that older doctors do. They often seek a more balanced lifestyle—most want regular hours, little or no on-call hours, a reasonable number of free weekends, and time to enjoy life. This makes sense, but it also affects physician availability.

The implementation of primary health care reform models has bridged this issue somewhat. A team approach to health care, after-hours clinics, and Tele-health advice lines have helped doctors keep more reasonable hours.

Decline in the Number of Physicians Choosing Family Medicine

A majority of medical graduates are choosing to enter specialties outside of family medicine for several reasons, including insufficient exposure to family medicine in medical school and changes to the old system of rotating intern-ship that enabled a new graduate to practise family medicine immediately after completing an internship. Practising family medicine now requires a postgradu-ate education. As well, many doctors perceive family medicine to be harder work requiring longer hours for less money. Rural and northern regions of the country suffer most from doctor shortages. Few physicians choose to practise in northern or rural areas, preferring urban settings. Figure 10.2 shows that, in 2006, almost a third more family or general practice physicians practised in urban rather than in rural Canada. (Manitoba was the only province with more rural than urban general practitioners.)

Aging Doctors

In 2007, the average age of all doctors was just over 49 years; for general practi-tioners, it was 50.5 years. According to an article by Shelley Martin, the average age that Canadian physicians plan to retire at is 63 years. She notes, however, distinct differences among demographic groups. Female physicians, for example, tend to aim to retire earlier than their male colleagues (i.e., at age 60 versus age 64) (Martin, 2000).

Acutely aware of the impact that large numbers of retiring doctors will have on Canadians, some older physicians attempt to reduce their client load rather than retiring. One doctor held a lottery to identify which 800 clients he would discharge from his practice, feeling that was the only fair way to do it (CIHI, 2007b). The retirement of just one general practitioner may well leave upward of 2000 patients without a family doctor (Canadian Broadcasting Corporation, 2005).

It is difficult—sometimes impossible—for retiring physicians to find some-one to assume their practice. Many family doctors continue working, caught between wanting to retire and not wanting to abandon their patients. For

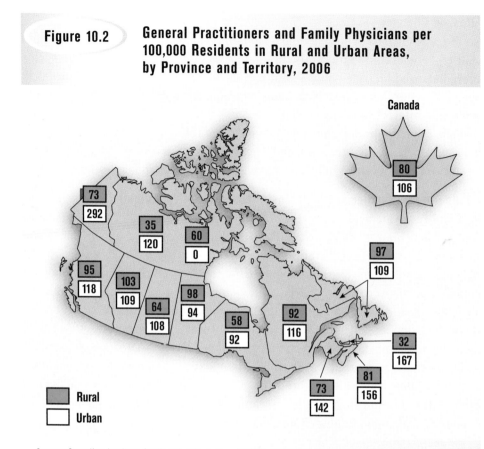

Figure 10.2   **General Practitioners and Family Physicians per 100,000 Residents in Rural and Urban Areas, by Province and Territory, 2006**

Source: Canadian Institute for Health Information. (2008). *Health care in Canada 2008*. Ottawa: Author, p. 17. Retrieved October 29, 2009 from http://secure.cihi.ca/cihiweb/products/HCIC_2008_e.pdf

example, Dr. Douglas Thompson, a family physician who has practised for 33 years in Stratford, Ontario, states that it would be "morally and ethically against [his] principles to walk away, leaving [his] patients without a physician" (D. Thompson, personal communication).

The 2008 downturn in the economy contributed to many physicians' choosing to continue to practise, as they wait for their investment portfolios to bounce back so that they can be assured financially stability once they do retire.

Impact of the Shortage

A physician shortage affects access to care as well as quality of care. To illustrate, consider the effect of Canada's shortage of pathologists (specialists who study tissue). Estimates suggest Canada requires another 200 to 500 specialists in this field; however, only about 30 new pathologists graduate from Canadian medical schools each year (Weeks & Leeder, 2008). Of Canada's 32,000 specialist physicians, just more than 1000 practise as pathologists (Weeks & Leeder, 2008). A shortage of these specialists—combined with financial cutbacks, new and complex diagnostic techniques, poorly trained technicians, and inadequate staffing—has contributed to quality-control issues in laboratories across the country, resulting in numerous cases of misdiagnosis, sometimes with deadly results.

In the **News**   **The Consequences of Misdiagnosis**

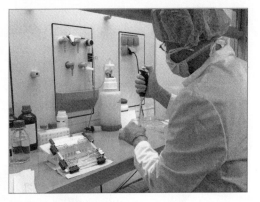

In March 2008, it was discovered that nearly 400 women with breast cancer had received inaccurate test results at Newfoundland and Labrador's main medical laboratory over an eight-year period. More than 40% of 763 samples of breast cancer tumours taken from living clients had been mistakenly identified as hormone-receptor negative, resulting in misdiagnoses, inappropriate treatments, or lack of treatment, and the deaths of more than 100 women.

Testing a client's hormone-receptor status provides an oncologist with valuable information regarding the type of treatment a cancer client should receive. Problems with the testing at this laboratory were first identified in the spring of 2005, when doctors questioned the hormone-receptor test results of a client who had an invasive form of lobular breast cancer. The woman, who originally tested negative, was retested and found to be positive. In a report released in March 2009, the justice minister noted, "the whole of the health system, to varying degrees, can be said to have failed the ER/PR [estrogen receptor/progesterone receptor] patients." According to a CBC News report, investigations released early in 2008 cited staff incompetence, poor quality control, imperfect procedures, and a general negligence in keeping up with the evolution of this subspecialty of pathology.

The justice minister delivered 60 recommendations, including more training and ongoing education for technologists, clinicians, and other health care professionals and more accurate and efficient record keeping and external reporting.

Source: Canadian Broadcasting Company. (2008, April 28). Cancer misdiagnosed. Anatomy of Newfoundland's cancer-testing scandal. *CBC News.* Retrieved May 29, 2009, from http://www.cbc.ca/news/background/cancer/misdiagnosed.html

Photo credit: © iStockphoto.com/thelinke.

Strategies for the Future

Increased Enrolment in Medical Schools

Medical schools have increased enrolment, but Canadians will not see the effects for several years. As well, jurisdictions across Canada have implemented strategies to attract more foreign-trained physicians and to speed up the eligibility process for them to practise medicine in Canada.

A recent measure attempts to draw individuals from underserviced areas into medicine in the hopes that they will return to their communities to practise. High schools now offer programs to stimulate interest in medicine, and universities offer prospective students the opportunity to study medicine close to where they live. For example, the Northern Ontario School of Medicine—a joint venture between Lakehead University and Laurentian University—has recently opened in Ontario, with a curriculum focused on medical care in northern communities. Much of the learning occurs in smaller communities throughout Northern Ontario using electronic linkage.

In 2009, the Ontario government funded an additional 100 seats in medical schools at five universities, to be phased in over a three-year period. In 2002, the British Columbia government announced an investment of $134 million to expand facilities and add new seats for medical students at the University of British Columbia (UBC). UBC's medical school now accepts 256 students annually and provides training at more than 80 health care facilities throughout the province, allowing medical students to receive their education closer to where they live (BC Liberals, 2008).

Promoting Family Medicine

Provinces and territories have created incentive packages to attract medical graduates to family medicine and to make it worth their while to practise—at least initially—in underserviced areas.

Primary health care reform has helped to change practice settings and to encourage new graduates to look twice at family medicine. The team approach to client care enables physicians to share the workload and makes a balanced lifestyle possible. As well, many primary health care reform groups offer practising physicians more vacation time—sometimes six weeks or more—since other physicians are available to look after the clients of those on holidays. These clinics are managed by physicians on a rotating basis. Over 60% of doctors currently work in group practice (National Physician Survey, 2007).

Help for Northern and Rural Communities

Attracting doctors to northern and rural areas remains a challenge. Telehealth, which uses communication and information technology to deliver health care services over long distances, has eased the situation somewhat. (See Chapter 7 for more information about Telehealth.)

Although many rural and northern communities are underserviced, other areas lack physicians as well. Communities of varying sizes across Canada are doing what they can to attract doctors, especially new graduates. Sometimes communities bid against each other for doctors, organizing workshops and incentive weekends with free accommodation, tours around the community, gala dinners, and other activities to woo physicians. Some even offer physicians considerable amounts of money and a moving allowance to settle in a community. Most offer turnkey operations—practices complete with clients, electronic medical records systems, and administrative and nursing staff. Many of these practices operate under the umbrella of a primary health care reform group.

Current Situation

Slowly, the number of physicians in Canada is increasing. The number of general practitioners grew by almost 6% between 2002 and 2006, while the number of specialists grew a modest 4% (National Physician Survey, 2007). Despite these increases, a shortage remains. Canadians without doctors are making do with visits to walk-in clinics, urgent care clinics, and emergency rooms. Some jurisdictions have introduced special clinics for designated groups needing health care, such as pregnant women. The women will receive routine care and then be referred, when timely, to an obstetrician. Frequently, a family doctor will then assume care for the family.

Thinking It Through

A significant number of foreign-trained physicians live in Canada but are unqualified to practise medicine here. The process to obtain a licence to practise in Canada is gruelling and lengthy but is currently under review. Some support making the process to obtain a licence less demanding and lowering the standards to speed up the process. What do you think about this idea?

HOME AND CONTINUING CARE

Home care includes a variety of services provided both at home and in the community. Continuing care provides similar services to individuals discharged from hospital but who nevertheless require support, usually only for a short term. Home care services are categorized as either professional (e.g., nursing care, physiotherapy, speech therapy, social services) or nonprofessional (e.g., house-work, meal preparation, personal care, shopping). For the most part, home care includes health promotion and health teaching, curative and restorative care, supportive, palliative, and rehabilitation services, and support for caregivers. Although the majority of individuals using home care are over the age of 65, people of any age may receive home care services. Home care clients include people who are discharged early from hospital; those with chronic conditions who are not sick enough to remain in an institution or hospital but who cannot manage independently; and those who, because of age or a disability, cannot manage to live independently but can get by with a little help. Home care has also become a viable option for persons wishing to die at home.

Although the provision of home care is not mandated under the *Canada Health Act*, with the 2004 Accord, all levels of government agreed to certain principles, including two weeks of coverage for acute care patients discharged from hospital (e.g., pain control, IV therapy, dressing checks/changes); two weeks of community care for people with acute mental illness; and palliative care. Outside of these principles, home care services, fees, and co-payments vary across the country since no national standards exist for home care.

Currently, fulfilling home care services needs across Canada presents challenges, in part due to a lack of human resources. The type and extent of services a client receives are based on an assessment of his or her needs. For the most part, basic needs can be met, but clients who feel they require additional help may purchase additional services (if available). However, the shortage of trained individuals to provide home care services and the cost of these services sometimes present barriers to care. As the demand for home care services increases, providing adequate services will become even more of a challenge. According to the Canadian Home Care Association (CHCA), the use of home care services increased a startling 51% between 1997 and 2007. In 2008–9 alone, an estimated 1 million Canadians received home care services. The CHCA predicts that the number of older Canadians with chronic conditions who require home care will increase by 33% by 2017 (Canadian Home Care Association, 2008).

Growing numbers of private, for-profit organizations offer home care services. We Care, one of the largest, with branches across Canada, offers nursing, personal support, homemaking, cleaning, and companionship services 24 hours a day, 7 days a week.

How vital is home care? Home care is recognized as a critical component of primary health care, particularly considering the emphasis the Canadian health care system now places on community- and home-based care. The current philosophy holds that individuals can receive better and more cost-effective care at home. As well, people cared for in the home appear to recover faster and are less likely to acquire an institution-based infection. For the future, the CHCA maintains that

> *Without additional investment, the home care sector will not be able to meet the needs of our aging population with chronic conditions. This deficit will result in seniors accessing health care in more expensive facility-based care or increased visits to emergency departments. The costs of providing care will rise, the choice and independence of seniors will be limited and the future of the health care system will be jeopardized. (Canadian Home Care Association, 2008)*

THE PROBLEMS

With a population living longer and more people coping with chronic diseases, the demand for home care is growing at an alarming rate. Yet, many home services remain outside of provincial or territorial health plan coverage. For example, many people require assistance with housekeeping or household maintenance—items not covered by insured services. Other concerns regarding home care include poor coordination of services, insufficient human resources, inconsistent care, and poor-quality care. These concerns vary from community to community, as well as among jurisdictions across the country.

FUNDING

Even though home care services are not mandated by the *Canada Health Act*, provincial and territorial governments, and sometimes municipal governments, provide funding for home care. Most jurisdictions will offer an individual home care up to a maximum dollar value per month or a stipulated number of hours per week. Since no one is denied care, those with limited incomes can usually receive further government funding.

As mentioned earlier, because they are not mandated under the *Canada Health Act*, home care services vary considerably from one jurisdiction to another in terms of access, services offered, and delivery. In Canada, home care is provided by a mix of public (i.e., government), for-profit, and not-for-profit organizations. For example, Manitoba, Ontario, New Brunswick, and Prince Edward Island charge co-payments for certain services, whereas others are entirely covered (up to a predetermined limit). Home care programs in British Columbia, Nunavut, and the Northwest Territories impose no ceiling or limits on services. Alberta offers home care services based on client need, authorizing regional health authorities to perform the necessary assessments. In New Brunswick, too, the government covers costs based on need. Precisely how many hours of home care and which services are publicly funded vary widely across the country, as does the cost of services.

Public funding for home care, when available, is often based on a certain number of hours of care per client per week. As a rule, when an applicant registers for home care services, he or she undergoes a formal assessment to determine the number of hours of care the provincial or territorial plan will cover. Most often, the individual requires more hours than provincial or territorial insurance will pay for. To receive the extra time and services, clients must pay the full amount for some services and a co-payment for others. Home care, therefore, can be costly and out of reach for many Canadians, particularly for those requiring nonprofessional services, the cost of which, if not provided by volunteer organizations, is usually the care recipient's responsibility. Even some volunteer-dominated services (e.g., Meals on Wheels) come with a cost.

THE FUTURE

Organizations and stakeholders, including the Canadian Medical Association (CMA), have asked the federal government to expand Medicare to include home care. As an alternative to reopening the *Canada Health Act* (which is unlikely to happen), the CMA has proposed a *Canada Extended Health Services Act* to cover home care and other extended health services. Currently, the government has shown no serious consideration of this request.

Provincial and territorial governments are working toward extending funding for certain aspects of home care, including, for example, short-term home care services for individuals discharged from hospital and short-term community-based mental health care (including case management and critical response services).

In addition to—or in some cases, in place of—home care assistance, each year, 26% of Canadians provide care for a seriously ill friend or relative (Health Council of Canada, 2008a). Some jurisdictions have legislated a compassionate leave, which allows individuals to take time from their workplace to care for a loved one without fear of losing their job.

DRUG COVERAGE

THE PROBLEM

Prescription drugs compose the fastest growing health care cost, with some people taking more than 10 to 15 pills daily for a variety of conditions. The number of Canadians being prescribed drugs is increasing, but, unfortunately, a large portion of these people cannot pay for the medications they need. Since Canadians are surviving longer, often with several health problems, they tend to need more medications as they age.

FUNDING

The Romanow and Kirby reports (see Chapter 3) cite the lack of public drug coverage for Canadians as a major flaw in our health care system. All provinces and territories provide some coverage to low-income individuals, older adults, and people with overwhelming drug costs in relation to their income. As well, the federal government provides coverage for Aboriginal peoples. Drug formulary lists (see Chapter 5) help provincial and territorial governments to control the cost of publicly insured medications. (Drug coverage is discussed further in Chapter 6.)

Still, many Canadians carry no private drug insurance and suffer financial hardship when they need medications. Furthermore, some fall through the cracks in the public plans, resulting in no coverage at all.

THE FUTURE

Although the need for providing a national drug plan has been recognized, no immediate strategy has resulted. In the meantime, provinces and territories do their best to ensure that no one goes without the drugs they need and that no one endures significant financial hardship because of drug costs. A national and comprehensive drug program would cost the federal, territorial, and provincial governments hundreds of millions of dollars—more money than the system appears to have.

Thinking It **Through**

Calls for public health insurance plans to add comprehensive home care services and medications to insured services are increasing. However, these additions will cost enormous amounts of money that will compromise funding for other services.

1. Do you think funding home care services and prescription drugs is a good idea?

2. Can you see a workable compromise?

WAIT TIMES AND ACCESS TO MEDICAL CARE

Access to health care is not an issue exclusive to Canada. Americans, for example, experience similar access problems, but for different reasons. Access to health care in the United States is largely limited by clients' finances, while, in Canada, the problem stems mostly from long wait lists for select health care services.

The causes of these long waits vary across the country, although the following common themes exist in all jurisdictions:

- An increase in the number of people requiring services
- A shortage of human health resources
- Limited access to required diagnostic services
- Lack of coordination of services
- Limited access to operating rooms and operating time for surgeons, often because of hospital operating costs (e.g., hospitals may close operating rooms as a cost-saving measure)

Services that clients often have to wait for include gaining access to specialists; having diagnostic tests performed, especially magnetic resonance imaging (MRI) and computed axial tomography (CT) scans; visiting a general practitioner for routine medical care; and, in the case of disabled individuals, seeking help with daily routines. Aside from seeing a family doctor, the five major health care services Canadians have difficulty accessing in a reasonable period of time are:

1. Diagnostic imaging
2. Cancer treatment
3. Cardiac surgery
4. Eye surgery (particularly cataract)
5. Joint replacements

The length of time Canadians must wait for these services varies even among hospitals. Most provinces and territories host Web sites outlining the approximate wait for each service. Updated monthly, these Web sites inform individuals of their wait time and, in some cases, may suggest they seek the service elsewhere. In general, wait times range from 4 to 18 weeks, depending on the location and the service required. Table 10.2 provides an overview of reporting from provincial wait times Web sites.

In 2009, national suggested "acceptable" wait times for surgery ranged from 2 to 26 weeks, depending on the individual case. Surgery for high-risk

Table 10.2   Overview of Reporting From Provincial Wait Times Web Sites

Province	Wait Times Web Sites	Joint Replacement	Sight Restoration	Cardiac	Cancer	Diagnostic Imaging	Reporting Includes All Facilities
Newfoundland and Labrador	www.releases.gov.nl.ca/releases/2006/health/0822no1.htm	•	•	•	•		Yes
Prince Edward Island*	www.gov.pe.ca/index.php3?number=news&lang=E&newsnumber=4418	•	•		•	•	Yes
Nova Scotia	www.gov.ns.ca/health/waittimes/	•	•	•	•		Yes
New Brunswick	www1.gnb.ca/0217/surgicalwaittimes/index-e.aspx www.gnb.ca/0051/cancer/benchmarks-e.asp	•	•	•	•		Yes
Quebec†	www.msss.gouv.qc.ca/en/sujets/organisation/waiting_lists.html	•	•	•	•		Yes
Ontario‡	www.health.gov.on.ca/transformation/wait_times/wait_mn.html www.cancercare.on.ca/cms/One.aspx?portalId=1377&pageId=8836	•	•	•	•	•	No
Manitoba	www.gov.mb.ca/health/waitlist/index.html	•	•	•	•		Yes
Saskatchewan	www.sasksurgery.ca/wli-wait-list-info.htm www.saskcancer.ca	•	•	•	•		Yes
Alberta	www.ahw.gov.ab.ca/waitlist/WaitListPublicHome.jsp			•	•	•	No
British Columbia	www.healthservices.gov.bc.ca/waitlist/	•	•	•	•		Yes

* Prince Edward Island does not offer cardiac services; patients receive care out of province.

† Quebec does not monitor wait times but, rather, the percentage of procedures performed within recommended time frames.

‡ 82 hospital organizations (of the 150 in Ontario) report to the Wait Time Information System (WTIS); total surgical volume reported for cancer surgery, cataract surgery, and hip and knee replacement represents 65% of the total operating room surgical volume in the province.

Source: Canadian Institute for Health Information. (2009). *Wait times tables—A comparison by province, 2009* (Table 3, p. 5). Retrieved May 29, 2009, from http://secure.cihi.ca/cihiweb/products/wait_times_tables_aib_e.pdf

individuals should occur within 16 weeks; however, what constitutes "high risk" is subjective. No national benchmark time frame has been set for either MRI or CT scans, although Alberta, Ontario, and Prince Edward Island have developed their own wait times targets. See Web Resources at the end of this chapter for a link to view wait times for various procedures across the country.

ESTIMATING WAIT TIMES

Numerous, complex variables determine wait times. For example, if Paula needs a hip replacement, does her wait start when she makes an appointment with her family doctor, sees her family doctor, has her first visit to the specialist, or is booked for surgery?

Wait lists for services at hospitals vary for different reasons. Suppose the University of Alberta Hospital in Edmonton performed more emergency angioplasties than the Foothills Hospital in Calgary. The former hospital would, therefore, be unable to do as many nonurgent angioplasties.

IMPROVING WAIT TIMES

The federal government is leading and funding an initiative (at a cost of an estimated $4.5 billion) for the provinces and territories to establish "reasonable" guaranteed wait times by 2010. Each jurisdiction is working independently toward this goal.

The provinces and territories began by collaborating to produce what they term "benchmark" time frames for guaranteed maximum wait times. For example, a wait of no more than 4 weeks is considered reasonable for radiation therapy for cancer clients; 26 weeks for hip and knee replacements, with an exception made for emergencies such as hip fractures, for which the maximum wait is 48 hours (Case Example 10.1); and 16 weeks for cataract surgery for high-risk persons. Cardiac bypass surgery limits range from 2 to 26 weeks, depending on the client's condition (Health Canada, 2007a).

Case Example 10.1

John, age 82, is admitted to hospital through the ER, where he was diagnosed with a hip fracture resulting from a fall. The hospital must complete a hip replacement within a 48-hour time frame. John will be made comfortable until his surgery takes place.

Individual jurisdictions are prioritizing these services according to need and adjusting guaranteed wait times accordingly. For example, British Columbia, Alberta, Manitoba, New Brunswick, Nova Scotia, and Prince Edward Island have set as a priority access for cancer treatment—specifically, radiation therapy. Newfoundland and Labrador identified cardiac care as its priority; Quebec, joint replacements; the Northwest Territories, access to care; Nunavut, access to diagnostic imaging; and Yukon, access to mammography. With the exception of Manitoba, the target date for reducing wait times is 2010. (Manitoba met its goal by 2008.)

After determining the guaranteed wait times, each province and territory must provide clients with alternative treatment if the wait time guarantees are unmet. Case Example 10.2 illustrates this process.

It must be noted that people experiencing emergency or urgent medical situations are not subject to wait lists. Instead, with triage, they receive care as soon as possible. Across Canada, most Canadians report that when they urgently need care, they get it.

Case Example 10.2

Aisha, who lives in Alberta, has breast cancer. She was guaranteed a wait of no more than 8 weeks to begin receiving her radiation treatments. After 10 weeks without treatment, the Alberta government sought treatment for her in the United States and covered the cost.

IMPROVING EMERGENCY ROOM WAIT TIMES

Approximately 14 million Canadians use emergency room (ER) services annually. Lower-income Canadians and those in rural centres are most likely to use ER services. Males and females visit the ER with about the same frequency. Infants compose the age group seen most (Statistics Canada, 2008b).

Canadians accessing an ER should be prepared to wait from 2 to 12 hours to receive treatment, after which they will either be discharged or be admitted to hospital. The reasons for these waits include an uneducated public (i.e., people using the ER for nonessential reasons), a shortage of family doctors, fully booked family doctors or those with limited available hours, a shortage of ER staff, the closure or reduced services of emergency departments, and insufficient numbers of hospital beds.

Many Canadians view the ER as a reasonable place to seek after-hours health care. Some use the ER for convenience—for example, if their doctor's office is closed by the time they get off work, if they neglected to make an appointment, or if they did not want to take time away from work to see their doctor. Orphan patients may not know where else to turn, or they may not have reasonable geographic access to an walk-in or urgent care clinic. The number of clients (with and without family doctors) that clog the ER system for minor complaints such as colds, sore throats, rashes, headaches, and stomach aches remains overwhelming. Many do not realize how much money a visit to the ER costs the system compared with a visit to their family doctor. Others simply do not care.

The inability to access family doctors in a timely manner presents a real issue that results in increasing numbers of nonacute cases being seen in the ER. A person may phone for an appointment, only to be told he or she cannot be seen for several days. Whether the complaint is urgent or not, that person may decide to go to the ER to seek prompt attention. In most cases, however, family doctors will see a client the same day for anything considered urgent (or refer the client accordingly). Many family doctors are also trying to teach their clients not to use the ER as a convenience and not to seek care there for nonurgent conditions.

After-hours access to family doctors has improved across Canada with the implementation of primary health care reform groups. Most of these groups offer after-hours telephone advice as well as evening and Saturday clinics (some only for rostered clients). All jurisdictions have province- or territory-funded telephone access to health advice.

Physician shortages have forced many ERs to reduce services or, in some cases, to close outright. Usually, such situations are reversed as soon as staffing issues are resolved. To ease the problem, many ERs now hire nurse practitioners or physician assistants to see nonurgent cases.

One of the most effective measures for reducing ER wait times for individuals with more serious health problems has been assessing and triaging clients as soon as they arrive. Many hospitals have also created transitional care beds for people waiting for placement in long-term care facilities, thereby freeing up space for those who come into the ER with complex conditions that require extended care.

Triage

In the past, most clients in the ER got care on a first come, first served basis, barring a clear emergency. Today, clients are assessed for priority needs. As they register in an ER, a physician or other health care professional assesses them. Those arriving by ambulance often receive priority.

A standardized tool developed to triage clients, called the Canadian Triage and Acuity Scale, has increased assessment effectiveness. The scale standardizes the assessment of cases and provides the foundation for effective triage. Clients assessed at I or II on the scale are seen sooner than those assessed at III or IV.

Wait times in an ER vary widely. In general, clients visiting an ER of a larger hospital or a teaching hospital in an area with a high-density population have to wait longer than do individuals visiting an ER in an area of lower-density population.

Thinking It **Through**

You have an extremely sore throat and a bad cough. You think you might need an antibiotic. It is Friday morning, you have plans to go away for the weekend, and you work until 17:00—the time that your family doctor's office closes. What would you do?

ABORIGINAL HEALTH CARE

For the most part, the plight of the Aboriginal population, although serious, makes headlines only when a significant event occurs, such as drinking water contamination on a **reserve**, a rash of suicides within a community, or something draws sudden attention to substance abuse.

Reserve

Land set aside by the Crown for Aboriginal people to live on. Reserves came about through treaties signed in the 1800s and remain in existence today.

In June 2008, Statistics Canada released the first analysis of data on Aboriginal people from the 2006 census. It showed that Canada's Aboriginal people, who include First Nations, Inuit, and Métis, constitute a total population of approximately 1,172,790. The largest population gain was among the Métis for a total population number of 389,785; Canada's First Nations population (status and non-status) was reported at 698,025 (a 29% increase since 2006), and the Inuit population increased by 26% to 50,485. Eight of every 10 Aboriginal people live in Ontario, Manitoba, Saskatchewan, Alberta, or British Columbia. Just over 108,000 live in Quebec, mostly in the north. Most of the Métis population inhabits Western Canada; 70% of these individuals live in urban areas, with a large population in Winnipeg, Manitoba (Statistics Canada, 2006).

The federal government first became involved in the health care of Aboriginal people in the mid-1940s. Providing fair, high-quality health care to these populations presents several challenges, discussed below.

THE PROBLEMS

First Nations, Inuit, and Métis people suffer health problems that extend beyond those experienced by other Canadians. Injuries, suicide, diabetes, cardiovascular disease, and alcohol and substance abuse count among the leading causes of death of these populations. They endure poverty, inadequate housing, contaminated drinking water, and suffer from poor self-esteem and feelings of isolation. The federal, provincial, and territorial governments have jointly initiated strategies to improve housing, sanitation, and access to prenatal care, as well as facilities and counselling to deal with substance abuse—but with limited success.

Aboriginal people have a higher morbidity and mortality rate than the rest of Canadians. Whereas the Canadian average life expectancy is 76 years for men and 83 years for women, males in the First Nations population can expect to live 68.9 years, and females, 76.6 years,(Health Canada, 2005; Health Council of Canada, 2005). The most common causes of death of Aboriginal persons between the ages of 1 year and 44 years of age are injury (specifically, fire, drowning, and motor vehicle accidents) and poisoning. Suicide and self-inflicted injuries are the most common cause of death of youth and adults.

First Nations people have higher rates of pertussis (whooping cough), rubella, and tuberculosis. Rates for some sexually transmitted infections (STIs) are up to seven times higher than for the rest of Canada. AIDS is becoming prevalent among these populations. Mental health, too, is emerging as a critical issue—often contributing to or causing other problems, such as depression, family abuse, suicide, and drug or alcohol abuse (Health Canada, 2005; Health Council of Canada, 2005).

STRATEGIES FOR IMPROVEMENT

To address these issues, the Health Council of Canada has introduced the following initiatives:

- A collaborative population health approach involving the federal, provincial, and territorial governments and stakeholders within Inuit, First Nations, and Métis communities. The first step is drafting a tool for gathering essential health information, which will contribute to designing health care reforms.

- A population health model of care and services that will effectively address the health problems unique to Aboriginal communities. For this approach to prove successful, health care professionals must show sensitivity to the needs of the population, considering the unique lifestyle, beliefs, culture, and traditions of Aboriginal peoples. As well, Aboriginals themselves must be involved at all levels of health care—from identifying health problems to participating in solutions for appropriate care.

Canada needs more Aboriginal health care professionals. In 2002, Aboriginal students represented a stark 0.9% of all first-year medical students in Canada. As part of a strategy to increase the numbers of Aboriginals in health care fields, health care professionals working with Aboriginals have been encouraged to suggest careers in health care to Aboriginal youth. Opportunities to train Aboriginal people in all aspects of health care must be made more geographically accessible, which can be achieved through distance education, videoconferencing, and the Internet. Such educational opportunities must have the flexible financial support of federal, provincial, and territorial governments.

The Indigenous Physicians Association of Canada and the Association of Faculties of Medicine of Canada are currently collaborating to introduce to universities programs that specifically address Aboriginal health concerns. In 2008, the groups launched the First Nations, Inuit, and Métis Health Core Competencies, a curriculum framework for undergraduate medical education. As well, the National Aboriginal Health Organization (NAHO), funded by Health Canada, implements strategies to improve the health of the people it represents through such activities as research, education, and the promotion of culturally relevant approaches to health care.

SYSTEMS OF DELIVERY OF HEALTH CARE FOR ABORIGINALS

Health Canada and its First Nations and Inuit Health Branch assume most of the responsibilities for the health care of Aboriginal peoples, with intervention and additional services provided by other designated organizations and stakeholders, such as the Public Health Agency of Canada.

Stakeholders disagree over the best approach. Many communities feel that health care would be best controlled and managed locally. Depending on local and provincial or territorial agreements, some Aboriginal groups have the option of withdrawing from government control over their health matters and managing their own health care programs. A large number of communities have taken on this responsibility, with varying degrees of success. The concept bears a resemblance to regional health authorities, which were founded on the belief that the people within a given community best understand the health care services required in that community. As well, individuals from the community can better motivate and direct fellow members of the community to accept help, adopt balanced lifestyles, and participate in disease prevention and health promotion.

No short-term solution exists for Aboriginal health issues. To bring about progress, Aboriginals must, with the assistance and support of all Canadians, find a balance between a balanced lifestyle, health, and prosperity and their culture, traditions, and way of life. As well, the independence and dignity of Aboriginal peoples must be restored and honoured.

The document *The Health Status of Canada's First Nations, Métis and Inuit Peoples* (see the Web Resources section at the end of this chapter) will provide you with an excellent overview of health issues related to the Aboriginal population.

THE HEALTH CARE SYSTEM: GOING ELECTRONIC

The electronic exchange of information has expanded enormously in the past decade, with computerization changing the face of business and industry worldwide. However, despite the high volume of health information created, accessed, and exchanged on a daily basis in health care offices and facilities across the country, the health care system, as a whole, has lagged behind technological advances.

The federal government formally initiated the use of computers to connect Canada's health care professionals and health care services in 2001. Connectivity in the health care sector provides health care professionals with links to information resources, electronically stored health-related educational information, other professionals (in health care and other disciplines), laboratories and diagnostic services, pharmacies, and, most important, clients' **electronic health records (EHRs)** and **electronic medical records (EMRs)**. Technology offers all health care professionals endless options, including the opportunity to view the charts, X-rays, and test results of hospitalized clients from their home or office and the ability to fax documents via computers, which both reduces the opportunity for misplaced documents and reduces the carbon footprint. In many jurisdictions, physicians can also complete and send prescriptions directly to a client's pharmacy.

EHRs and EMRs provide health care professionals the ability to access the health information of a client at any point of care. Instant retrieval of such information aids them in making an informed diagnosis and in developing an appropriate treatment plan for the client.

USE OF ELECTRONIC TECHNOLOGY

Hospitals

Most hospitals in Canada either fully or partially use electronic systems. In general, lab and diagnostic tests are now ordered electronically, as are other components of physician orders. Client charts, though primarily computerized, have some components that are still kept as hard copy. For example, many hospitals keep handwritten physicians' orders in clients' charts. Likewise, although electronically generated by the pharmacy department in many facilities, medication administration records are kept in clients' charts or in a medication administration binder. Consent forms are also kept in hard copy.

Doctors

Contrary to popular belief, the majority of Canadian physicians do not yet have a fully electronic office, nor will they in the near future. Most use computers for functional purposes (e.g., scheduling and billing) but not for electronic medical records and networking. Some physicians also use more advanced features related to scheduling. For example, a system introduced in Ontario in 2007 features a self-registration kiosk that can track the length of time a client has been waiting and update client information through prompts. The system, which offers five languages for clients to choose from, uses colour-coding to alert the office administrator that the client has arrived and registered. This system is used extensively across Ontario.

Although much of the groundwork has been laid for network integration and the use of electronic records, technical and political challenges remain. A little over 10% of Canadian physicians are using EMRs (National Physician Survey, 2007). Converting to electronic systems in the health care sector remains a slow process for a number of reasons, including the following:

- Software must meet certain electronic standards and be capable of networking with provincial or territorial systems—and choosing an appropriate program from a reliable vendor remains a challenge. Few jurisdictions have standardized options in place.

- Such systems are expensive. Although most governments provide some funding for health care professionals (but particularly physicians) to convert to EMRs, they rarely provide enough.

- Many health care professionals (notoriously physicians), especially older ones, have only a limited comfort level with computers, although this situation is changing. Estimates suggest that physicians under the age of 35 are most likely to convert to electronic charts (National Physician Survey, 2007). In 2007, only 30% of physicians were electronically connected with diagnostic and laboratory facilities, and less than 5% with pharmacies.

- Because fully networked health information will be available to a variety of health care professionals, confidentiality concerns present a barrier for some physicians unwilling to fully embrace the technology.

Jurisdictions that provide government funding for EMR initiatives for physicians are moving ahead more rapidly with implementations of the systems than jurisdictions that do not (i.e., Newfoundland and Labrador, Prince Edward

Island, New Brunswick, and the territories). See Web Resources at the end of this chapter for a link to information about provincial EMR programs.

Computerization and EHRs will eventually exist across the country, and health care professionals in all disciplines will ultimately have no choice but to "join the movement."

NATIONAL INITIATIVES TO PROMOTE ELECTRONIC SYSTEMS

The federal, provincial, and territorial governments are committed to establishing a pan-Canadian electronic health system within the next 10 years. Working collaboratively with all levels of government, regional health authorities, health care facilities, and other stakeholders, the Canada Health Infoway (CHI) is leading the transition to electronic health systems. Through this organization, electronic health information systems and EHR projects are approved, funded, and implemented. CHI projects include digitizing diagnostic imaging, expanding drug and laboratory information systems, and expanding and promoting the **interoperable EHR** program. See Web Resources at the end of this chapter for a link to a graphic representation of how interoperable EHRs work.

By 2008, CHI had already approved more than 230 projects across the country, bringing the total cumulative value of CHI's investments to $1.457 billion (which accounts for 89% of the $1.6 billion provided by the federal government) (Canada Health Infoway, 2008).

Each province and territory has an organization that supports (i.e., provides direction and sometimes funding) the implementation of electronic health systems within its jurisdiction (Box 10.1).

Interoperable EHR
Connected EHR systems that will enable authorized health care professionals to view and, in some cases, update a client's essential health information.

Box 10.1   Ontario Integrates E-Health Activities

Smart Systems for Health Agency, a provincially funded e-health network in Ontario, created and managed electronic networks promoting the sharing of health information among health care professionals. In September 2008, the Ontario government announced the integration of the Smart Systems for Health Agency and the province's e-health program into an organization called eHealth Ontario. This new agency manages all aspects of e-health in the province and works in partnership with a physician-based organization (Ontario MD) to ease the way toward the use of information technology among Ontario physicians. One of the organization's priorities is the implementation of electronic health records for all Ontario residents.

Inasmuch as eHealth Ontario has facilitated electronic connectivity of the medical community, problems have plagued the organization since 2009. Accusations of eHealth awarding untendered contracts (i.e., contracts awarded without a bidding process) and paying large bonuses and extraordinary salaries are only part of the organization's troubles.

Source: Ministry of Health and Long-Term Care. (2008, September 29). *Ontario integrates e-health activities under one agency* [News release]. Retrieved May 29, 2009, from http://www.health.gov.on.ca/english/media/news_releases/archives/nr_08/sep/e_health_nr_20080929.pdf

The pan-Canadian establishment of EHRs and EMRs will:

- Allow family doctors' offices to connect with specialists' offices, determine appointment availability, and choose the shortest wait time and most suitable appointment for their client while the client is still in the office.

- Facilitate the prompt delivery of laboratory tests to a family doctor, hospital, specialist, or other health care professional, which will, for example, allow physicians to adjust medications or order more blood work in a timely manner.

- Enable clients to access their medical records through an electronic portal, allowing them to view lab reports and physician updates and to participate in their own health care management as directed by health care professionals.

- Improve access to home care facilities and services by using an integrated approach to prioritizing and organizing required care and by managing elements of medical treatment assisted by electronic information exchange.

- Facilitate a drug information system that will allow a health care professional to view a client's medications. For example, in an ER, an attending physician or nurse can immediately access the drug profile of a recently admitted client and provide prompt and more effective treatment, while also avoiding drug-to-drug interactions, side effects, and overdoses.

- Enable implementation of public health tracking systems that allow prompt identification of individuals who may have had contact with someone with an infectious disease, allowing for timely exchange of advice to those involved and the implementation of appropriate containment strategies, if appropriate. (British Columbia is leading Canada in this area of electronic development.)

CHALLENGES

The goal of providing Canada with a workable and nationwide system is ambitious, and the challenges immense. The initiative will require the following:

- The commitment of all stakeholders to share in the vision and to embrace the technology

- Collaborative efforts by all levels of government and health care organizations

- Continual financing for provincial and territorial initiatives, including funds to encourage all stakeholders to go electronic (converting to an electronic environment is costly for small community organizations and physicians because they must purchase equipment, train staff, maintain skills and equipment, and access computer and software support)

- A public that trusts that their health information will be managed respectfully and securely

- Foolproof tracking and security systems that can identify who accesses what information in case of security breaches, and laws that specifically address privacy violations

- Computer software programs that talk to each other without connectivity difficulties

- Support systems at the federal, provincial, territorial, and municipal levels that work together to ensure seamless information exchange

- A uniform vocabulary of technical language to increase the effectiveness of system use

- Clearly defined laws governing the use and exchange of health information across provincial and territorial boundaries, including specific guidelines to clarify who bears responsibility for the information and what fees are charged for services provided

NEXT STEPS

The implementation of EHRs in Canada is just beginning. The CHI and other stakeholders have strategies in place and goals to reach. Short-term goals include having 50% of Canadian doctors using EMRs in 2010–11 and, by 2015, having EMRs in all physicians' offices across the country (Canada Health Infoway, 2008).

The vision for establishing electronic health systems includes implementing Telehealth solutions to enhance services in remote areas. By 2010, Canadians residing in northern and rural regions will have improved Telehealth access to larger centres and a variety of physicians to provide distance-based assessment of and solutions to their health care issues. This technology will enable individuals to receive care within their own communities and will improve access to coordinated community health services.

THE FUTURE OF PRIMARY HEALTH CARE REFORM

The current trend toward community-based health care and the collaboration of health care groups to offer that care will continue. This team approach to health care embraces the objective of offering *all* Canadians timely access to primary health care services. Health care teams will expand to include family doctors, optometrists, specialists, nurses, pharmacists, dietitians, social workers, nurse practitioners, physician assistants, physiotherapists, respiratory therapists, and other professionals. Alternative health care professionals are also likely to become a critical part of these teams, balancing a holistic lifestyle and treatments with the medical model of care. The focus on preventive care will become more clearly defined and efficiently implemented; for example, ensuring that all those required have access to mammograms, colorectal screening, immunizations, and Pap smears. The increased use of the team approach will improve access and quality of care as illustrated in Case Example 10.3.

Case Example 10.3

At the beginning of the chapter, you learned about Merle, who suffers from congestive heart failure, hypertension, diabetes, osteoarthritis, and chronic pain. Merle also wears glasses and must see an optometrist regularly because of the damage diabetes can cause to her eyes. Instead of relying on her family doctor to treat all of her medical problems, a team approach would benefit Merle in the following ways:

- The dietitian could help monitor her blood sugar levels and provide diet counselling.

- The nurse practitioner could manage a significant portion of Merle's medical complaints, including, for example, her arthritis, pain, and hypertension.

- The nurse practitioner could also work with the dietitian to better regulate Merle's blood sugar levels, suggesting Merle visit her family doctor or referring her to a specialist if necessary.

- The optometrist can assess her vision at regular intervals, referring her to an ophthalmologist if the need arises.

- If Merle wishes to see a chiropractor, an acupuncturist, a massage therapist, or another alternative health care professional for pain control,

Continued on next page

for example, she can discuss the matter with her nurse practitioner or physician, a referral can be made, and Merle may be able to reduce the amount of pain medication she takes.

Through the health care team approach, a wider population base can access effective, high-quality health care from a variety of health care professionals. The responsibility for keeping Merle as healthy as possible is more effectively distributed to individuals who have knowledge in specific areas.

Primary health care reform includes providing the public with 24/7 access to health information and advice through telephone helplines and providing appropriate follow-up care for those who call and do need doctors. For the continuous flow of health information and to ensure appropriate follow-up care, a system must be in place to notify family doctors when their clients have received care elsewhere. Read more about primary health care reform in Chapter 7.

Monitoring Health Care Initiatives

An independent body established and funded by the government of Canada, the Health Council of Canada provides objective reporting to Canadians on health matters and promotes both transparency and accountability regarding the progress of health care initiatives outlined in first ministers' accords. The Council collaborates with Quebec's Council on Health and Well-Being.

The Health Council of Canada has completed a new strategic plan to guide its future work. The following are the Council's strategies for 2008 to 2013:

- "Deepen public understanding of the features of a sustainable and high-performing health care system"

- "Support the health care community in its pursuit of high-potential opportunities to achieve a sustainable and high-performing health care system"

- "Monitor and report on successes and challenges in achieving a sustainable and high-performing health care" (Health Council of Canada, 2008b, p. 9)

SUMMARY

❖ Despite strategies that have been implemented to address the issues facing our health care system, problems remain. An aging population, high-volume demands for limited services, a shortage of human health resources, and insufficient funds to "fix" the problems remain as barriers to achieving an improved health care system.

❖ Some would argue that the principles of the *Canada Health Act* are outdated and must be revised for public health care to meet the needs of Canadians in the twenty-first century. Certain services (e.g., home care and drug benefits) are not mandated under the Act. Although most jurisdictions cover these expenses, they also enforce limitations, resulting in uneven coverage across the country. As a result, many Canadians go without or receive inferior care because of cost.

❖ Health care services for the mentally ill also remain inadequate. Although implementing community-based care for the mentally ill appeared, in theory, to be a positive change, this care model has proven both costly and difficult. Issues of insufficient funding for community programs and too few adequately trained professionals to coordinate this care must be addressed.

❖ Although the situation is improving slowly, the shortage of human health resources across the country affects every level and type of health care. Doctors, nurses, and other health care professionals are aging right along with a chunk of the Canadian population—and inadequate numbers of health care professionals exist to take their places. Strategies to address this shortage include the introduction of new levels of health care practitioners (e.g., physician assistant, nurse practitioner) and a redefinition of the roles of others.

❖ The health issues facing Canada's Aboriginal population surpass those facing other Canadians. Aboriginals have higher mortality and morbidity rates, more problems with alcohol and drug abuse, a lower standard of living, more mental health issues, and more problems related to isolation. The federal, provincial, and territorial governments have implemented many strategies to improve Aboriginal health care over the years with little gain. Governments are working toward increasing the involvement of Aboriginals in managing their own health care and educating health care professionals in delivering culturally sensitive care.

❖ The implementation of electronic health records—a measure expected to improve health care at all levels—is currently underway in Canada.

REVIEW QUESTIONS

1. Briefly identify three factors that affect a person's mental health.

2. List three factors contributing to Canada's aging population.

3. What two professions are most affected by Canada's human health resources shortage?

4. Who are Canada's baby boomers?

5. State two reasons for Canada's shortage of doctors.

6. What two general categories of health care workers provide home care services?

7. How is home care funded, and by whom?

8. Outline four areas in which the health of Aboriginal Canadians falls below national standards.

9. Why do some Canadians have no drug coverage?

10. List three benefits of electronic health records.

DISCUSSION QUESTIONS

1. Read the Kirby report *Out of the Shadows at Last*. Discuss the current issues (e.g., homelessness, the effectiveness of community-based care) facing the mentally ill in your community and in your province or territory. Research the support that your province or territory provides, including community resources. Are the problems in your jurisdiction similar to those described in Kirby's report?

2. Research your province's or territory's wait times for joint surgery, eye surgery, cancer treatment, cardiac surgery, family doctor appointments, referrals to specialists, lab and diagnostic tests, and test results. Have these times improved over the past five years? What strategies has your province or territory implemented to deal with wait times?

3. Identify the for-profit and not-for-profit home care services in your community. Find out how home care is paid for and by whom, how much it costs, and what services are covered. Research how

individuals in your province or territory obtain referrals for home care, how many people use home care, and the top two reasons they use it.

4. Working with two or three other students, choose a significant health care "problem" in your community, city, or region (e.g., long waits in the ER, inability to find a family doctor, shortage of nursing staff in a hospital). Construct a survey of 10 to 12 questions about that problem or issue. Each student must then distribute 10 surveys to either a target or random population group. Analyze your respondents' answers and present your findings in class.

5. If you were a provincial or territorial minister of health, what strategies would you put in place to improve the health of the Aboriginal population in your jurisdiction? Use the links in Web Resources to gain a more in-depth understanding of Aboriginal health issues and current strategies for health care reform.

WEB RESOURCES

The Health Status of Canada's First Nations, Métis and Inuit Peoples

http://healthcouncilcanada.ca.c9.previewyoursite.com/docs/papers/2005/BkgrdHealthyCdnsENG.pdf

This 2005 report by the Health Council of Canada presents a detailed account of the current health status of the First Nations, Métis, and Inuit peoples in Canada.

Find a Mental Health Professional in Canada

http://www.mentalhealthcanada.com/main.asp?lang=e

This page on the Mental Health Canada Web site provides an interactive map to help Canadians locate a mental health professional. Acting as the link between the public and mental health professionals, Mental Health Canada alerts the public about available mental health services across the country.

The Human Face of Mental Health in Canada

http://www.phac-aspc.gc.ca/publicat/human-humain06/pdf/human_face_e.pdf

This 2006 report, published by the Government of Canada, was designed to increase public awareness of mental illness and mental health. It explores both mental health and mental illness, a biological condition that more than one in five Canadians face at some point in their lives.

Health Human Resources Strategy

http://www.hc-sc.gc.ca/hcs-sss/hhr-rhs/strateg/index-eng.php

This Health Canada Web page provides information about strategies to address human resources shortages in the health care industry.

Wait Times for Health Care in Canada

http://canadaonline.about.com/od/healthcarewaittimes/Wait_Times_for_Health_Care_in_Canada.htm

This Web page provides links to wait times for select health care services in each province and territory across Canada.

Beyond Good Intentions: Accelerating the Electronic Health Record in Canada

http://www.healthcouncilcanada.ca/docs/papers/2006/infoway.pdf

Pages 8, 9, and 10 of this document summarize the benefits of the electronic health record to the health care system.

Canadian EMR: Provincial Programs

http://www.canadianemr.ca/index.aspx?PID=50

This Web page provides information about available funding for the implementation of electronic medical records.

Interoperable EHR

http://www.infoway-inforoute.ca/lang-en/about-infoway/approach/investment-programs/interoperable-ehr

This Web page links to a graphic representation of an interoperable EHR.

Moving to an All-Degree Nursing Profession at Registration

http://www.kcl.ac.uk/content/1/c6/04/47/23/PolicyIssue14.pdf

This article discusses how moving to an all-degree nursing profession in the United Kingdom might affect the nursing workforce and quality of care.

Province Invests $15 Million to Support Nursing in B.C.

http://www.bcliberals.com/?section_id=1332&section_copy_id=11789

This article from the BC Liberals discusses a 2008 strategy implemented to recruit, train, and retain quality nurses in British Columbia.

Strengthening Health Care in Newfoundland and Labrador

http://www.releases.gov.nl.ca/releases/2008/health/0429n04.htm

This news release discusses the government of Newfoundland and Labrador's investment in health care facilities, equipment, and its health care workforce; support for regional and community health authorities and long-term care; and the development of the electronic health record.

WEB RESOURCES

McGuinty Government Investing in Quality Nursing Care

http://www.health.gov.on.ca/english/media/news_
releases/archives/nr_06/jan/nr_012606.html

This news release discusses a 2006 Ontario initiative to provide funding for nurses in order to expand their knowledge and training, in turn, allowing vacancies to be filled, improving access to full-time employment opportunities, and enhancing working conditions. The initiative aimed to deliver on three key priorities of the Ontario health care system: providing better access to nurses and doctors, keeping residents healthy, and reducing wait times.

ADDITIONAL RESOURCES

Guillemette, Y., and Robson, W.B.P. (2006). No elixir of
   youth: Immigration cannot keep Canada young.
   C.D. Howe Institute Backgrounder 96, 3–4. Toronto:
   C.D. Howe Institute.

REFERENCES

BC Liberals. (2008, May 20). *Record number of doctors
   graduate in B.C.* Retrieved September 26, 2009,
   from http://www.bcliberals.com/news/health_care_
   and_health_prevention/record_number_of_doctors_
   graduate_in_b.c

Brennan, R.J. (2009, March 7). Mental illness rife in
   prisons. *The Toronto Star.* Retrieved May 29, 2009, from
   http://mentalhealthfamilyguide.ca/news.php?id=70

Canada Health Infoway. (2008). The e-volution of health
   care: Making a difference. *Canada Health Infoway
   Annual Report 2007–2008.* Retrieved May 29, 2009,
   from http://www.infoway-inforoute.ca

Canadian Broadcasting Corporation. (2005, May 12).
   Family doctors. *CBC News.* Retrieved May 29, 2009,
   from http://www.cbc.ca/news/background/healthcare/
   familydoctors.html

Canadian Broadcasting Corporation. (2007, August 31).
   Homeless hospitalized more often for mental illness:
   Study. *CBC News.* Retrieved May 29, 2009, from
http://www.cbc.ca/canada/ottawa/story/
   2007/08/30/homeless-illness.html

Canadian Broadcasting Corporation. (2009, May 8).
   60 new beds in Alberta for mental health, addiction
   treatment. *CBC News.* Retrieved May 29, 2009, from
   http://www.cbc.ca/health/story/2009/05/08/
   calgary-alberta-mental-health-beds.html

Canadian Health Services Research Foundation. (2001).
   Myth: The aging population will overwhelm the
   healthcare system. *MythBusters.* Retrieved May 29,
   2009, from http://www.chsrf.ca/mythbusters/pdf/
   myth5_e.pdf

Canadian Home Care Association. (2008). *Home care:
   Meeting the needs of an aging population.* Retrieved
   May 29, 2009, from http://www.cdnhomecare.ca/
   media.php?mid=1914

Canadian Institute for Health Information. (2007a).
   *Improving the health of Canadians: Mental health and
   homelessness.* Ottawa: CIHI. Retrieved May 29, 2009,

REFERENCES

from http://secure.cihi.ca/cihiweb/products/mental_ health_report_aug22_2007_e.pdf

Canadian Institute for Health Information. (2007b). *Supply, distribution, and migration of Canadian physicians, 2007*. Ottawa: CIHI. Retrieved May 29, 2009, from http://secure.cihi.ca/cihiweb/products/ SupDistandMigCanPhysic_2007_e.pdf

Canadian Institute for Health Information. (2008a). *Health care in Canada*. Retrieved May 29, 2009, from http://secure.cihi.ca/cihiweb/products/ HCIC_2008_e.pdf

Canadian Institute for Health Information. (2008b). *National health expenditure trends, 1975–2008*. Retrieved May 29, 2009, from http://secure.cihi.ca/ cihiweb/products/nhex_2008_en.pdf

Canadian Institute for Health Information. (2008c). *Regulated nurses: Trends, 2003 to 2007*. Ottawa: CIHI. Retrieved May 29, 2009, from http://secure.cihi. ca/cihiweb/products/nursing_report_2003_to_2007_ e.pdf

Canadian Mental Health Association. (n.d.a). *Justice and mental health*. Retrieved September 25, 2009, from http://www.ontario.cmha.ca/justice.asp

Canadian Mental Health Association. (n.d.b). *Police record checks*. Retrieved May 29, 2009, from http://www.ontario.cmha.ca/policy_and_research. asp?cID=25813

Canadian Mental Health Association. (2005). *Sub-standard treatment of mentally ill inmates is criminal: Experts* [News release]. Retrieved September 26, 2009, from http://www.cmha.ca/bins/content_page. asp?cid=6-20-21-965-773

Canadian Mental Health Association. (2009). *Canadian Mental Health Association urges governments to develop more appropriate solutions for the mentally ill housed in today's prisons*. Retrieved May 29, 2009, from http://www.cmha.ca/bins/content_page. asp?cid=6-20-21-2614-2615&lang=1

CanWest News Service. (2008, March 17). *Women poised to dominate doctors' offices*. Retrieved May 29, 2009, from http://www.scwist.ca/index.php/main/entry/ women-poised-to-dominate-doctors-offices/

Citizenship and Immigration Canada. (2008). *Minister Kenney announces immigration levels for 2009; issues instructions on processing federal skilled workers*. Retrieved May 29, 2009, from http://www.cic.gc.ca/ english/DEPARTMENT/MEDIA/releases/2008/ 2008-11-28.asp

Dewa, C.S., Lesage, A., Goering, P., & Caveen, M. (2004). Nature and prevalence of mental illness in the workplace. *Healthcare Papers, 5*(2), 12–25.

Gulli, C., & Lunau, K. (2008, January 14). Canada's doctor shortage worsening. *Maclean's*. Retrieved May 29, 2009, from http://www.thecanadianencyclopedia.com/ index.cfm?PgNm=TCE&Params=M1ARTM0013191

Health Canada. (2002). *A report on mental illnesses in Canada*. Retrieved May 29, 2009, from http://www. phac-aspc.gc.ca/publicat/miic-mmac/pdf/men_ill_ e.pdf

Health Canada. (2005). *First Nations comparable health indicators*. Retrieved May 29, 2009, from http://www. hc-sc.gc.ca/fniah-spnia/diseases-maladies/ 2005-01_health-sante_indicat-eng.php#life_expect

Health Canada. (2007a). *Wait times in Canada*. Retrieved May 29, 2009, from http://www.hc-sc.gc.ca/hcs-sss/ qual/acces/wait-attente/index-eng.php

Health Canada. (2007b). *The working conditions of nurses: Confronting the challenges*. Retrieved May 29, 2009, from http://www.hc-sc.gc.ca/sr-sr/pubs/ hpr-rpms/bull/2007-nurses-infirmieres/7-eng.php

Health Council of Canada. (2005). *The health status of Canada's First Nations, Métis and Inuit peoples*. Retrieved May 29, 2009, from http://healthcouncilcanada.ca.c9.previewyoursite.com/ docs/papers/2005/BkgrdHealthyCdnsENG.pdf

Health Council of Canada. (2008a). *Fixing the foundation: An update on primary health care and home care*

REFERENCES

renewal in Canada. Retrieved May 29, 2009, from http://healthcouncilcanada.ca/docs/rpts/2008/phc/HCC_PHC_Main_web_E.pdf

Health Council of Canada. (2008b). *Strategic plan 2008/2009–2012/2013. Taking the pulse toward improved health and health care in Canada*. Retrieved May 29, 2009, from http://www.healthcouncilcanada.ca/docs/rpts/2008/HCCStratplan2008to2013.pdf

Here to Help. (2006). *Economic costs of mental disorders and addictions*. Retrieved September 25, 2009, from http://www.heretohelp.bc.ca/publications/factsheets/costs

Human Resources and Skills Development Canada. (2007). *Looking-ahead: A 10-year outlook for the Canadian labour market (2006–2015)*. Retrieved May 29, 2009, from http://www.hrsdc.gc.ca/eng/publications_resources/research/categories/labour_market_e/sp_615_10_06/page03.shtml

Human Resources and Skills Development Canada. (2009). *Health—Life expectancy at birth*. Retrieved May 29, 2009, from http://www4.hrsdc.gc.ca/.3ndic.1t.4r@-eng.jsp?iid=3

Kanchier, C. (2006, January 8). Depression: A self-help guide to lift the blues. *The Vancouver Sun*. Retrieved May 29, 2009, from http://www.canada.com/vancouversun/story.html?id=d2f1119b-6100-4230-8e9b-06ab1bf922f5

Kirby, M.J.L., & Keon, W.J. (2006). *Out of the shadows at last: Highlights and recommendations from the Kirby Report*. Final report of the Standing Senate Committee on Social Affairs, Science and Technology. Ottawa, ON. Retrieved May 29, 2009, from http://www.parl.gc.ca/39/1/parlbus/commbus/senate/com-e/soci-e/rep-e/pdf/rep02may06high-e.pdf

Lunau, K. (2008, May 14). Overworked nurses mess up patients' meds: A nurse responds to StatsCan report. *Maclean's*. Retrieved May 29, 2009, from http://www2.macleans.ca/tag/nursing-shortage/

Martin, S. (2000). "Freedom 55" closer to age 65 for physicians. *Canadian Medical Association Journal, 163*(11). Retrieved May 29, 2009, from http://www.cmaj.ca/cgi/content/full/163/11/1499-a

Mental Health Commission of Canada. (n.d.). *About the commission*. Retrieved May 29, 2009, from http://www.mentalhealthcommission.ca/English/Pages/default.aspx

Mental Health Commission of Canada. (2007, October 17). *A submission to the Mental Health Commission of Canada*. Vancouver: Canadian Mental Health Association, BC Division.

National Alliance on Mental Illness. (2009). *The global burden of disease stresses the global burden of mental illness*. Retrieved May 29, 2009, from http://www.nami.org/Template.cfm?Section=Bipolar_Disorder&template=/ContentManagement/ContentDisplay.cfm&ContentID=28739

National Physician Survey. (2007). *2007 national physician survey*. Retrieved May 29, 2009, from http://www.nationalphysiciansurvey.ca/nps/2007_Survey/2007nps-e.asp

NationTalk. (2008, April 28). *Health: Mental Health Commission of Canada outlines startling statistics at public forum on homelessness & mental illness*. Retrieved September 24, 2009, from http://www.nationtalk.ca/modules/news/article.php?storyid=895

Office of the Correctional Investigator. (2009, March 3). Backgrounder: "A preventable death." Retrieved September 25, 2009, from http://www.oci-bec.gc.ca/rpt/oth-aut/oth-aut20080620info-eng.aspx

Romanow, R. (2002). *Building on values: The future of health care in Canada*. Retrieved May 29, 2009, from http://www.cbc.ca/healthcare/final_report.pdf

Statistics Canada. (2001). The Vietnamese community in Canada. *Profiles of Ethnic Communities in Canada, 2006*(2). (No. 89-621-XWE.) Ottawa, ON: Author. Retrieved May 29, 2009, from http://www.statcan.gc.ca/pub/89-621-x/89-621-x2006002-eng.htm

REFERENCES

Statistics Canada. (2004). Canadian community health survey, 2003. *The Daily.* Ottawa, ON: Author. Retrieved May 29, 2009, from http://www.statcan.gc.ca/daily-quotidien/040615/dq040615b-eng.htm

Statistics Canada. (2006). *Aboriginal peoples in Canada in 2006: Inuit, Métis and First Nations, 2006 census.* (No. 97-558-XWE2006001). Ottawa, ON: Author. Retrieved May 29, 2009, from http://www.statcan.gc.ca/bsolc/olc-cel/olc-cel?catno=97-558-XWE2006001&lang=eng

Statistics Canada. (2007). Depression and work impairment. *Health Reports, 18*(1). (No. 82-003). Ottawa, ON: Author. Retrieved May 29, 2009, from http://www.statcan.gc.ca/pub/82-003-x/2006001/article/depress/82-003-x2006001-eng.pdf

Statistics Canada. (2008a, June 25). Canada's population estimates. *The Daily.* Ottawa, ON: Author. Retrieved May 29, 2009, from http://www.statcan.gc.ca/daily-quotidien/080625/dq080625b-eng.htm

Statistics Canada. (2008b, June 18). Canadian community health survey. *The Daily*. Ottawa, ON: Author. Retrieved May 29, 2009, from http://www.statcan.gc.ca/daily-quotidien/080618/dq080618a-eng.htm

Statistics Canada. (2009, January 15). Canada's population by age and sex. *The Daily*. Retrieved May 29, 2009, from http://www.statcan.gc.ca/daily-quotidien/090115/dq090115c-eng.htm

Steed, J. (2008, November 15). 10 innovative fixes for what ails us. *The Toronto Star.* Retrieved May 29, 2009, from http://www.thestar.com/printArticle/537348

UNICEF. (2004). *At a glance: Canada*. Retrieved May 29, 2009, from http://www.unicef.org/infobycountry/canada_statistics.html

Weeks, C., & Leeder, J. (2008, March 18). Quality of cancer testing a "nightmare." *The Globe and Mail*. Retrieved from http://www.theglobeandmail.com/servlet/story/RTGAM.20080318.wcancer18/BNStory/specialScienceandHealth/home

Glossary

Aboriginal peoples
Broadly, individuals indigenous to a country or region. In Canada, the term applies to First Nations, Inuit, and Métis people.

Accord
An agreement between two or more parties.

Act
A usually comprehensive body of laws passed by Parliament or a provincial or territorial legislature.

Active euthanasia
Death caused by taking deliberate steps.

Active ingredients
Those ingredients in a drug that have therapeutic value meant to cure, palliate, or otherwise treat a health problem.

Advance directive
A set of instructions outlining the nature and level of treatment a person wants to receive in the event that he or she becomes unable to make such decisions at the necessary time.

Affiliating body
An association that provides, among other things, direction, support, continuing education, and networking opportunities for its professional members (who may be regulated or nonregulated).

Age of majority
The age at which a person is considered an adult; depending on the province or territory, age 18 or 19.

Aseptic technique
A procedure performed under sterile conditions to reduce the risk of infection.

Atherosclerosis
A disease resulting from fatty deposits building up on the inner lining of arteries, eventually forming a mass called plaque. The artery may ultimately close completely, causing a heart attack or stroke.

Autonomy
A person's right to self-determination. In health care, autonomy refers to a client's right to make decisions without coercion.

Beneficence
An ethical principle encompassing the duty to prevent harm, the duty to remove harm, and the duty to promote good.

Best practice
The most current and effective methods of reaching a goal.

Block transfer
One payment to cover all services.

Branch
A division of a main office offering extended or supportive functions.

Bureau
Government department responsible for a specific entity or duty.

Canada Health Act
Legislation passed in 1984 that governs and guides the delivery of prepaid, medically necessary health care to Canadians.

Capitation-based funding
A funding formula to pay physicians who participate in some type of primary health care reform group. The doctor receives a set amount (determined by

the age and health status of each client) for each rostered client per year.

Cardiovascular disease
Disease that affects the heart and vascular system (i.e., blood vessels).

Catastrophic drug costs
Prescription drug costs that cause undue burden on individuals suffering with serious health conditions or illnesses.

Central agency
An organization or department with the authority to direct or intervene in the activities of other departments. Central agencies aid with policy development and the coordination of activities.

Chronic obstructive pulmonary disease (COPD)
Persistent lung disease that interferes with normal breathing, including both chronic bronchitis (i.e., permanent inflammation of the main airways in the lungs) and emphysema (i.e., enlargement of the air sacs in the lungs).

Circle of care
The individuals and health care professionals legitimately involved in rendering a client's care.

Civil law
A legal system in which laws governing civil rights, relationships within society and between people and property, and family relationships are written rather than being determined by judges.

Clinic
A setting in which multiple health care professionals work collaboratively, usually in a similar field, to provide cost-effective, client-centred health care.

Code of ethics
A set of values and responsibilities serving to guide the behaviour of the members of an organization or a profession.

Common law
Law resulting from the decisions of judges, based on precedents.

Community-based care
Care provided for the client in the home (e.g., incorporating visits from nurses or physiotherapists) or on an outpatient basis rather than in the hospital or another health care facility.

Compassionate interference
The act of imposing treatment against a client's will when deemed in the best interests of the client.

Compensation
That part of the health–illness continuum in which a person is neither in good nor poor health, is able to accommodate a malady, and is continuing on with daily life.

Confidentiality
In health care, the moral obligation of a health care professional to keep a client's health information private.

Conflict of interest
The possible clash of two or more concerns. For example, a personal financial interest in a business may influence one's professional decisions.

Congenital
Present at birth but not attributed to hereditary factors; a condition that may have developed during pregnancy due to a variety of factors.

Constitutional law
The area of law dealing with legislation derived from or related to Canada's Constitution.

Consumer price index (CPI)
A method of determining changes in the cost of goods and services through the monitoring of select items (e.g., food, rent, mortgages, gasoline) across Canada. Used to measure inflation,

the CPI may affect such payments as social security, spousal support, and rent, which are periodically adjusted to reflect the CPI.

Continuity of care
Health care based on the treating practitioners' having all required information to optimize the care the client receives; this requires their having access to the individual's health records and maintaining excellent communication among all parties involved in the client's care.

Contract law
Law that concerns legally binding contracts, whether expressed or implied.

Controlled act
A potentially harmful act that must be performed only by trained members of a particular profession.

Controlled Drugs and Substances Act
Federal legislation addressing Canada's drug laws, including a classification system for drugs.

Co-payment
A predetermined dollar amount or percentage of the cost of a health care service or medication that an individual must pay.

Criminal law
The field of law dealing with crimes against the state or against society. Criminal law defines offences and controls the regulations concerning the apprehension, charging, and trying of those believed to have committed a criminal offence.

Culture
Common elements of a social group, including its beliefs, practices, behaviours, values, and attitudes. Culture can relate to a society or sub-groups within a society.

Deductible
The amount of money that an individual or family is required to pay toward health care costs before an insurance plan will take over.

Delegated act
An act, treatment, or intervention performed by a health care professional that is outside of that person's scope of practice but is allowed in certain circumstances and, in many cases, under direct supervision.

Delisted
The removal of an item from a list or a registry. In Canada, the term is frequently used when a medical service is no longer considered medically necessary and is removed from the government's list of insured services.

Deontological theory
An ethical theory based on a duty to do the "right" (i.e., moral) thing, regardless of consequences.

Deregulated
No longer covered under the provincial or territorial health plan.

Determinants of health
The conditions (economic, social, environmental, etc.) in which people live that affect their current and future health.

Disability
A physical or mental incapacity that differs from what is perceived as normal function. A disability can result from an illness or accident or be genetic in nature.

Disease
A disorder affecting a system or organ, which can be mental, physical, or genetic in origin. *Disease* also refers to a change in, or deviation from, how the body normally functions.

Disease burden
The impact of a health problem, measured by financial cost, mortality, morbidity, or other indicators.

Disease prevention
Although used in conjunction with health promotion, disease prevention is a separate entity. It seeks to stop the development of a disease or to detect and treat a disease as early as possible when it does occur to control its spread and reduce the chances of it returning.

Dispensing fee
A service fee charged by a pharmacy for dispensing a prescription medication (i.e., reading the prescription and preparing the medication for the client).

Divine command ethics
An ethical theory whereby decisions are made according to rules set out by a higher power—for example, through the Bible, the Koran, or the Torah.

Double effect
An ethical principle requiring a person to choose the option that causes the least harm.

Drug identification number (DIN)
A unique number assigned to each medication approved by Health Canada for use in Canada.

Drug-seeking behaviour
A behaviour or activity focused on obtaining access to addictive controlled substances.

Duties
Obligations a person has in response to another's claims on them. A duty may result from a professional or personal obligation or may relate to one's own morals or values.

Duty of care
The obligation to act in a competent manner according to the standards of practice.

Electronic health record (EHR)
A secure accumulation of essential information about a client that is accessed electronically at different points of service (e.g., doctor's office, dentist's office, chiropractor's office, and a pharmacy) for purposes of client care.

Electronic medical record (EMR)
Health information obtained and stored at one facility, perhaps a dentist's, chiropractor's, or doctor's office.

Eligible
To be qualified for something by meeting certain criteria or requirements.

Emotional wellness
Displaying an ability to understand oneself, to recognize personal strengths and limitations, and to accept these realities.

Empirical studies
Studies based on observation and experience.

Enhanced services
Allows patients to pay for enhanced or optional health services such as, choice in hospital rooms, enhanced medical goods and services, and the ability to purchase services not covered by a province's public health insurance system.

Environmental wellness
Engaging in a lifestyle that shows respect for one's environment.

Epidemiology
Research into what causes diseases, how they are spread, and how they are controlled. It includes the study of the effects of disease on various populations, including a population's susceptibility or resistance to disease.

Ethical principle

An acceptable, usually highly valued and moral, standard of human behaviour—for example, honesty, truthfulness, and fairness.

Ethical theory

A framework of ideas that provides a template for making decisions to justify a set of actions.

Ethics

The philosophical study of standards accepted by society that determine what is right and wrong in human behaviour.

Etiology

The study of causes. In medicine, *etiology* refers to the origin or cause of a disease.

Evidence-based

Proven, through high-quality scientific studies, to be effective.

Exacerbation

A period of time when a disease (usually chronic) is active and the person has symptoms. *Exacerbation* may also refer to an increase in the severity of a disease.

Fidelity

The ethical principle of faithfulness, which includes carrying out one's obligations and duties and keeping commitments to employers, clients, and peers.

Fiduciary duty

A duty binding physicians and other health care professionals to act with honesty and integrity, and in the best interests of their clients, with regard to their professional practice.

Fiduciary relationship

A relationship based on trust.

First ministers

The premiers of the provinces and territories.

First Nations

A Canadian term of ethnicity referring to indigenous Canadians. The First Nations comprise a group (usually registered as "Indians" under the *Indian Act*) of 633 First Nations bands, representing 52 cultural groups and more than 50 languages. Other terms used include *Aboriginal*, *Native*, or *indigenous people*.

Forensic psychiatric hospitals

Hospitals that serve individuals referred by the Canadian courts for treatment and assessment and that provide treatment and support for individuals requiring a secure inpatient facility due to their risk of harm to self and/or others.

Formulary list

A list of prescription medications (often generic brands) selected for coverage by a public or private health insurance plan.

Geriatrics

The branch of medicine dealing with the physiologic characteristics of aging and the diagnosis and treatment of diseases affecting the aged.

Gestation

The period of time from a baby's conception until its delivery.

Good Samaritan law

A law protecting individuals who attempt to offer help to a person in distress.

Gross national product (GNP)

The total value of all the goods and services produced by a country within a year.

Health behaviour

The activities and actions a person engages in to acquire and maintain good physical and psychological health.

Health beliefs

What a person believes to be true about his or her health and susceptibility to illness, and about illness, prevention, and treatment in general.

Health–illness continuum

A method of measuring one's state of health at any given point in time. A person's health state may range from optimum health at one end to death at the other end.

Health indicators

Measurements that help to gauge the state of health and wellness of a population.

Health promotion

Initiatives that inform people about things they can do to prevent disease and illness. These include the principles outlined in the *Ottawa Charter for Health Promotion*: building healthy public policy, creating supportive environments, strengthening community action, developing personal skills, and reorienting health services. Imparting such knowledge helps individuals take responsibility for their own well-being.

Hemochromatosis

A condition that causes the body to absorb and store excessive amounts of iron and that, if untreated, can cause the major body organs to fail.

Holistic

Whole. In health care, a holistic approach treats the whole person, not an individual part of the person. For example, a holistic approach to treating a person with a heart condition would consider the client's emotional state, diet, and fitness level, not just his or her heart problem.

Hydrocephalus

Abnormal accumulation of cerebrospinal fluid (CSF) in the brain. The cause is usually genetic.

Hypoglycemic

Pertaining to low blood sugar.

Hypoglycemic reaction

A response to a drop in blood sugar levels. The symptoms may include mild weakness or dizziness; headache; cold, clammy, or sweaty skin; problems concentrating; shakiness; uncoordinated movements or staggering; blurred vision; irritability; hunger; fainting; and loss of consciousness.

Illness

The presence of a disease affecting the body or the mind, or the state of feeling unhealthy, even if no disease is present.

Implied consent

Consent assumed by the client's actions, such as his or her seeking out the care of a health care professional or his or her failure to resist or protest.

Incident report

A legal document outlining all relevant information concerning any negative occurrence in the workplace.

Inequities in health

Unfair and unequal distribution of health resources in relation to resources available and the population involved.

Infant mortality

The death of an infant (i.e., within the first year of life).

Informed consent

Legally and ethically, clients must be given all relevant information about a treatment before agreeing to undergo the treatment. A client's consent without full disclosure of information is not considered informed consent.

Innu

Naskapi and Montagnais First Nations (Indian) peoples who live in Northern Quebec and Labrador.

Inpatient

A person admitted to, and staying in, a hospital for one or more nights.

Intellectual wellness

Displaying an ability to make informed decisions that are appropriate and beneficial.

Interoperable EHR

Connected EHR systems that will enable authorized health care professionals to view and, in some cases, update a patient's essential health information.

Intersectoral cooperation

Joint action among the public, the government, and nongovernment or community-based organizations.

Intubate

To pass a tube into a person's trachea to facilitate breathing.

Inuit

Aboriginal people in northern Canada living generally above the treeline in the Northwest Territories, Northern Quebec, and Labrador.

Involuntary euthanasia

Ending the life of an ill person without that person's consent.

Jurisdiction

Authority over specific geographic and legislative areas.

Laparoscopic surgery

A type of surgical procedure in which a small incision is made in the body, through which a viewing tube (laparoscope) is inserted. A small camera in the laparoscope allows the doctor to examine internal organs. Other small incisions may be made to insert instruments to perform surgery.

Legislation

Laws made by a provincial or territorial legislature or by Parliament. To become law, a bill (i.e., proposed legislation) that has been introduced to Parliament requires the agreement of the House of Commons, the Senate, and the Crown (i.e., the Governor General, the representative of the British monarch in Canada).

Life expectancy

The number of years a population or parts of a population is expected to live as determined by statistics.

Malpractice

A civil wrong that occurs when any professional fails to fulfill his or her duty to meet the reasonable standard of care or practice. Also called *negligence*.

Medically necessary

A clinical judgement made by a physician regarding a service provided under a provincial or territorial health plan that is necessary to maintain, restore, or palliate (i.e., ease symptoms, such as pain, without curing the underlying disease).

Medicare

The informal name for Canada's national health insurance plan. Note that the term's use in Canada differs from that in the United States, where *Medicare* refers to a federally sponsored program for individuals over the age of 65.

Methicillin-resistant *Staphylococcus aureus* (MRSA)

A strain of *Staphylococcus aureus* that has become resistant to the antibiotic methicillin.

Minor

A person under the age of majority in a particular province or territory.

Modalities

Prescribed methods or techniques.

Morality

A code of conduct put forward by a society or some other group, such as a religion; also, a code of conduct accepted by an individual to guide his or her own behaviour, or one that, given specified conditions, would be put forward by all rational persons.

Morals

What a person believes to be right and wrong pertaining to how to act, how to treat others, and how to behave in an organized society.

Morbidity

Disease, the occurrence of disease, or impairment resulting from accidents or environmental causes that adversely affects health.

Mortality

Death or the occurrence of deaths resulting from disease, accidents, or environmental causes.

Negligence

A civil wrong that occurs when any professional fails to fulfill his or her duty to meet the reasonable standard of care or practice. Also called *malpractice*.

Nonmaleficence

An ethical principle encompassing the duty to refrain from harming another person.

Nonprofit

Not seeking or producing a profit.

Nursing home

A facility or part of a facility that provides accommodation to persons usually over the age of 16 requiring intensive personal care under the supervision of a registered nurse.

Obesity

Excessive accumulation of body fat to the point that an individual's health is at risk; sometimes objectively defined as a person's weighing more than 30% of his or her ideal body weight as determined by individual height and build.

Oral consent

A binding agreement to treatment made in person or over the phone.

Organisation for Economic Co-operation and Development (OECD)

Established in 1961 and now representing 30 countries, the OECD provides a setting in which member governments compare policy experiences, seek answers to common problems, identify best practices, and coordinate domestic and international policies.

Orphan patient

A person without a family doctor.

Palliative care

Care for the dying. Palliative care services, offered in the home or another facility (e.g., palliative care unit in a hospital or a hospice), may include nursing care, counselling, and pain management and may involve those close to the client.

Pandemic

A sustained, worldwide human-to-human transmission of disease.

Passive euthanasia

Death caused by removing life support or life-sustaining treatment.

Patented drugs

Drugs that are legally protected from generic production for a period of 20 years from the date of filing.

Paternalism

The attempt to control or influence another's decision regarding medical care. Paternalism does not honour the client's right to autonomy.

Personal Information Protection and Electronic Documents Act (PIPEDA)

A federal act ensuring the protection of personal information in the private sector.

Physical wellness

Maintaining a healthy body by eating a nutritious, balanced diet, exercising regularly, making intelligent, informed decisions about one's health, and seeking medical assistance when necessary.

Physician-assisted suicide

A physician providing the means by which a client can end his or her own life.

Placebo effect

An improvement in a person's condition without any actual treatment. Some evidence suggests that if people believe a specific treatment (e.g., a pill, which may be only a sugar pill) will cure them, a biochemical effect can minimize or alleviate symptoms.

Population-based surveillance

The collection and analysis of data that are needed to plan, implement, and evaluate population health initiatives.

Population health

A framework for gathering and analyzing information about conditions that affect the health of a population. The aim is to both maintain and improve the health of the entire population and to reduce inequities in health status among population groups.

Power of attorney

A legal document naming a specific person or persons to act on behalf of another in matters concerning personal care, personal estate, or both.

Prepaid health care

Access to medically necessary hospital and physician services on a prepaid basis, and on uniform terms and conditions.

Primary care

Front-line care, direction, and advice provided by multidisciplinary health care teams. Primary health care also involves initiatives that seek to improve access to, quality of, and continuity of care; client and health care professional satisfaction; and cost-effectiveness of health care services.

Primary health care

Health care with an emphasis on individuals and their communities. Primary health care includes essential medical and curative care received at the primary, secondary, or tertiary levels and involves health care professionals, as well as community members, delivering care within the community that is cost-effective, comprehensive, and collaborative (i.e., uses a team approach).

Primary health care reform

Changes to the delivery of primary health care with the goal of providing all Canadians access to an appropriate health care professional 24 hours a day, 7 days a week, no matter where they live.

Privacy

The client's right to control access to their body and personal information.

Profession

An occupation that involves some branch of advanced learning.

Professional

A person practising an occupation that involves some branch of advanced learning.

Professional misconduct

Behaviour or some act or omission that falls short of what would be proper in the circumstances. Examples include deviating from a profession's standards of practice or violating the boundaries of a professional–client relationship.

Professionalism

A standard of skill and behaviour appropriate for a specific profession.

Proxy consent

Consent given by a person authorized by a health care client to give consent on his or her behalf.

Public health

Public health uses health information to improve the health of communities. Public health programs often carry out recommendations made by population health studies, so they tend to focus more on applying measures than on gathering and analyzing information.

Qualitative research

A method of research that examines the way a population group thinks and behaves. The analysis is largely subjective in nature.

Quantitative research

A method of objective research that deals with the measurement of data, such as the number of deaths from cancer.

Quarantine

The act of isolating people having, or suspected of having, a contagious disease.

Quarantine Act

Updated in 2005, this legislation gives the federal government powers to assess individuals and possibly detain those who may pose a health risk to Canadians.

Refraction

Testing of the eyes to evaluate their ability to see. An ophthalmologist or optometrist does a refraction to determine the type of lens a client needs in his or her glasses to maximize vision.

Refugee claimants

People who, feeling unsafe in their home country, seek protection in another country.

Regulation

A form of law, made by persons or organizations (e.g., an administrative agency) awarded such authority within an act (whether federal, provincial, or territorial), that has the binding legal power of an act.

Regulatory law

Laws made not by Parliament or by a legislature but by authorized persons or organizations to govern a particular group; these laws are ultimately subject to the provincial, territorial, or federal act that governs the administrative body, organization, or tribunal.

Remission

A period of time during which a chronic disease is neither active nor acute and the person has no obvious symptoms.

Renal dialysis

A mechanical process to remove unwanted elements normally taken from the blood by the kidneys. This process becomes necessary when a person's kidneys are not functioning.

Reserve

Land set aside by the Crown for Aboriginal people to live on. Reserves came about through treaties signed in the 1800s and remain in existence today.

Rights in health care

Entitlements, things that can and should be expected of health care professionals and the health care system. Rights may be tangible (e.g., the right to receive a vaccination covered under the provincial or territorial plan) or intangible (the right to be treated with respect).

Role fidelity

In health care, meeting the reasonable expectations of members of the health care team, clients, their families, and employers by being loyal, truthful, and faithful, by showing respect, and by earning and maintaining trust.

Rostering

The registering of a client in a primary health care reform group. Clients sign a form, which is nonbinding, stating that they will seek care only from a specific doctor.

Royal assent

The final stage a bill passes through before becoming law. Largely symbolic in nature, this approval is given by the Governor General as a representative of the Crown.

Scope of practice

A range of skills, learned in school or through on-the-job training, that a practitioner can perform competently and safely. From a professional perspective, legal parameters usually (but not always) dictate what a practitioner may or may not do, based on the profession's education, training, and licensure.

Self-determination

The freedom to make one's own decisions.

Self-imposed risk behaviours

Actions (such as smoking) that a person willfully engages in despite knowing they pose a danger to his or her health.

SES gradient

A measurement of health or health inequalities as they relate to a person's or population's socioeconomic circumstances.

Severe acute respiratory syndrome (SARS)

A severe form of pneumonia that first swept across parts of Asia and the Far East before spreading worldwide in 2003.

Sick role behaviour

A person's response to disease or illness. Removed from normal societal expectations and responsibilities, the sick person may respond to situations differently from when he or she is well. Sick role behaviour is usually temporary in nature.

Signs

Those things related to an illness that a person or examiner can see (e.g., a rash).

Social movements

Advancements by advocacy or interest groups to promote a common interest by acting together to influence public policy.

Social wellness

Relating effectively to others, including being able to form close, loving relationships, to laugh, to communicate effectively and empathically, to be a good listener, and to respond appropriately.

Specialist

A physician trained in a specific field, usually concerning body systems or organs—for example, cardiology, internal medicine, orthopedic surgery—

although some specialties (e.g., geriatrics) have a socioeconomic focus.

Spiritual wellness
Seeking to contribute to society; may, but does not necessarily, include a commitment to a religion or a higher power that evokes a sense of belonging to something greater than self.

Statutory law
A law or act passed by Parliament or a provincial or territorial legislature.

Subdural hematomas
A type of brain injury in which blood collects between the outer protective covering of the brain (i.e., the dura) and the middle layers of the brain covering (i.e., the meninges), most often caused by torn, bleeding veins on the inside of the dura as a result of a blow to the head.

Symptoms
Those things that a person feels that may relate to an illness (e.g., fatigue, a headache).

Telehealth
A telephone help system, usually available 24/7 and funded by the provincial or territorial government, used to provide professional health care advice to Canadians who cannot readily access a doctor or other primary care provider.

Teleological theory
An ethical theory based on acting to bring about the most benefit for the most people. Also called *consequence-based theory*.

Title protection
Legal protection of a professional title and the legal right to use that title.

Tort
A civil wrong committed against a person or his or her property.

Upstream investments
Actions that can be taken to improve the health of a population or to prevent illness when the potential for a problem is first recognized.

Urodynamic
Referring to tests and assessments done to measure the function of the bladder and urinary tract.

Values
Beliefs that a person holds dear and that guide that person's decisions and behaviour or conduct.

Values history form
A comprehensive document used to determine and record treatment options people would or would not want if they were unable to make their own decisions.

Vancomycin-resistant *Enterococcus* (VRE)
A form of the bacteria *Enterococcus* that has become resistant to many antibiotics, including vancomycin—one of the most effective antibiotics to treat enterococcal infections.

Vancomycin-resistant *Staphylococcus aureus* (VRSA)
A strain of *Staphylococcus aureus* that has become resistant to the antibiotic vancomycin.

Virtue ethics
An ethical theory based on the assumption that if the person making the decision is of high moral character, his or her decision will be wise and just.

Voluntary euthanasia
Ending the life of an ill person with that person's consent.

Wellness

The way a person feels about his or her health and quality of life. People with a disability or a chronic disease may still consider themselves to be well and enjoying a good quality of life.

Whistleblower

A current or past employee or member of an organization who reports another's misconduct to people or entities with the power and presumed willingness to take corrective action.

WHMIS legislation

National legislation for health and safety that applies to all Canadian workplaces in which identified hazardous materials are used.

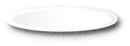

APPENDIX

DECLARATION OF ALMA-ATA

Declaration of Alma-Ata: International Conference on Primary Health Care, Alma-Ata, USSR, 6–12 September 1978

The International Conference on Primary Health Care, meeting in Alma-Ata this twelfth day of September in the year nineteen hundred and seventy-eight, expressing the need for urgent action by all governments, all health and development workers, and the world community to protect and promote the health of all the people of the world, hereby makes the following Declaration:

I

The Conference strongly reaffirms that health, which is a state of complete physical, mental and social wellbeing, and not merely the absence of disease or infirmity, is a fundamental human right and that the attainment of the highest possible level of health is a most important world-wide social goal whose realization requires the action of many other social and economic sectors in addition to the health sector.

II

The existing gross inequality in the health status of the people particularly between developed and developing countries as well as within countries is politically, socially and economically unacceptable and is, therefore, of common concern to all countries.

III

Economic and social development, based on a New International Economic Order, is of basic importance to the fullest attainment of health for all and to the reduction of the gap between the health status of the developing and developed countries. The promotion and protection of the health of the people is essential to sustained economic and social development and contributes to a better quality of life and to world peace.

IV

The people have the right and duty to participate individually and collectively in the planning and implementation of their health care.

V

Governments have a responsibility for the health of their people, which can be fulfilled only by the provision of adequate health and social measures. A main social target of governments, international organizations and the whole world community in the coming decades should be the attainment by all peoples of the world by the year 2000 of a level of health that will permit them to lead a socially and economically productive life. Primary health care is the key to attaining this target as part of development in the spirit of social justice.

VI

Primary health care is essential health care based on practical, scientifically sound and socially acceptable methods and technology made universally accessible to individuals and families in the community through their full participation and at a cost that the community and country can afford to maintain at every stage of their development in the spirit of self-reliance and self-determination. It forms an integral part both of the country's health system, of which it is the central function and main focus, and of the overall social and economic development of the community. It is the first level of contact of individuals, the family and community with the national health system, bringing health care as close as possible to where people live and work, and constitutes the first element of a continuing health care process.

VII

Primary health care:

1. reflects and evolves from the economic conditions and sociocultural and political characteristics of the country and its communities and is based on the application of the relevant results of social, biomedical and health services research and public health experience;

2. addresses the main health problems in the community, providing promotive, preventive, curative and rehabilitative services accordingly;

3. includes at least: education concerning prevailing health problems and the methods of preventing and controlling them; promotion of food supply and proper nutrition; an adequate supply of safe water and basic sanitation; maternal and child health care, including family planning; immunization against the major infectious diseases; prevention and control of locally endemic diseases; appropriate treatment of common diseases and injuries; and provision of essential drugs;

4. involves, in addition to the health sector, all related sectors and aspects of national and community development, in particular agriculture, animal husbandry, food, industry, education, housing, public works, communications and other sectors; and demands the coordinated efforts of all those sectors;

5. requires and promotes maximum community and individual self-reliance and participation in the planning, organization, operation and control of primary health care, making fullest use of local, national and other available resources; and to this end develops through appropriate education the ability of communities to participate;

6. should be sustained by integrated, functional and mutually supportive referral systems, leading to the progressive improvement of comprehensive health care for all and giving priority to those most in need;

7. relies, at local and referral levels, on health workers, including physicians, nurses, midwives, auxiliaries and community workers as applicable, as well as traditional practitioners as needed, suitably trained socially and technically to work as a health team and to respond to the expressed health needs of the community.

VIII

All governments should formulate national policies, strategies and plans of action to launch and sustain primary health care as part of a comprehensive national health system and in coordination with other sectors. To this end, it will be necessary to exercise political will, to mobilize the country's resources and to use available external resources rationally.

IX

All countries should cooperate in a spirit of partnership and service to ensure primary health care for all people since the attainment of health by people in any one country directly concerns and benefits every other country. In this context, the joint WHO/UNICEF report on primary health care constitutes a solid basis for the further development and operation of primary health care throughout the world.

X

An acceptable level of health for all the people of the world by the year 2000 can be attained through a fuller and better use of the world's resources, a considerable part of which is now spent on armaments and military conflicts. A genuine policy of independence, peace, détente and disarmament could and should release additional resources that could well be devoted to peaceful aims and in particular to the acceleration of social and economic development of which primary health care, as an essential part, should be allotted its proper share.

The International Conference on Primary Health Care calls for urgent and effective national and international action to develop and implement primary health care throughout the world and particularly in developing countries in a spirit of technical cooperation and in keeping with a New International Economic Order. It urges governments, WHO and UNICEF, and other international organizations, as well as multilateral and bilateral agencies, nongovernmental organizations, funding agencies, all health workers and the whole world community to support national and international commitment to primary health care and to channel increased technical and financial support to it, particularly in developing countries. The Conference calls on all the aforementioned to collaborate in introducing, developing and maintaining primary health care in accordance with the spirit and content of this Declaration.

Source: World Health Organization. (1978). *Declaration of Alma-Ata/: International conference on primary health care, Alma-Ata, USSR, 6–12 September 1978.* Retrieved May 29, 2009, from http://www.who.int/publications/almaata_declaration_en.pdf. Reproduced by permission.

INDEX